Autism and Child Psychopathology Series

Series Editor

Johnny L. Matson, Baton Rouge, LA, USA

Brief Overview

The purpose of this series is to advance knowledge in the broad multidisciplinary fields of autism and various forms of psychopathology (e.g., anxiety and depression). Volumes synthesize research on a range of rapidly expanding topics on assessment, treatment, and etiology.

Description

The **Autism and Child Psychopathology Series** explores a wide range of research and professional methods, procedures, and theories used to enhance positive development and outcomes across the lifespan. Developments in education, medicine, psychology, and applied behavior analysis as well as child and adolescent development across home, school, hospital, and community settings are the focus of this series. Series volumes are both authored and edited, and they provide critical reviews of evidence-based methods. As such, these books serve as a critical reference source for researchers and professionals who deal with developmental disorders and disabilities, most notably autism, intellectual disabilities, challenging behaviors, anxiety, depression, ADHD, developmental coordination disorder, communication disorders, and other common childhood problems. The series addresses important mental health and development difficulties that children and youth, their caregivers, and the professionals who treat them must face. Each volume in the series provides an analysis of methods and procedures that may assist in effectively treating these developmental problems.

Michael P. Kranak
Editor

Behavioral Treatments for Individuals with Autism

Promoting Longevity and Durability

Springer

Editor
Michael P. Kranak
Oakland University and Oakland University Center for Autism
Rochester, MI, USA

Department of Human Development and Child Studies
Oakland University Center for Autism
Rochester, MI, USA

ISSN 2192-922X ISSN 2192-9238 (electronic)
Autism and Child Psychopathology Series
ISBN 978-3-031-91964-0 ISBN 978-3-031-91965-7 (eBook)
https://doi.org/10.1007/978-3-031-91965-7

This Springer imprint is published by the registered company Springer Nature Switzerland AG
The registered company address is: Gewerbestrasse 11, 6330 Cham, Switzerland

An Introduction to *Behavioral Treatments for Individuals with Autism: Promoting Longevity and Durability*

Behavior analysts and related professionals have a long-standing history of working with individuals with intellectual and developmental disabilities, including those with autism. When working with individuals with autism, intervention agents like behavior analysts aim to rearrange the environment in such a way that decreases the likelihood problem behavior[1] (e.g., aggression, self-injury) will occur and increases the likelihood that a more desirable alternative behavior (e.g., communication response) will occur. In other words, behavior analysts work to equip individuals with the skills they need to communicate their wants and needs in a safe, effective, and efficient manner, all towards the goals of improving their qualities of life and increasing their autonomy. Indeed, there is substantial evidence that behavior-analytic treatments are both efficacious and effective at reducing problem behavior and increasing adaptive, communicative behavior (e.g., Howard et al., 2005; Kurtz et al., 2011; Reichow et al., 2018; Richman et al., 2015; Rooker et al., 2013).

One hallmark of truly desirable treatment outcomes is the extent to which treatment effects last (1) over extended periods of time, (2) when treatments are implemented in a variety of settings, and (3) when treatment implementation occurs under conditions different from the initial treatment setting (e.g., different care providers, potential momentary and inadvertent modifications). That is, the effects of treatment must have generalization and generality outside of the initial treatment setting when implemented under ideal conditions, such as perfect levels of procedural fidelity and when implemented by highly trained intervention agents (see Hagopian, 2020 for a discussion on generality). Put simply, the treatments we design for problem behavior displayed by individuals with autism—or any individual that engages in problem behavior—and the resulting behavior change must be *durable*.

[1] There is currently no consensus for the collective terminology used to describe behaviors such as aggression, self-injury, or pica engaged in by individuals with autism that could lead to harm of either themselves or others, or negatively impact those individuals' quality of life. Throughout the book, authors use terms such as "problem behavior," "challenging behavior," and "destructive behavior" interchangeably. Please note that those terms all refer to generally the same types of behavior.

The concept of *durability* in the treatment of problem behavior largely refers to the extent to which desirable behavior persists and problem behavior remains abated in the face of treatment challenges (e.g., procedural fidelity errors; Greer & Shahan, 2019; Wacker et al., 2011). Durability of treatment effects goes beyond effects that maintain across a few days or weeks or those that generalize to new settings, but effects that last and endure under less-than-desirable environments. When problem behavior returns as a result of some treatment challenge, this is a phenomenon known as relapse[2] (e.g., Falligant et al., 2022; Kranak & Falligant, 2021; Mitteer et al., 2022). Unfortunately, relapse can lead to treatment failure, necessitate more intensive or restrictive components, or result in potentially starting treatment over from the beginning. Thus, ensuring treatments are durable is of critical importance to clinicians, regardless of the functional class of behavior (see Kimball et al., 2023).

In short, the goal of this book is to provide clinicians with the relevant information and strategies necessary to design durable behavioral treatments. Majority of the content focuses on the most relevant forms of relapse as they pertain to the assessment and treatment of problem behavior—resurgence, renewal, and reacquisition and reinstatement (see Wathen & Podlesnik, 2018). Specifically, there are two chapters per each of the aforementioned forms of relapse. For each form of relapse, one respective chapter first describes basic (and when applicable, translational) research and variables that impact that type of relapse, with the content written towards clinicians. The other respective chapter per form of relapse describes applied research and mitigation strategies that can readily be adopted in one's own practice. A reader might wonder, "why do I need to understand or consume basic research if I work in only applied settings?" Or, "how could these basic chapters be applicable to my clients and their treatments?" Those are very reasonable questions.

Consider the following analogies. Suppose an engineer was developing a plan for constructing a bridge or building. The engineer could readily follow general design principles and build structures. However, without comprehending the underlying physics of force, stress, and motion, the engineer would not know *why* or *how* a bridge holds up. Or, the engineer might not understand why the building could fail under certain conditions. Therefore, it is likely the engineer would be able to problem-solve or identify the root causes of structural issues, for example. Similarly, a cook might be able to follow recipes, which usually result in good meals. However, without understanding the chemistry involved in food science, they would likely struggle to troubleshoot issues (e.g., lack of bread rising, incorrect balances of marinades for certain cuts of meat), resulting in inedible or incorrectly prepared dishes. These analogies help explain why applied clinicians need to understand the basic principles underlying relapse, and, ultimately, durable behavior change. Clinicians that have a sound comprehension of basic behavior-analytic principles are better equipped to troubleshoot, adapt, and solve complex challenges related to treatment durability.

---

[2] For descriptions on specific forms of relapse, readers are directed to the respective chapters in this volume.

Along with a basic and applied chapter on relevant forms of relapse, there are additional chapters that highlight some nuanced issues related to ensuring treatment durability or otherwise unique clinical situations. These chapters focus on the topics of (a) durability of treatments for inappropriate mealtime behavior, (b) promoting the persistence of desirable behavior, (c) ensuring safety during the treatment process, and (d) comprehensive discharge planning, such that clinicians can make every effort to promote successful transfer of treatment to their clients' natural environments (e.g., homes and schools). All of the chapters are authored by, from my perspective, some of the leading authorities in their respective content areas. It is my sincere hope that this book improves readers' clinical practice and related skills, as well as positively impacts the lives of the individuals they serve.

Finally, I want to thank (a) all of the authors for their contributions, time, and efforts related to the book; (b) my students and colleagues for their assistance and contributions; and (c) my wife Sarah for her unwavering support in my professional endeavors, and my son Jack for sleeping just long enough at night to give me the time necessary to write this introduction.

Department of Human
Development and Child Studies
Oakland University
and Oakland University Center for Autism
Rochester, MI, USA

Michael P. Kranak

Author Note
Chapter preparation was supported in part by Grants 1R21HD113794-01A1 and 1R21HD113881-01 from the Eunice K. Shriver National Institute of Child Health and Human Development (NICHD). Its contents are solely the responsibility of the authors and do not necessarily represent the official views of the NICHD.

References

Falligant, J. M., Chin, M. D., & Kurtz, P. F. (2022). Renewal and resurgence of severe problem behavior in an intensive outpatient setting: Prevalence, magnitude, and implications for practice. *Behavioral Interventions, 37*(3) 909–924. https://doi.org/10.1002/bin.1878

Greer, B. D., & Shahan, T. A. (2019). Resurgence as Choice: Implications for promoting durable behavior change. *Journal of Applied Behavior Analysis, 52*(3), 816–846. https://doi.org/10.1002/jaba.573

Hagopian, L. P. (2020). The consecutive controlled case series: Design, data-analytics, and reporting methods supporting the study of generality. *Journal of Applied Behavior Analysis, 53*(2), 596–619. https://doi.org/10.1002/jaba.691

Hagopian, L. P., Rooker, G. W., & Zarcone, J. R. (2015). Assessment and treatment of severe problem behavior. *Journal of Applied Behavior Analysis, 48*(2), 405–418. https://doi.org/10.1002/jaba.76

Howard, J, S, Sparkman, C. R., Cohen, H. G., Green, G., & Stanislaw, H. (2005). A comparison of intensive behavior analytic and eclectic treatments for young children with autism. *Research in Developmental Disabilities, 26*, 359–383. https://doi.org/10.1016/j.ridd.2004.09.005

Kimball, R. T., Greer, B. D., Fuhrman, A. M., & Lamber, J. M. (2023). Relapse and its mitigation: Towards behavioral inoculation. *Journal of Applied Behavior Analysis, 56*(2), 282–301. https://doi.org/10.1002/jaba.971

Kranak, M. P., & Falligant, J. M. (2021). Further investigation of resurgence following schedule thinning: Extension to an inpatient setting. *Behavioral Interventions, 36*(4), 1003–1012. https://doi.org/10.1002/bin.1831

Kurtz, P. F., Boelter, E. W., Jarmolowicz, D. P., Chin, M. D., & Hagopian, L. P. (2011). An analysis of functional analysis outcomes among individuals with autism spectrum disorders. *Research in Developmental Disabilities, 32*(5), 1809–1824. https://doi.org/10.1016/j.ridd.2011.03.021

Mitteer, D. R., Greer, B. D., Randall, K. R., & Haney, S. D. (2022). On the scope and characteristics of relapse when treating severe destructive behavior. *Journal of Applied Behavior Analysis, 55*(3), 688–703. https://doi.org/10.1002/jaba.912

Reichow, B., Hume, K., Barton, E. E., & Boyd, B. A. (2018). Early intensive behavioral intervention (EIBI) for young children with autism spectrum disorders (ASD). *The Cochrane Database of Systematic Reviews, 5*(5), CD009260. https://doi.org/10.1002/14651858.CD009260.pub3

Richman, D. M., Barnard-Brak, L., Grubb, L., Bosch, A., & Abby, L. (2015). Meta-analysis of noncontingent reinforcement effects on problem behavior. *Journal of Applied Behavior Analysis, 48*(1), 131–152. https://doi.org/10.1002/jaba.189

Wacker, D. P., Harding, J. W., Berg, W. K., Lee, J. F., Schieltz, K. M., Padilla, Y. C., Nevin, J. A., & Shahan, T. A. (2011). An evaluation of persistence of treatment effects during long-term treatment of destructive behavior. *Journal of the Experimental Analysis of Behavior, 96*(2), 261–282. https://doi.org/10.1901/jeab.2011.96-261

Wathen, S. N., & Podlesnik, C. A. (2018). Laboratory models of treatment relapse and mitigation techniques. *Behavior Analysis: Research and Practice, 18*(4), 362–387. https://doi.org/10.1037/bar0000119

Contents

Chapter 1
Basic Laboratory Research on Resurgence

Courtney Mauzy IV, Sean Smith, Beatriz Arroyo Antunez, Jacqueline DeBartelo, Thanh Nguyen, Leondra Tyler, Henry Roane, William Sullivan, and Andrew Craig

In the last few decades, there has been a dramatic increase in basic studies (i.e., those conducted with nonhuman animals) analyzing the mechanisms behind the recurrence of behaviors targeted for elimination (Epstein, 2015; Kimball et al., 2023; Lattal et al., 2017). Studying behavioral relapse is important because it may inform both our understanding of basic behavioral processes and clinical practices. Relapse shows us how histories of reinforcement that may have occurred in the distant past are carried forward to affect ongoing operant behavior, including and ranging from behaviors such as lever presses to clinically significant behavior (e.g., drug use, aggression). Moreover, understanding why a behavior recurs presents opportunities to understand how to prevent or avoid its recurrence. The operant laboratory has long served as an especially suitable context for studying behavioral processes like relapse. Among the various models of relapse, resurgence—generally defined as the return of a previously reinforced behavior after a worsening of reinforcement conditions, usually for an alternative behavior—has garnered particular attention for its relevance to both basic and applied settings.

Resurgence is directly related to relapse occurring in the context of behavioral interventions programmed to decrease challenging or undesired behaviors because these interventions typically include reinforcement of alternative, more socially appropriate behaviors (e.g., Tiger et al., 2008). Resurgence of challenging behavior is likely when reinforcement conditions worsen in the natural environment (e.g., when treatment fidelity errors occur or conditions of alternative reinforcement are

C. Mauzy IV (✉) · S. Smith · B. A. Antunez · J. DeBartelo · T. Nguyen · H. Roane · W. Sullivan · A. Craig
SUNY Upstate Medical University, Syracuse, NY, USA
e-mail: mauzyc@upstate.edu

L. Tyler
Syracuse University, Syracuse, NY, USA

M. P. Kranak (ed.), *Behavioral Treatments for Individuals with Autism*, Autism and Child Psychopathology Series,
https://doi.org/10.1007/978-3-031-91965-7_1

thinned, see Briggs et al., 2018; Haney et al., 2022; Muething et al., 2021; Volkert et al., 2009). Therefore, resurgence appears to be an issue that is common across a variety of clinical settings and socially significant behaviors, and evaluating and understanding the underlying processes that contribute to resurgence in preclinical research may directly facilitate the development of more durable treatments that minimize the likelihood of resurgence.

This chapter will discuss the historical progression of basic laboratory research with nonhuman animals on resurgence and the development of experimental arrangements commonly employed to evaluate this phenomenon. We will provide an overview of the common dependent variables and measures used in these experiments, review elements of a formal contemporary definition of resurgence, and highlight research on the effects of specific variables that affect resurgence. Finally, we will conclude with an outline of quantitative frameworks that attempt to explain the relations among these variables.

Historical Studies of Resurgence

Early Demonstrations

Although the general phenomenon of relapse has been a topic of many research studies throughout history, Hull's (1934) study on speed gradients in rats running through a maze is considered one of the first demonstrations of operant resurgence. Specifically, in a 40-foot maze, he noted that the rats would start traversing the maze slowly, gaining speed as they approached the end of the maze (with food provided for completing the maze). Therefore, he attempted to train a group of rats to run at a consistently fast pace by first providing the food upon completing half of the maze (20 feet). After exhibiting high speeds in the 20-foot maze, he moved the food to the end of the entire 40-foot maze, which resulted in rats running the entire maze faster than they were in baseline. He then withheld reinforcement altogether for one group and fed another group of rats prior to conducting sessions (i.e., presession feeding). During this final phase, rats in both groups exhibited similar patterns and speeds of running as they did in the initial baseline phase. Although Hull was interested in the reasons for the original gradients and not factors that affected their reemergence, this experiment represents an early demonstration of behavior returning after a period of suppression because of a degradation in reinforcement conditions for an alternative pattern of responding.

Several other early studies produced patterns of behavioral reemergence that could be loosely interpreted as resurgence (see Epstein, 2015), but Carey (1951) conducted the first direct experimental analysis evaluating relapse of a target behavior in what has become the standard paradigm for studying resurgence. Carey was evaluating the impact of response complexity and recency of training on the "restoration" of an alternative behavior. Carey trained two groups of rats to engage in either a "single" (Group 1) or "double" (Group 2) bar press during an initial phase. Subsequently, he conducted a second phase where the opposite type of response than what had been trained in the initial phase (i.e., "double" for Group 1, "single" for Group 2) produced reinforcement. In a third phase, extinction was implemented for all bar pressing. During extinction, the response trained during Phase 1 reemerged. This study was the first to present the three main elements that comprise the most commonly used resurgence paradigm in current research: (1) training a target response, (2) suppressing the target response while training an alternative response, and (3) withholding reinforcement for both target and alternative responses to evaluate the return of the target response.

Leitenberg and his colleagues were the first to incorporate the elements from Carey's three-phase procedure to explicitly evaluate return of target responding in the context of behavior analytic interventions in the early 1970s. Their research was an early example of the translational research on relapse because their experiments were specifically designed to evaluate questions related to clinical treatments that use differential reinforcement for an alternative behavior (DRA) and extinction. Many of their studies explicitly examined the impact of training an alternative response on suppression of target behavior in combination with extinction compared to implementing extinction alone. Observing relapse during extinction was a byproduct of their experimental design.

For example, Leitenberg et al. (1975) trained a target lever press in rats using a variable-interval (VI) 30-s schedule for food reinforcers during Phase 1. During Phase 2, pressing a separate lever produced reinforcement according to a fixed ratio (FR) 10 schedule while the target lever press was placed on extinction. After target responding was suppressed and alternative responding was stable, reinforcement was withheld for both responses during Phase 3. This resulted in increases in target responding above baseline levels. The extinction phase for both groups produced an initial increase in target responding, followed by a progressive decline with continued exposure of the target response to extinction. Although still not explicitly labeled resurgence, this study contributed to systematic formalization of the three-phase preparation to study resurgence that is most commonly used to this day by applying these procedures in the context of DRA and extinction (Wathen & Podlesnik, 2018).

Epstein and Skinner (1980) were the first to use the term "resurgence" in a scientific journal when they described the perplexing return of pigeons' key pecking observed in an autoshaping experiment. During an initial phase, a light on the wall of the chamber slowly moved towards the food hopper, and food was delivered when the light reached the feeder. Pigeons exhibited stable rates of pecking at the light on the wall. Subsequently, Epstein and Skinner conducted a phase designed to suppress pecking by presenting reinforcement independent of the light's movement or position. This resulted in an overall decrease in responding; however, two pigeons continued to peck the dot at low rates. Epstein (2015) later described how his curiosity about the lingering low rates of responding led to him identifying an outcome he later called resurgence:

> [That pigeons continued to peck the key] bothered me. So I went to the lab the next night, I disconnected the feeder. Presenting the spot alone would, I reasoned, get rid of those last few pecks, which might have been maintained, I thought, by the occasional coincidental pairing of pecking with food delivery… Over the next few minutes I heard a few clicks from the relay racks, indicating that the pigeons were continuing to peck the spot at a low rate. But about 10 min into the session, one pigeon started pecking the spot continuously and at a fairly high rate. A few minutes later, the second pigeon started doing the same thing. (p. 22)

The discussed studies all contributed to a well-defined, three-phase experimental arrangement for studying resurgence. Phase 1 involves establishing a target response with reinforcement, usually on a dense schedule. Phase 2 involves target response suppression, and the introduction of reinforcement for an alternative response. Phase 3 represents the test for resurgence of target responding by worsening the reinforcement conditions for the alternative response, usually through extinction. Subsequent researchers have used versions of this preparation to study resurgence across a wide range of species, responses, and environments (see Podlesnik et al., 2022a for review).

Variations to Three-Phase Procedure

The three-phase procedure described above is a common method for evaluating resurgence. Other procedural variations, however, also are used. In this section, we will describe some of those variations.

Elimination Procedures

In the standard three-phase resurgence procedure, the target response is suppressed through the reinforcement of, and corresponding shift in response allocation to, an alternative response. Some researchers suggest this only nominally eliminates the target response (e.g., Leitenberg et al., 1975). Specifically, it is unclear whether the response suppression is due to (a) the functional extinction of target behavior as the contingency between the response and reinforcer is broken or (b) response competition introduced by alternative reinforcement. To ensure *extinction* of the target response prior to resurgence testing, some studies have used a four-phase resurgence procedure, which includes a phase wherein target responding is placed on extinction prior to the phase that introduces reinforcement for an alternative response (e.g., Cleland et al., 2000; Epstein, 1983; Lieving & Lattal, 2003). Importantly, removing alternative reinforcement also caused resurgence in these studies, demonstrating that prevention of functional extinction by response competition is not a suitable mechanism by which to explain resurgence.

Although the above elimination methods are the most common in the literature, Podlesnik et al. (2022) identified at least seven other ways researchers have reduced target behavior (see their Table 13). The most common variation involves programming differential reinforcement of other behavior (DRO) during Phase 2 rather than a DRA (da Silva et al., 2008; Doughty et al., 2007). In this approach, the target response is eliminated by creating sufficiently long periods without target responding to meet the DRO interval. Other experiments reinforced different response sequences (e.g., Galizio et al., 2020), or provided reinforcement independent of responding (e.g., Trask & Bouton, 2016). Despite the inclusion of this wide variety of elimination procedures, more research directly comparing different elimination methods is needed to understand any potential effect on the subsequent resurgence.

Compound Schedules

A frequently employed design element in resurgence preparations is the implementation of compound schedules, particularly multiple and concurrent schedules. Using compound schedules enables the comparison of the effects of two or more independent variables, or manipulations of the independent variable, on resurgence during Phase 3. In a *multiple schedule* of reinforcement, two or more basic schedules of reinforcement, extinction, or punishment are associated with schedule-correlated stimuli and alternate across time (Ferster & Skinner, 1957). For example, Doughty et al. (2007, Experiment 1) used a multiple schedule arrangement to compare the effect of different target response elimination strategies during Phase 2 on the resurgence of key pecking in pigeons. For all pigeons, a light above the key alternated between blue (component 1) or green (component 2) every 3 min across the three phases of the resurgence preparation. In Phase 2, with the target key on extinction, one component included a DRO schedule, while the other component included an alternative key that produced reinforcement on a VI schedule. In Phase 3, both components were associated with extinction of the target key with no additional reinforcement contingencies. By comparing levels of resurgence during Phase 3 across components, the authors observed greater and more immediate resurgence in the component associated with the DRO schedule.

Similar to the use of multiple schedules, some studies used *concurrent schedules* to make direct comparisons of the impact of different variables on resurgence (Epstein, 1983; da Silva et al., 2008). For example, da Silva et al. (2008, Experiment 1b) sought to compare the effects of two different reinforcement schedules on the resurgence of two responses. During Phase 1, pigeons' peck to either of two keys concurrently produced reinforcement according to either a VI 1-min or VI 6-min schedule. After placing pecks to both keys on extinction, the authors trained a third key peck during Phase 2 using a VI 3-min schedule of reinforcement, the experimenters compared response rates on the target keys during Phase 3 in relation to the different schedules of reinforcement programed in Phase 1. During Phase 3, key pecking occurred more frequently on the key associated with the richer schedule of reinforcement in Phase 1. This finding should be interpreted with caution, however, because this effect was not replicated when the experimenters controlled for the response rates produced during Phase 1. Nevertheless, this study represents an example of how researchers can incorporate concurrent schedules in evaluations of resurgence.

Within-Session Analyses

Some researchers use procedures to evaluate resurgence within individual sessions, rather than across conditions spanning multiple sessions (e.g., Bai et al., 2017; Cook & Lattal, 2019; Kincaid et al., 2015). Repeating the process that produces resurgence multiple times with a single participant or subject can produce a baseline against which to compare the effects of variables on resurgence within the individual in a relatively short period of time. For example, Cook and Lattal (2019, Experiment 3) evaluated the validity of a within-session resurgence arrangement by attempting to replicate the effects of rich and lean target and alternative reinforcement rates on resurgence. They used pigeons as subjects, divided each session into three 30-min phases, and programmed a three-phase arrangement within a session. Additionally, they trained responding to the target and alternative keys under different VI schedules signaled by specific key colors. Each color represented one of four conditions associated with rich or lean baseline or alternative reinforcement rates. The authors compared levels of resurgence across the four conditions for each subject. Consistent with previous findings, levels of resurgence were sensitive to the different rates of reinforcement arranged during Phases 1 and 2. Although this experiment represents a promising demonstration of a within-session evaluation, this methodology requires extension to other common outcomes across a variety of dependent measures to better understand its utility.

Dependent Variables and Measures Used to Evaluate Resurgence

In the previous section, we discussed common experimental preparations used in basic resurgence research. Now, we will examine the key responses involved in these experiments (i.e., target, alternative, and inactive control responses) and review common measures used to evaluate these dependent variables.

Responses

Resurgence preparations typically evaluate three different types of responses: the target response, the alternative response, and the inactive control response. The *target response* is the primary dependent variable relevant to resurgence. In basic research, this response is established with an experimentally programmed reinforcement schedule to ensure each subject has a specific history of reinforcement. It is the initial response that is trained during Phase 1, suppressed during Phase 2, and subsequently evaluated for its reemergence when conditions of reinforcement worsen in Phase 3. This behavior is often conceptualized as an analog for a clinically relevant behavior that (a) has been established by a history of reinforcement (b) is targeted for reduction, but (c) is at risk for relapse in real-world situations. In research on resurgence, the defining features of the target response are its establishment in the subject's behavioral repertoire by a history of reinforcement and its suppression prior to the resurgence phase (Lattal & St. Peter Pipkin, 2009; Lattal et al., 2017).

The *alternative response* is a separate behavior that typically begins producing reinforcement during Phase 2. Often, the alternative response is not available (e.g., response lever is not present in the chamber) or eligible for reinforcement during Phase 1. The reinforcement conditions for the alternative response are degraded or completely removed during Phase 3, setting the occasion for resurgence of the target response. The alternative response is often conceptualized as representing a more desirable behavior than the target response and is learned during treatment. For example, an alternative response could represent a functional communicative response that would be taught during a functional communication training intervention designed to decrease destructive behavior (e.g., aggression, self-injury; Brown et al., 2020) or engagement in behaviors other than drug taking in the case of treatments for substance use disorders (e.g., Brown & DeFulio, 2020; Silverman et al., 1999).

The *inactive control response* is a response that is available for engagement throughout all phases of the resurgence evaluation; however, the inactive control response typically does not produce reinforcement at any point during the experiment. Lattal and Oliver (2020) compared the inactive control response to a behavioral barometer, designed to provide an index of what level of behavioral return can be contributed to resurgence rather than extinction-induced variability. Since the inactive control response produces no programmed reinforcement in the resurgence evaluation, elevated rates of inactive control responding during Phase 3 may be a product of extinction-induced variability (Bolívar et al., 2017; Saini et al., 2021; Sweeney & Shahan, 2016). Therefore, some researchers suggest including an inactive control response as the recurrence of target responding should only be considered resurgence if it occurs to a greater extent than this inactive control response (see Lattal & Oliver, 2020 for a more comprehensive discussion).

The specific topography of these three responses varies depending on the species and context. For example, with rats and mice as subjects, common responses include lever pressing, a nose poke, or a chain pull (e.g., Craig et al., 2017, 2020; Kestner et al., 2015; Nist & Shahan, 2023; Podlesnik et al., 2006; Shahan et al., 2015; Sweeney & Shahan, 2013). For pigeons, target and alternative responses are often pecking different keys (e.g., "key A" is the target response and "key B" is the alternative response; Cook & Lattal, 2019; Jarmolowicz & Lattal, 2014; Oliver et al., 2018, Experiment 1) or treadle-press responses (e.g., Doughty et al., 2007; Lieving & Lattal, 2003). Studies using species of fish often use approaching different sensors as the target and alternative responses (e.g., Kuroda et al., 2017a, b). In experiments with human participants, common target and alternative responses include clicking different symbols or completing response chains on computer interfaces or manipulating physical objects like buttons or microswitches in lower-tech arrangements (e.g., Kuroda et al., 2016; Ritchey et al., 2021; Saini et al., 2021; Smith et al., 2017; Smith & Greer, 2022a, b).

Measures to Evaluate Resurgence

Resurgence is typically reported as a change in some dimension of target responding when reinforcement conditions worsen for the alternative response in the transition from Phase 2 to Phase 3. This change in target responding can be quantified in various ways. Each quantification provides specific information about different properties of resurgence. The following section will outline measures commonly used to quantify resurgence that have been reported in previous research.

Response Rate

The most common measurement used to evaluate resurgence is response rate (Cançado et al., 2017). Response rate is the number of occurrences with respect to the amount of time when the response could have occurred. A response rate provides an absolute measure of how many responses occurred during a certain amount of time, typically the test of resurgence (Phase 3). As Skinner (1938, 1950) argued, response rate often serves as the fundamental datum for understanding and predicting behavior as it provides insights into the probability of a response at any given time and permits exploration to the conditions that determine that probability. Therefore, target response rates are often used as the main measure to determine the level of resurgence. Although target response rates during the resurgence test (i.e., Phase 3) is a measure of the amount of resurgence that occurred, many studies report target response rates across all experimental phases, which permits comparisons between target response rates at the beginning of Phase 3 to target response rates at other times during the experiment (e.g., the end of Phases 1 and 2).

Cumulative Responses

Another measurement commonly used to evaluate resurgence is cumulative responses across time in the resurgence test. This measure provides a moment-by-moment aggregated total of responses over a period of time, yielding an interpretable slope that is directly related to momentary changes in response rate. Like response rates, cumulative responses provide a measure of the absolute amount of target behavior that occurred across the phases of a resurgence preparation. However, cumulative responses allow for evaluating within session changes in resurgence. This enables researchers to observe the progression of resurgence over time on a more molecular level (e.g., on a second-by-second basis) than evaluating response rates (e.g., on a session-by-session basis). Typically, cumulative responses are graphically depicted as a line that increases along on the *y*-axis according to the number of cumulative responses that have occurred at each time point in an experiment, which is depicted along the *x*-axis. Thus, a line with 0 slope is indicative of no responses whereas a line with a positive slope indicates responding. Differential responding is determined by evaluating the slope of the line. Steeper slopes suggest higher response rates.

For example, Shahan et al. (2015) used cumulative responses as the primary measure to evaluate the resurgence of sucrose (Experiment 1) and cocaine (Experiment 2) seeking in rats in two experiments. In the first phase of Experiment 1, rats received sucrose reinforcers on a VI 45-s schedule for target lever presses. Alternative nose pokes produced no reinforcers in Phase 1. In Phase 2, target lever presses no longer produced reinforcement. Instead, the alternative nose pokes generated sucrose deliveries on a VI 10-s schedule of reinforcement prior to testing for resurgence in Phase 3. Shahan et al. examined the cumulative sucrose lever presses (target response) in 5-min bins for the last session of Phase 2 and each session in Phase 3 to compare resurgence of sucrose lever presses across sessions. Figure 1.1 presents cumulative responding for one subject, with each line representing a specific session of the resurgence test. The bolded solid line shows responding during the last session of Phase 2 for comparison. Visual inspection of the data suggests resurgence of sucrose seeking (target responding) occurred during the initial sessions of Phase 3.

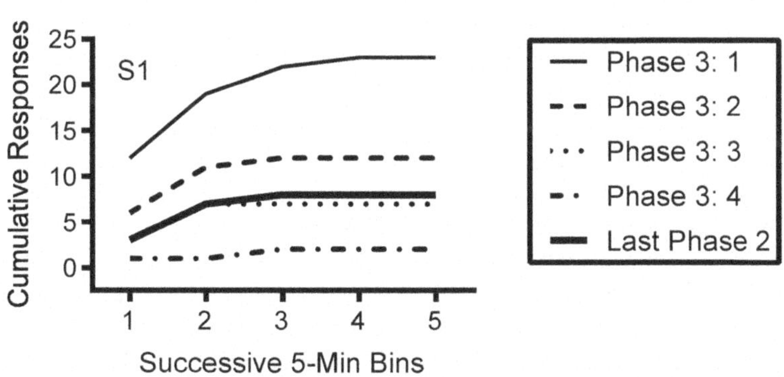

Fig. 1.1 Cumulative responding from Shahan et al. (2015). *Note.* Cumulative lever presses for sucrose across successive 5-min bins for the last session of Phase 2 and the four sessions of the resurgence test (i.e., Phase 3) for one subject from Shahan et al. (2015)

Proportional Response Rate

One limitation of absolute measures, like response rate or cumulative responses, is they fail to account for differences in baseline response rates across conditions or participants (e.g., Cançado et al., 2016). Without this context, absolute measures can lead to misleading conclusions about the magnitude of resurgence. Imagine two participants who demonstrate similar target response rates during Phase 3 of a resurgence evaluation. The most obvious conclusion is that these participants showed similar magnitudes of resurgence. However, if one participant exhibited higher rates of target responding during baseline, that participant may tend to engage in more overall responding compared to the other participant. Thus, one would expect that this participant would also engage in more target responding compared to the other participant when resurgence occurs. Further, research has demonstrated that baseline response rates can have important effects on behavioral persistence and relapse irrespective of other variable manipulations (see Craig, 2023; Craig & Shahan, 2016; Sweeney & Shahan, 2013). For these reasons, it can be important for researchers to account for between-subject variance in overall and baseline response rates when evaluating resurgence.

Calculating response rates as a proportion of the response rate that occurred during baseline is a commonly used strategy to account for such differences (e.g., Nevin & Shahan, 2011; Podlesnik & Shahan, 2010; Shahan & Sweeney, 2011). Proportion of baseline is typically calculated by dividing the obtained response rate from a given session by response rates from the end of Phase 1 (from either a single session or an average across multiple sessions). This measure is commonly used to compare the magnitude of resurgence effects because it accounts for differences in response rates across participants and conditions within the comparison, which allows researchers to compare differences in resurgence while controlling for this potentially confounding variable.

Reporting response rates or proportional response rates can lead to different conclusions when comparing the amount of resurgence between participants, groups, or conditions. To illustrate this point, Fig. 1.2 depicts the data reported for one participant from Fisher et al. (Fisher et al., 2020, Experiment 1). This study observed differentially greater rates of resurgence of children's challenging behavior in conditions associated with higher rates of baseline reinforcement (VI 2 s) relative to a leaner schedule (VI 14 s) that were compared using a multiple schedule. As the authors highlighted, reporting proportion of baseline controls for differing response rates that are associated with specific multiple-schedule components. During baseline, this participant engaged in consistently higher rates of destructive behavior during the lean condition relative to the dense condition. Therefore, although the absolute rates of responding were higher in lean condition in Phase 3 (i.e., the "Extinction Challenge" in the top panel of Fig. 1.2), resurgence of destructive behavior in the dense condition recurred to a greater extent as the first three data points were greater than any given session during baseline.

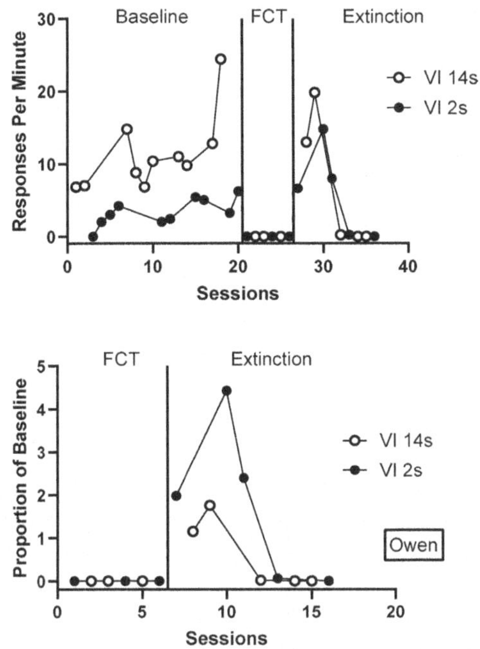

Fig. 1.2 Destructive behavior from Fisher et al. (2020). *Note.* The top panel depicts rate of destructive behavior across the three-phase arrangement. The bottom panel reports destructive behavior as a proportion of baseline responding across sessions of Phase 2 and 3

Proportion of Alternative-Reinforcement Phase

Another common practice is reporting resurgence as a proportion of response rates during the last session or sessions of the Phase 2. This approach offers insight into the magnitude of resurgence relative to the immediately preceding phase, designed to suppress the target response, rather than comparing it to the baseline reinforcement phase. However, because response rates during the final sessions of Phase 2 are often very low or near zero, even small differences between groups or conditions in Phase 2 can lead to exaggerated differences in proportional resurgence.

Table 1.1 depicts hypothetical data illustrating the difference between proportional rates when using the rates representative of the last session of Phase 2 responding in the left panel relative to the last session of Phase 1 in the right panel. During the resurgence test, both groups exhibited identical response rates. Comparing proportional rates between groups in Experiment 1 suggests markedly greater resurgence for Group 2; however, the proportional rates are nearly identical between groups of Experiment 2. The low levels of responding used in calculating the proportional rates make this measure particularly sensitive to any differences in average response rates.

Table 1.1 Hypothetical data from two experiments

Hypothetical data					
Experiment 1			Experiment 2		
	Group 1	Group 2		Group 1	Group 2
	Average RPM	Average RPM		Average RPM	Average RPM
Last phase 2	1.2	0.2	Last phase 1	100	90
First phase 3	30	30	First phase 3	30	30
Proportional rate	25	150	Proportional rate	0.3	0.33

Note. Absolute response rates of the first session of the resurgence test as a proportion of the last session of Phase 2 (left panel), or Phase 1 (right panel)

Target Response Duration

Another dimension of behavior sometimes reported in basic studies of resurgence is the duration of the response (e.g., Baum, 2012; Bruzek et al., 2009; Cançado et al., 2017). For behaviors that are not best represented by a discrete frequency count, such as reading, exercising, or eating, time allocated to that behavior is a more appropriate measure. In general, the literature on response duration suggests similar patterns of resurgence as response frequency. For example, within a human operant preparation, Benavides and Escobar (2017) evaluated the resurgence of button-press durations (short and long response durations) with graduate students. The response duration was recorded via two buttons on a controller. Using a computer program, participants were exposed to a two-component multiple schedule (blue and gray screens) with a chained VI 30 s, VR 3 schedule of reinforcement active in both components. The final link in the chain required either long or short durations of the number of responses dictated by the VR schedule. For example, in a terminal link in the short response component with a ratio of 2, two short responses resulted in reinforcement. In Phase 1, one component of the multiple schedule (blue) produced reinforcement (points) for shorter durations of button presses (0.1–0.5 s) and the second component (gray) produced points when the individual held the button for longer durations (2–8 s). Phase 2 reversed the two components. During Phase 3, no programmed consequences were provided across components, which produced resurgence of response durations above levels observed during the last sessions of Phase 2. Notably, participants engaged in greater rates of target behavior during the short duration component. This finding highlights how response duration, much like frequency, can resurge when reinforcement conditions change.

Other Measures

Although the previously discussed measures are the most prominent in the literature, studies have reported a variety of less traditional dependent variables as well. For instance, Bachá-Méndez et al. (2007) established, and subsequently observed resurgence of lever press sequences in rats. Furthermore, studies evaluating behavior variability as an operant often include response sequences as the main dependent variable. In a human operant evaluation of the resurgence of response variability, Galizio et al. (2020) provided reinforcement during Phase 1 each time a participant constructed a new rectangle that varied across a target dimension (i.e., size or location). During Phase 2, participants produced reinforcement when constructing rectangles that varied across an alternative dimension. Reinforcement was withheld for all new rectangles during Phase 3. The authors reported the U-value (e.g., Page & Neuringer, 1985) to assess for behavior variability across phases, which showed some evidence of resurgence of a target dimension of variability. Other direct measures noted in the literature to evaluating resurgence include the number of intervals in which the target, alternative, and inactive responses occurred during the resurgence test in Phase 3 (Cook & Lattal, 2019; Experiments 1 and 2) and the latency to the first target response during the resurgence test (Frye et al., 2018).

Defining Features of Resurgence

Having outlined the procedures and dependent variables typically used in basic laboratories when studying resurgence, the following section discusses a more formal definition of the term *resurgence*. Lattal et al. (2017) reviewed research on resurgence to develop a comprehensive definition. Ultimately, they formulated the following definition designed to encompass this broad area of research: resurgence is "the transient recurrence, with consideration of the stimulus context, of some dimension of previously established but not currently occurring activity when reinforcement conditions of current behavior are worsened." To explore this definition more thoroughly, we list each part of the definition as a separate subheading and discuss the meaning of that part of the definition and why it is an important feature of resurgence.

"Previously Established…Activity"

When Lattal et al. (2017) refer to "previously established…activity," they are referring to a target behavior with a known history of producing reinforcement. As noted previously, researchers typically study resurgence using a three-phase arrangement, so this history of reinforcement is typically established by providing reinforcers contingent on target responses during the first phase of an experiment. Further, this phase usually continues until the rate of target responding stabilizes, suggesting that the response is firmly established in the organism's repertoire, before moving to the next phase.

This feature of resurgence is important because it helps delineate resurgence as a separate phenomenon from both extinction-induced variability and extinction bursting. Previous research has demonstrated that suspending reinforcement often causes organisms to engage in a wide range of behaviors that have not produced reinforcement previously (i.e., extinction-induced variability, e.g., Neuringer et al., 2001, see Lattal et al., 2013, for discussion). Resurgence is distinguished from this phenomenon by the presence of a specific history of reinforcement for the target behavior. Thus, under extinction conditions, the previous history of reinforcement for a target response causes the target response to occur to a greater extent than other responses that have not produced reinforcement previously. Said another way, when all reinforcement is suspended, a previous history of reinforcement for target responding (e.g., during the first phase of an experiment) causes the target response to occur more frequently than other extinction-induced behaviors which do not have a specific history of reinforcement. The greater recurrence of the target response relative to other behaviors is resurgence (see Lattal & Oliver, 2020, for an in-depth discussion of measuring resurgence in terms of comparing rates of target responding to rates of an inactive control response).

Further, suspending reinforcement can evoke increased frequencies of the behavior, in general (i.e., extinction bursting, Fisher et al., 2023). This differs from resurgence in that increases in target responding during Phase 3 represent a recurrence or reemergence of behavior relative to a previous period of its suppression. Extinction bursting is characterized by an increase relative to a previous period of reinforcement associated with stable rates of target responding. This delineation between resurgence and other extinction-induced behavior is conceptually important because it demonstrates that an organism's history of reinforcement is carried through time and continues to affect their ongoing response patterns, even following its temporary suppression. Thus, studying resurgence is an important avenue for evaluating how temporally distal behavioral histories continue to influence an organism's behavior.

Another important point regarding this part of the definition provided by Lattal et al. (2017) is that they use the term "activity," rather than "response" or "behavior." This terminology is used to emphasize that, although researchers often measure resurgence in terms of response frequencies, resurgence can be measured in terms of time allocation and other dimensions of behavior, as well.

"But Not Currently Occurring Activity"

This feature of resurgence means that, after the target behavior is established, the target behavior needs to decrease such that it is "not currently occurring." Although the definition that Lattal et al. (2017) provide may seem to imply that the target behavior needs to decrease to an extent that it is not occurring at all, there are no firm rules suggesting exactly how much the target behavior needs to reduce prior to testing for resurgence. For example, in a comprehensive review of basic and preclinical research on resurgence conducted from 1970–2020, Podlesnik et al. (2022) identified that 66% of studies began resurgence testing independent of specific performance-based criteria. That is, instead of beginning resurgence testing after a specific amount of reduction in target responding, researchers tend to begin testing after a fixed amount of time, sessions, trials, or reinforcers that are earned. Although there is good reason for researchers to begin resurgence testing independent of specific criteria related to the reduction of target responding (e.g., to facilitate between-group comparisons), this demonstrates that there is no clear rule regarding how much a target behavior must be reduced prior to resurgence testing. Despite the lack of a clear consensus on the objective amount of reduction necessary to study resurgence, an important consideration is that target behavior needs to be reduced to levels that permit the behavior to increase during resurgence testing. Greater reductions in target responding allow researchers to detect subsequent increases during resurgence testing more easily. In turn, this can make it easier for researchers to detect differences in the amount of resurgence that occurs across independent variable manipulations, as well.

"When Reinforcement Conditions of Current Behavior"

As noted in the previous section, target behavior needs to decrease. The "when reinforcement conditions of current behavior" feature of the resurgence definition implies that researchers must use specific procedures to decrease target responding for subsequent recurrences of behavior to be considered resurgence. Specifically, while target behavior is being reduced, some form of reinforcement must remain available. The availability of reinforcement during target response reduction is essential because it permits the experimenter to implement a subsequent "worsening" of reinforcement conditions that causes target responding to recur (see "Are Worsened" section below for further discussion). This procedure is a critical feature of resurgence because it delineates resurgence from other forms of relapse (e.g., renewal), which may be related to different behavioral processes (e.g., generalization; see "Context Theory" section for elaboration).

"Are Worsened"

The definition provided by Lattal et al. (2017) says that resurgence occurs when reinforcement conditions for current behavior "are worsened." A "worsening" of conditions encompasses a broad set of stimulus changes such as introducing extinction (e.g., Epstein, 1983); reducing the rate (e.g., Shahan et al., 2020), magnitude (e.g., Craig et al., 2017), or immediacy (e.g., Nighbor et al., 2020) of reinforcement; introducing punishment (e.g., Fontes et al., 2018); or increasing the response effort of responses that produce reinforcement (see Haney et al., 2022, for discussion). Any of these situations, which make the conditions of reinforcement worse, are likely to cause target behavior to recur.

"Transient Recurrence"

According to Lattal et al. (2017), another critical feature of resurgence is that it is transient. Specifically, target behavior typically increases during the first session of Phase 3 when the worsening occurs. Often, but not always, the target behavior will remain elevated or continue to increase for a relatively short period of time (Podlesnik & Kelley, 2015). Then, because target behavior typically remains unreinforced, it will begin decreasing and return to levels that are similar to those observed prior to the worsening of conditions. Although the transient nature of resurgence is not uniform across all individual organisms, patterns that deviate from this typical pattern may be due to factors (e.g., the organism's normal amount of variability, confounding variables) unrelated to the worsening of conditions, so the increase in target behavior may not be a demonstration of resurgence.

"Some Dimension"

Although resurgence is most commonly measured in terms of increases in the frequency or rate of a target response, resurgence can also be quantified along other dimensions of behavior. As described later, research has demonstrated resurgence of several dimensions of behavior (e.g., frequency, duration) which follow similar patterns to response rates, suggesting that conditions that tend to produce resurgence of response frequency could potentially produce resurgence of other dimensions of behavior (e.g., duration, latency, intensity), as well.

"With Consideration of the Stimulus Context"

As noted in the following section, a history of reinforcement for target responding is a defining feature of resurgence, and an organism's history of reinforcement is carried through time, continuing to affect its ongoing behavior. It is also important to recognize that this reinforcement history always occurs within a specific stimulus context, so the stimulus contexts where learning occurs will also continue to affect an organism's ongoing behavior and the resurgence of its previously established behaviors. Perhaps the clearest examples of the effects of stimulus context on resurgence are in experiments using multiple schedules as part of the experimental design (e.g., Cançado & Lattal, 2011; Reed & Morgan, 2007).[1] Several studies have used these within-subject designs to (a) establish two different learning histories for

[1] Multielement designs, which also use different stimulus contexts to signal different conditions, are also commonly used to study resurgence in more translational and applied experiments (e.g., Fisher et al., 2019, 2020).

individual organisms in the context of two different components of a multiple schedule, and then (b) produce differential amounts of resurgence across the two different stimulus contexts in the presence of the same worsening of reinforcement conditions. From these studies, in which the amount of resurgence differed in relation to the different stimulus contexts in the multiple schedules, it is evident that stimulus context can play an important role in relation to resurgence, and the nuances of this important relation is discussed further in the "Context Theory" section later in this chapter.

Variables That Influence Resurgence

Knowing how resurgence has been conceptualized, experimentally evaluated, and redefined over time lends to a discussion of how different variables can impact the likelihood and magnitude of resurgence. In the following section, we will discuss relevant research that has manipulated variables that fall into two categories: (1) variables related to consequences and (2) variables related to the response.

Consequence-Based Variables

Reinforcement Rate

Reinforcement rate, the frequency with which reinforcement is delivered, has been extensively studied for its effects on resurgence. Research consistently shows that higher reinforcement rates for alternative responding during Phase 2 lead to greater suppression of target responding and, subsequently, higher levels of resurgence in Phase 3. For example, Leitenberg et al. (1975, Experiment 3) demonstrated this effect in pigeons using a three-phase resurgence preparation. Pigeons exposed to a dense reinforcement schedule (VI 30 s) during Phase 2 exhibited greater suppression of target-key pecking and higher levels of resurgence in Phase 3 than pigeons exposed to a lean schedule (VI 240 s) or no reinforcement at all. This finding has been replicated by other studies (e.g., Bouton & Trask, 2016; Cançado et al., 2016; Craig & Shahan, 2016; Craig et al., 2016, 2020; Shahan et al., 2020, Winterbauer & Bouton, 2010), and with human participants in human operant settings using arbitrary responses (e.g., Smith et al., 2017, Podlesnik et al., 2022, Experiment 1).

The impact of reinforcer rates for target responding during Phase 1 on the level of resurgence is less well understood. Some studies suggest a similar relation as alternative reinforcement rates such that greater rates of reinforcement during Phase 1 lead to greater magnitudes of resurgence (e.g., Kuroda et al., 2016; Podlesnik & Shahan, 2009). However, this relation is not universally supported (see Craig & Shahan, 2016).

Another interesting finding related to manipulations of reinforcement rate is that decreasing the reinforcement rate progressively over Phase 2 (i.e., schedule thinning), may result in lower levels of resurgence compared to an "overall" richer schedule. Sweeney and Shahan (2013) explored the effects of schedule thinning by exposing rats to different alternative reinforcement schedules during Phase 2. Researchers compared either a dense, low, or progressively thinned (i.e., thinning) schedule of reinforcement. Interestingly, rats in the thinning condition showed reduced levels of resurgence compared to those in a consistently dense reinforcement schedule, suggesting that gradual reductions in reinforcement may serve as a mitigation strategy when attempting to reach lower schedules of reinforcement that might more closely mimic clinical treatment goals.

Other manipulations to reinforcement rate have also been explored, as studies have evaluated the speed of schedule thinning and the impact of rate downshifts on resurgence (see Lieving & Lattal, 2003; Shahan et al., 2020; Winterbauer & Bouton, 2012). Taken together, studies evaluating the impact of response rates in the context of resurgence show greater reinforcement rates for alternative responding during Phase 2 lead to greater target response suppression but higher levels of resurgence during Phase 3.

Reinforcement Magnitude

Another important variable explored in resurgence literature is magnitude of reinforcement. Reinforcement magnitude is defined as the amount or intensity of reinforcement delivered (e.g., number of reinforcers or duration of time reinforcement is available; Catania, 1963). Craig et al. (2017, Experiment 1) manipulated magnitude of reinforcement for the alternative response in a resurgence preparation with three groups of rats. During Phase 2, while experimenters placed target responses (lever pressing) on extinction, pressing a different lever allowed the rats to gain either five pellets (i.e., high-magnitude group), one pellet (i.e., low-magnitude group), or zero pellets (i.e., extinction group). Rats in the high-magnitude group exhibited greater target response suppression during Phase 2 and greater levels of resurgence relative to the other groups, indicating resurgence shows similar sensitivities to reinforcement magnitude as reinforcement rate. Interestingly, during Experiment 2, rats exhibited similar levels of resurgence when experiencing decreases in alternative reinforcement magnitude as when encountering total response extinction during Phase 3. As mentioned above, manipulating magnitude through the duration of reinforcement, rather than number of reinforcers, results in similar suppression of target responding in Phase 2 and similar increases in resurgence during Phase 3 (e.g., Oliver et al., 2018).

Additionally, Browning et al. (2022) explored schedule thinning in conjunction with different magnitudes of reinforcement. Using procedures similar to those of Sweeney and Shahan (2013), they exposed three groups of rats—high, low, and thinning—to varying reinforcement magnitudes (rather than reinforcement rates) for engaging in the alternative response. The results indicated that the group experiencing higher magnitudes of reinforcement exhibited the greatest decrease in target responding during Phase 2, followed by thinning and low magnitudes of reinforcement. Additionally higher magnitudes were associated with greater levels of resurgence compared to the thinning and low magnitude groups.

Interestingly, although the effects of reinforcement rate have been systematically replicated across a wide range of species and preparations, the effects of reinforcement magnitude with human participants have produced mixed results. For example, Podlesnik et al. (2022, Experiments 2 and 3) reported the use of similar manipulations of reinforcement magnitude in a human operant arrangement using a computer-based task. However, their results suggested a lack of differential target response suppression during Phase 2, as well as a lack of differential rates of resurgence between groups during Phase 3. Podlesnik et al. suggested that the behavior of their participants might not have been particularly sensitive to the specific manipulations of reinforcer magnitude they arranged. Nevertheless, it is unclear why magnitude may differentially impact levels of resurgence across species, and more research is warranted to better understand this variable with humans in a controlled setting.

Reinforcement Quality

Quality of reinforcement is another dimension of reinforcement that has been explored in basic research on resurgence. Quality refers to characteristics of a given stimulus that can be manipulated to enhance its value, resulting in greater response allocation (Hollard & Davison, 1971). Research on reinforcer quality suggests higher-quality reinforcement results in greater levels of resurgence. For example, Shahan et al. (2024) explored the impact of reinforcement quality (using food as the high-quality reinforcer and sucrose as the low-quality reinforcer) on resurgence with rats. Specifically, the authors examined the effects of increasing (Experiment 1) or decreasing (Experiment 2) the quality of reinforcement for alternative responding during Phase 2 relative to reinforcement for the target response in Phase 1. Results of a three-phase resurgence evaluation showed slight differences in target response suppression between experiments, with greater suppression for rats that received higher quality reinforcement for the alternative response in Phase 2. Additionally, rats receiving higher-quality reinforcement during Phase 2 demonstrated greater levels of resurgence. Similarly, when rats experienced a downshift in quality from food pellet deliveries in Phase 1 to sucrose solution deliveries during Phase 2, they exhibited less target behavior suppression, but less overall target responding during the test for resurgence, than the group that received the same high-quality reinforcers across phases.

Of note, the previously mentioned study is one of a scarce literature base evaluating the effects of reinforcer quality on resurgence. This is potentially due to the additional steps needed to demonstrate differences in stimulus quality (e.g., conducting choice assessments to ensure differences in quality). Further research on quality has explored the effects of reinforcer type on the degree of resurgence, across a variety of reinforcers including the comparison of food to drug reinforcers (e.g., Craig et al., 2016; Podlesnik et al., 2006; Quick et al., 2011; Shahan et al., 2015). Although these studies suggest an effect of quality on resurgence, additional research is needed, particularly exploring methods to assess quality across contexts.

Delays to Reinforcement

Although delays to reinforcement are commonly evaluated in basic research, their impact on resurgence remains relatively underexplored. A delay to reinforcement is defined as the time required for a reinforcer to be obtained after engaging in the response. Jarmolowicz and Lattal (2014) provided one of the first examinations of the effects of delayed reinforcement in a resurgence preparation, in which they exposed four pigeons to a four-phase resurgence procedure. After the target response was trained (i.e., Phase 1), the target response was then extinguished during Phase 2, followed by the reinforcement of the alternative response in Phase 3. During the resurgence test (i.e., Phase 4), responses to the alternative key produced reinforcement after progressively increasing, un-signaled delays. Three of four pigeons exhibited resurgence of target key pecking as the delays became progressively longer, suggesting more resurgence tended to occur with longer delays to reinforcement. Similarly, Nighbor et al. (2020) manipulated delays to reinforcement in a typical three-phase procedure using signaled delays during the test for resurgence. Results of this study supported the notion that greater delays to reinforcement produce more resurgence; however, the use of signaled versus un-signaled delays make direct comparisons between the Jarmolowicz and Lattal and Nighbor et al. data challenging. Further research is required to draw firmer conclusions regarding the generality of these effects.

Response Parameters

Although the majority of research focuses on manipulations to reinforcement parameters and their corresponding effect on resurgence, an increasing body of work targets manipulations to response characteristics.

Single Versus Multiple Responses

While standard resurgence preparations involve simply training a single alternative response, recent research has begun to examine the effects of training multiple alternative responses on resurgence. This approach may be considered more ecologically valid, as individuals in natural settings often have access to multiple response options to obtain reinforcers. Much of the research in this domain utilizes human operant arrangements to assess the effects of incorporating and teaching multiple responses on resurgence. Some evidence suggests training multiple alternative responses may reduce resurgence of target responding relative to only training a single alternative response. For example, Lambert et al. (2015) used a multiple schedule with a control and test component, reinforcing a designated target response in both components during Phase 1. During Phase 2, target responding was placed on extinction and one alternative response produced reinforcement in the control component. In the testing component, three alternative responses produced reinforcement according to a serial training schedule. Specifically, one response (i.e., A1) produced reinforcement until it reached a mastery criterion, at which point, a separate response (i.e., A2) produced reinforcement while A1 was placed on extinction and so forth. Results of the resurgence test indicated greater resurgence in the control component, potentially highlighting the use of multiple alternative responses to help mitigate resurgence.

Other studies have also provided promising support for the use of multiple alternative response options (e.g., Diaz-Salvat et al., 2020, Experiment 1). For example, Diaz-Salvat et al. (2020) found the mere presence of multiple options impacted resurgence, independent of how those options were trained. Specifically, when there were five response options available, authors observed no differences in levels of resurgence between a group that earned reinforcement for engaging in one specific response during the entirety of Phase 2 and a group who experienced a serial training procedure as described above (Experiment 2). Furthermore, greater resurgence occurred in conditions associated with fewer response options when the training type was held constant. Therefore, the authors concluded the simple presence and availability of additional alternative responses may reduce resurgence.

Although these studies present some interesting preliminary evidence in support of multiple alternative responses as a means of mitigating resurgence, several studies have failed to replicate this effect, calling into question the robustness of this outcome. For example, Nist and Shahan (2023) found no differences in resurgence between groups of rats that had access to several alternative response options compared to those that had single alternative options, regardless of whether the alternative options were reinforced according to concurrent, serial, or single arrangements. Furthermore, a recent review of this research suggested inconsistent results between the few studies directly evaluating expanded-operant training as a strategy for resurgence mitigation (Fuhrman et al., 2022). Nevertheless, future research should continue to evaluate the relation between expanded-operant arrangements and resurgence as it may represent a promising tool that clinicians can utilize to help mitigate resurgence.

Topography of Responses

As previously mentioned, basic and applied research tends to focus on resurgence due to its clear relation to the clinical treatment setting, particularly when it comes to the treatment of problem behavior using FCT. In the clinical context, the target and alternative behaviors differ in topography, but not function. For example, target responses may include challenging behavior, whereas alternative responses may include communication responses. In basic literature, there is less consistency when it comes to using topographically different responses for the target and alternative options. Podlesnik et al., (2022b) reported around 65% of studies used the same response topographies across phases (i.e., a key peck for the target, a different key peck for the alternative), although few studies directly evaluate the impact of different topographies on resurgence.

As one of the few examples, Doughty et al. (2007, Experiment 5) conducted a study with pigeons using a key peck as the target response, and either a key peck to a different key or a treadle press as the alternative response. Results showed greater resurgence in the pigeons who learned a topographically different alternative response relative to those for whom the target and alternative responses were of the same topography. Given the limited number of studies on this topic, additional research should explore whether these findings generalize to more applied settings, particularly where different topographies are used to replace problematic behaviors.

Response Effort

As mentioned by Wilson et al. (2016), response effort is another variable that has gained more recent attention in basic research on resurgence. For example, Walter and Dickson (2023, Experiment 1) conducted a study in a human operant setting with 10 participants engaging with a computer-based task with clicks to one of two moving circles as the target and alternative response. Both circles differed in color, shape, size, and speed, depending on the condition. Authors manipulated response effort in three different conditions, varying in difficulty from easy to difficult. In the intermediate condition, the circles were equal in size and speed and only differed in color. During the difficult condition, the stimulus for the target response was smaller and moved faster, while the stimulus for the alternative response moved slower and was of a bigger size. Lastly, during the "easy" condition, the stimulus for the target response was larger and slower, while the stimulus for the alternative response was smaller and faster. Results of the three-phase resurgence procedure showed greater resurgence during the easy condition, compared to the difficult condition. Replications of this effect are scarce (see Kestner et al., 2018, for a similar example), which should be taken into consideration for future studies.

Conceptual Analyses of Resurgence

The above discussion provided a brief overview of variables that impact resurgence. The effects of many of these variables are robust in that they have been replicated within and between species using a variety of different reinforcers and reinforcement contingencies. Given such regularities in how the environment affects behavior, it is reasonable to ask why those regularities exist. Fortunately, basic researchers have offered several conceptual approaches to explain why resurgence happens and the variables that affect it. This section will introduce three such analyses: behavioral momentum theory, context theory, and resurgence as choice. It is important to note that the purpose of this review is not to endorse one specific theoretical framework over another, nor is it to provide a critical analysis of the relative strengths and weaknesses of these frameworks (for such comparisons, see Craig, 2023; Shahan & Craig, 2017; Trask et al., 2015). Instead, this section attempts to provide an accessible introduction to the arguments put forward by these theories. In so doing, the goal is to equip readers with a repertoire that may be useful for identifying sources of resurgence in the natural environment and understanding how the decisions they make in their practice or research may affect resurgence.

Behavioral Momentum Theory

Tony Nevin and his colleagues (Nevin & Grace, 2000; Nevin et al., 1983) developed behavioral momentum theory to describe regularities in the relations between various reinforcement manipulations and the resistance to change of behavior they engendered. For example, Nevin (1974) trained pigeons to peck keys in a series of multiple schedules such that components signaled different rates, magnitudes, and immediacies of reinforcement. Nevin disrupted key pecking either by placing it on extinction or by presenting free reinforcers during the blackout periods that separated multiple-schedule components. He observed greater persistence of key pecking in the component associated with more (i.e., a higher rate or larger magnitude of) reinforcement, regardless of the reinforcer manipulation or the strategy he used to disrupt behavior.

According to behavioral momentum theory, how much behavior persists under conditions of disruption is a function of the Pavlovian relation between reinforcers and the context in which they were delivered prior to disruption (for reviews, see Craig et al., 2014, 2024). Higher rates and larger magnitudes of reinforcement produce stronger Pavlovian stimulus-reinforcer relations than lower rates or smaller magnitudes of reinforcement. Therefore, behavior is more likely to persist in a context associated with a stronger stimulus-reinforcer relation than in a context associated with a weaker stimulus-reinforcer relation.

There are parallels between the variables that have been shown to impact resistance to change and those shown to impact resurgence. For example, as described earlier, Leitenberg et al. (1975) observed higher rates of alternative reinforcement were associated with more resurgence than lower rates of alternative reinforcement (see also Bouton & Trask, 2016; Craig & Shahan, 2016). This outcome is similar to the greater persistence of operant behavior produced by higher relative to lower rates of pre-disruption reinforcement. Based on this similarity, Shahan and Sweeney (2011) developed a quantitative theory of resurgence based on behavioral momentum theory.

The behavioral-momentum theory of resurgence is expressed in the following equation:

$$\frac{B_t}{B_o} = 10^{\frac{-t(kR_a + c + d\Delta r)}{(r + R_a)^b}} \tag{1.1}$$

The left side of Eq. 1.1 is the dependent variable being modeled, proportion-of-baseline response rates during session t of extinction.[2] The right side of the equation argues that resurgence is the product of two opposing forces: disruptive factors that suppress operant responding (factors found in the numerator of the exponent) and response-strengthening factors that are affected by the stimulus-reinforcer relation in the conditioning situation and that support persistence (factors found in the denominator). Disruptive factors include the effects of suspending the response-reinforcer contingency during Phases 2 and 3 (c), generalization decrement produced by removing reinforcement for the target behavior during Phases 2 and 3 ($d\Delta r$, where Δr is the change in reinforcer rates, measured in reinforcers omitted per hour, between baseline and extinction; d is a scaling parameter), and provision of an alternative source of reinforcement during Phase 2 (kR_a, where R_a is the rate of alternative reinforcement in reinforcers per hour and k is a scaling parameter). The disruptive effects of these variables increase linearly with time in extinction (t, measured in sessions).

As expressed in the denominator of Eq. 1.1, the Pavlovian stimulus-reinforcer relation in the conditioning context is thought to be affected by all reinforcers that are delivered in a stimulus context, whether they be delivered contingently on the target behavior (r, in reinforcers delivered per hour) or the alternative behavior (R_a). The b parameter represents the individual's sensitivity to reinforcer rates. Moreover, once a source of reinforcement has been introduced, its contribution to the stimulus-reinforcer relation lingers over time, even if that source of reinforcement stops being productive during extinction. Resurgence happens because, when transitioning from Phase 2 to Phase 3, the disruptive impact of alternative reinforcement is removed from the numerator of the equation, but its response-strengthening effects linger in the denominator.

Figure 1.3 shows predictions of the behavioral-momentum model of resurgence over a range of values of r (top panel) and R_a (bottom panel) with k, c, d, and b fixed at 0.05, 1, 0.001, and 0.5, respectively. These are parameter values that are representative of those obtained from fits of Eq. 1.1 to obtained resurgence data (see Shahan & Sweeney, 2011; Craig & Shahan, 2016). In the top panel R_a was fixed at 180 reinforcers per hour, and in the bottom panel r was fixed at 180 reinforcers per hour. As the figure illustrates, increasing either r or R_a results in more resurgence during

[2] The dependent variable modeled by Eq. 1.1 is usually *log-transformed* proportion-of-baseline response rates, and the right side of the equation is usually not expressed as the exponent of 10. Setting both sides as the exponent of 10 expresses outcomes as raw proportion of baseline, a variable that may be more accessible to readers.

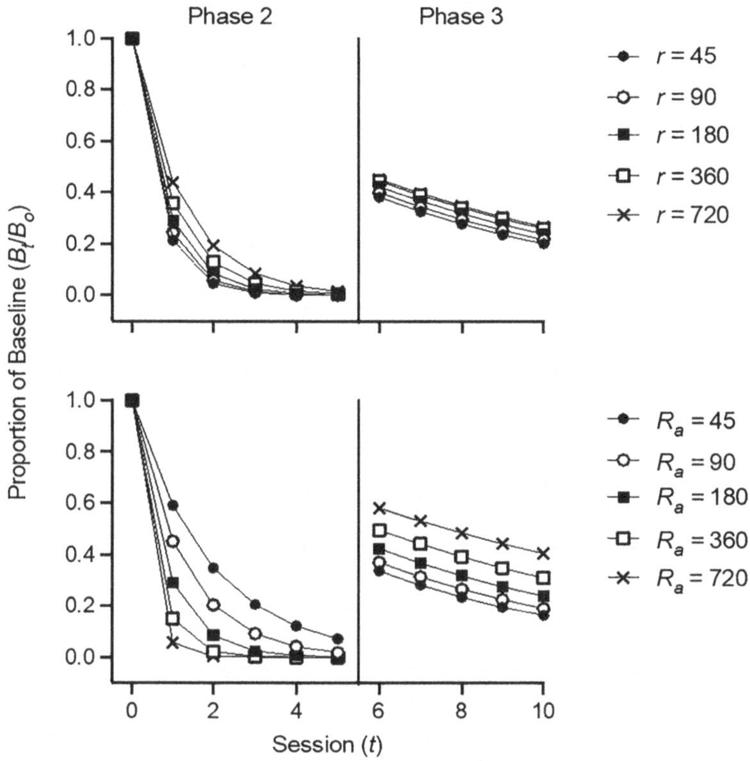

Fig. 1.3 Predictions of Eq. 1.1 (behavioral momentum theory) over a range of values for r and R_a. *Note.* $k = 0.05$, $c = 1$, $d = 0.001$, and $b = 0.5$. In the top panel, $R_a = 180$. In the bottom panel, $r = 180$

Phase 3, although the effects of R_a on resurgence are more pronounced than those of r. The positive relation between alternative-reinforcer rates and resurgence is well documented (e.g., Bouton & Trask, 2016; Craig & Shahan, 2016; Leitenberg et al., 1975), but the relation predicted by Eq. 1.1 between *target* reinforcer rates and resurgence is less robust, having been shown in some studies but not others (e.g., Craig & Shahan, 2016; Podlesnik & Shahan, 2009, 2010). Moreover, the r and R_a parameters have opposing effects on persistence of target behavior during Phase 2: increasing r promotes persistence, and increasing R_a reduces persistence, of target behavior. Presumably, manipulations to other dimensions of reinforcement, like its magnitude or quality, would impact r or R_a in a manner similar to reinforcer rate (see Craig et al., 2017), allowing the equation to describe the effects of diverse reinforcer dimensions on resurgence.

Context Theory

Bouton and colleagues (Bouton & Trask, 2016; Trask et al., 2015) provide an account of resurgence that couches it in terms of another form of relapse, *renewal*. Renewal is relapse that is occasioned by changing the context that was established during response elimination either to a context that was previously associated with reinforcement of the target behavior or to a completely novel context (see Chap. 3, Kimball et al., this volume). Like resurgence, renewal is studied in three phases. In Phase 1, the target behavior is reinforced, whereas it is extinguished in Phases 2 and 3. The major independent variable that is manipulated between phases is the context (e.g., physical stimuli in an operant chamber) that is arranged. Renewal has been demonstrated by manipulating the context across phases in several different ways.

Bouton and colleagues (Bouton, 2002, 2004) developed context theory to describe data from the literature on renewal of operantly and classically conditioned behavior (for the sake of simplicity, we will consider only operant renewal below). According to context theory, individuals develop excitatory, response-reinforcer associations when a target behavior is reinforced. When it is not reinforced, individuals develop inhibitory, response-no-reinforcer associations. Moreover, these associations come under the control of the context in the presence of which they are learned, but the extent to which these associations may generalize between contexts differs. On the one hand, excitatory learning, like the learning that occurs during Phase 1 of a renewal preparation, readily generalizes between contexts. On the other hand, inhibitory learning, like the learning that occurs during Phase 2 of renewal preparation, is context specific. When the context is changed in Phase 3, excitatory learning from Phase 1 readily generalizes to the Phase-3 context, but inhibitory learning does not. Therefore, behavior relapses.

Context theory argues that resurgence is simply another form of renewal wherein the response-elimination context is signaled by the availability of a source of alternative reinforcement during Phase 2. During Phase 3, removing or reducing the source of alternative reinforcement represents a context change that leaves behavior susceptible to relapse. Moreover, according to the theory, the salience of a context change should be positively related to the amount of relapse produced by the context change because inhibitory learning may be less likely to generalize between contexts that are less similar than between contexts that are more similar to each other (see Todd, 2013). As such, changes from higher rates or larger magnitudes of alternative reinforcement to no alternative reinforcement during Phase 3 of a resurgence preparation should produce less generalization of inhibitory learning, and thus more resurgence, than changes from lower rates or smaller magnitudes of alternative reinforcement (see Bouton & Trask, 2016).

Resurgence as Choice

The resurgence as choice model (RaC) proposed by Shahan and Craig et al. (2017) argues that resurgence is governed by the same basic processes that are through to govern choice. Like behavioral momentum theory, RaC offers a quantitative model that relates variables thought to affect resurgence to predicted response rates. The equation for behavioral output is based on Herrnstein's hyperbola (Herrnstein, 1970) and the concatenated matching law (Baum & Rachlin, 1969) and appears as follows:

$$B_t = \frac{kV_t}{V_t + V_\mathrm{a} + 1/A} \tag{1.2}$$

The left side of Eq. 1.2 is the dependent variable being modeled, the rate of the target behavior in responses per minute. In the numerator of the right side of the equation, k represents asymptotic response rates and V_t is the value of the source of reinforcement for the target response. In the denominator of Eq. 1.2, V_a is the value of the source of reinforcement for the alternative response, and A is arousal produced by reinforcer deliveries.

According to RaC, all of an organism's historical experiences with a source of reinforcement contribute that source's value, but they do so in a temporally weighted manner such that recent experiences influence value more strongly than experiences from the distant past. Quantitatively, the model uses a scaled version of the Devenports' (e.g., Devenport & Devenport, 1993) temporal weighting rule:

$$w_x = \frac{1/\left(t_x^c\right)}{\sum_{i=1}^{n} 1/t_i^c} \tag{1.3}$$

W_x is the weight assigned to experience x in the organism's behavior history. In the numerator of the right side of the equation, $1/t_x$ is the recency of experience x, where t_x is the amount of time (usually measured in sessions) that has passed since that experience. The denominator of the right side of the equation is all the relevant experiences in the organism's behavioral history that are being weighted. The c parameter represents how quickly the passage of time affects weighting. When $c = 0$, all events in the historical record receive equal weighting, and as c becomes larger, the amount of weight given to recent events increases and the amount of weight given to temporally distant experiences decreases. The c parameter is assumed to vary with reinforcer rates (r) as follows:

$$c = \lambda r + 1 \tag{1.4}$$

In Eq. 1.4, λ is a scaling parameter. Eq. 1.4 allows RaC to describe the partial-reinforcement extinction effect (see Gallistel, 2012; Mackintosh, 1974) by assuming that organisms weigh recent experiences more heavily (and temporally distant experiences less heavily) when reinforcer rates are higher than when they are low. Values of the target (Eq. 1.5a) and alternative (Eq. 1.5b) sources of reinforcement are calculated by multiplying the rates (*r*) and magnitudes (*m*) of reinforcement experienced at individual time points in the behavior history by their associated weights and summing across the series:

$$V_t = \sum_{i=1}^{n} w_i r_{ti} m_{ti} \tag{1.5a}$$

$$V_a = \sum_{i=1}^{n} w_i r_{ai} m_{ai} \tag{1.5b}$$

Arousal, *A*, is adopted from Killeen's (Killeen, 1994; Killeen & Sitomer, 2003) mathematical principles of reinforcement. As in its initial application, *A* in RaC is meant to capture the behaviorally invigorating effects of reinforcer deliveries and is a function of the summed, temporally weighted rates and magnitudes of reinforcement associated with the target and alternative options:

$$A = a\left(V_t + V_a\right) \tag{1.6}$$

In Eq. 1.6, *a* is a scaling parameter.

Figure 1.4 shows predictions of Eq. 1.2 over a range of r_t and r_a values. As with Eqs. 1.1 and 1.2 predicts that resurgence should be positively related to the rate of alternative reinforcement (r_a). Because rates and magnitudes of alternative reinforcement are treated equivalently by RaC (see Eqs. 1.5a and 1.5b), the equation would make the same ordinal predictions about alternative-reinforcer magnitude manipulations. Unlike Eq. 1.1, however, Eq. 1.2 predicts somewhat modest effects on resurgence of changes in rates of reinforcement for the target response (r_t). As described earlier, target reinforcer rates have been demonstrated to have inconsistent effects on resurgence in the literature. This is an area for future empirical work that may help to distinguish between predictions of Eqs. 1.1 and 1.2.

Summary and Conclusion

There are many conditions under which a behavior "comes back" or reemerges. This chapter specifically discussed the basic research evaluating the conditions when the reappearance of a behavior is classified as resurgence. This phenomenon has garnered particular interest from basic and translational researchers in behavior analysis because of its implications for clinical practice. This chapter discussed the historical development of procedures used to evaluate resurgence, the commonly used dependent measures reported in the basic literature, findings related to variables functionally related to resurgence effects, and description of the quantitative models developed to explain the fundamental behavioral processes underlying

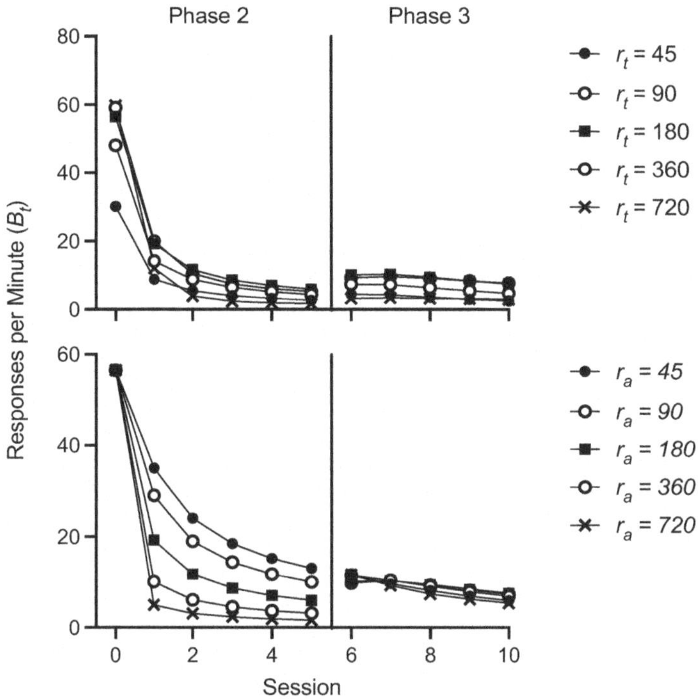

Fig. 1.4 Predictions of Eq. 1.2 (resurgence as choice) over a range of values for r_t and r_a. *Note.* $k = 60$, $\lambda = 0.006$, and $a = 0.0005$. Phases 1, 2, and 3 were all five sessions long. In the top panel, $r_a = 180$ during Phase 2. In the bottom panel, $r_t = 180$ during Phase 1

resurgence. In the next chapter, Norris et al. will discuss how the findings from basic literature have been applied to some of the clinical concerns described above.

As noted in the introduction and as can be seen throughout this chapter, basic researchers have made several significant contributions to our understanding of resurgence. Scientists and clinicians have a significantly greater understanding of the different variables that affect resurgence across a wide variety of species, behaviors, and contexts as a result of this research. The systematic review of the resurgence literature conducted by Podlesnik and his colleagues (2022) identified 200 experiments reported across 120 empirical articles, all contributing to our basic understanding of this form of relapse. These studies have served to help develop and test ways to prevent or mitigate resurgence and to create treatments that produce more sustainable and robust behavior change. Nevertheless, there remain gaps in the literature that need to be filled to fully flesh out the conditions under which resurgence may occur, and we have highlighted these gaps in this chapter. In order to provide the most comprehensive services based on the principles of the experimental analysis of behavior, basic laboratories are charged with continuing to develop a more complete understanding of the relevant variables and their relation to resurgence. We hope that interested readers will join in the effort to fill them.

References

Bachá-Méndez, G., Reid, A. K., & Mendoza-Soylovna, A. (2007). Resurgence of integrated behavioral units. *Journal of the Experimental Analysis of Behavior, 87*, 5–24. https://doi.org/10.1901/jeab.2007.55-05

Bai, J. Y., Cowie, S., & Podlesnik, C. A. (2017). Quantitative analysis of local-level resurgence. *Learning & Behavior, 45*(1), 76–88. https://doi.org/10.3758/s13420-016-0242-1

Baum, W. M. (2012). Rethinking reinforcement: Allocation, induction, and contingency. *Journal of the Experimental Analysis of Behavior, 97*(1), 101–124. https://doi.org/10.1901/jeab.2012.97-101

Baum, W. M., & Rachlin, H. C. (1969). Choice as time allocation. *Journal of the Experimental Analysis of Behavior, 12*, 861–874. https://doi.org/10.1901/jeab.1970.13-243

Benavides, R., & Escobar, R. (2017). Resurgence of response duration in human participants. *Behavioural Processes, 142*, 106–109. https://doi.org/10.1016/j.beproc.2017.06.010

Bolívar, H. A., Cox, D. J., Barlow, M. A., & Dallery, J. (2017). Evaluating resurgence procedures in a human operant laboratory. *Behavioural Processes, 140*, 150–160. https://doi.org/10.1016/j.beproc.2017.05.004

Bouton, M. E. (2002). Context, ambiguity, and unlearning: Sources of relapse after behavioral extinction. *Biological Psychiatry, 52*, 976–986. https://doi.org/10.1016/S0006-3223(02)01546-9

Bouton, M. E. (2004). Context and behavioral processes in extinction. *Learning and Memory, 11*, 485–494. https://doi.org/10.1101/lm.78804

Bouton, M. E., & Trask, S. (2016). Role of the discriminative properties of the reinforcer in resurgence. *Learning & Behavior, 44*(2), 137–150. https://doi.org/10.3758/s13420-015-0197-7

Briggs, A. M., Fisher, W. W., Greer, B. D., & Kimball, R. T. (2018). Prevalence of resurgence of destructive behavior when thinning reinforcement schedules during functional communication training. *Journal of Applied Behavior Analysis, 51*, 620–633. https://doi.org/10.1002/jaba.472

Brown, H. D., & DeFulio, A. (2020). Contingency management for the treatment of methamphetamine use disorder: A systematic review. *Drug and Alcohol Dependence, 216*, 108307. https://doi.org/10.1016/j.drugalcdep.2020.108307

Brown, K. R., Greer, B. D., Craig, A. R., Sullivan, W. E., Fisher, W. W., & Roane, H. S. (2020). Resurgence following differential reinforcement of alternative behavior implemented with and without extinction. *Journal of the Experimental Analysis of Behavior, 113*, 449–467. https://doi.org/10.1002/jeab.588

Browning, K. O., Sutton, G. M., Nist, A. N., & Shahan, T. A. (2022). The effects of large, small, and thinning magnitudes of alternative reinforcement on resurgence. *Behavioural Processes, 195*, 104586. https://doi.org/10.1016/j.beproc.2022.104586

Bruzek, J. L., Thompson, R. H., & Peters, L. C. (2009). Resurgence of infant caregiving responses. *Journal of the Experimental Analysis of Behavior, 92*(3), 327–343. https://doi.org/10.1901/jeab.2009-92-327

Cançado, C. R., & Lattal, K. A. (2011). Resurgence of temporal patterns of responding. *Journal of the Experimental Analysis of Behavior, 95*(3), 271–287. https://doi.org/10.1901/jeab.2011.95-271

Cançado, C. R. X., Abreu-Rodrigues, J., & Aló, R. M. (2016). A note on measuring recurrence. *Revista Mexicana de Análisis de La Conducta, 42*(1). 10.5514/rmac.v42.i1. https://doi.org/10.5514/rmac.v42.i1.56784

Cançado, C. R., Lattal, K. A., Carpenter, H. K., & Solley, E. A. (2017). Resurgence of time allocation. *Journal of the Experimental Analysis of Behavior, 108*(3), 398–413. https://doi.org/10.1002/jeab.288

Carey, J. P. (1951). Reinstatement of previously learned responses under conditions of extinction: A study of "regression" [Abstract]. *American Psychologist, 6*, 284.

Catania, A. C. (1963). Concurrent performances: A baseline for the study of reinforcement magnitude. *Journal of the Experimental Analysis of Behavior, 6*(2), 299–300. https://doi.org/10.1901/jeab.1963.6-299

Cleland, B. S., Foster, T. M., & Temple, W. (2000). Resurgence: The role of extinction. *Behavioural Processes, 52*(2-3), 117–129. https://doi.org/10.1016/s0376-6357(00)00131-5

Cook, J. E., & Lattal, K. A. (2019). Repeated, within-session resurgence: Repeated within-session resurgence. *Journal of the Experimental Analysis of Behavior, 111*(1), 28–47. https://doi.org/10.1002/jeab.496

Craig, A. R. (2023). Resistance to change, of behavior and of theory. *Journal of the Experimental Analysis of Behavior, 120*, 440–456. https://doi.org/10.1002/jeab.875

Craig, A. R., & Shahan, T. A. (2016). Behavioral momentum theory fails to account for the effects of reinforcement rate on resurgence. *Journal of the Experimental Analysis of Behavior, 105*(3), 375392. https://doi.org/10.1002/jeab.207

Craig, A. R., Nevin, J. A., & Odum, A. L. (2014). Behavioral momentum and resistance to change. In F. K. McSweeney & E. S. Murphy (Eds.), *The Wiley Blackwell handbook of operant and classical conditioning* (pp. 249–274). Wiley Blackwell. https://psycnet.apa.org/doi/10.1002/9781118468135.ch11

Craig, A. R., Nall, R. W., Madden, G. J., & Shahan, T. A. (2016). Higher rate alternative non-drug reinforcement produces faster suppression of cocaine seeking but more resurgence when removed. *Behavioral Brain Research, 306*, 48–51. https://doi.org/10.1016/j.bbr.2016.03.026

Craig, A. R., Browning, K. O., Nall, R. W., Marshall, C. M., & Shahan, T. A. (2017). Resurgence and alternative-reinforcer magnitude. *Journal of the Experimental Analysis of Behavior, 107*(2), 218–233. https://doi.org/10.1002/jeab.245

Craig, A. R., Sullivan, W. E., Derrenbacker, K., Rimal, A., DeRosa, N. M., & Roane, H. S. (2020). An evaluation of resurgence in mice. *Learning and Motivation, 72*, 101671. https://doi.org/10.1016/j.lmot.2020.101671

Craig, A. R., Ringdahl, J. E., & Sullivan, W. E. (2024). Resistance to change from bench to bedside (and back again). In H. S. Roane, A. R. Craig, V. Saini, & J. E. Ringdahl (Eds.), *Behavior analysis: Translational perspectives and clinical practice* (pp. 392–413). The Guilford Press.

da Silva, S. P. D., Maxwell, M. E., & Lattal, K. A. (2008). Concurrent resurgence and behavioral history. *Journal of the Experimental Analysis of Behavior, 90*(3), 313–331. https://doi.org/10.1901/jeab.2008.90-313

Devenport, J. A., & Devenport, L. D. (1993). Time-dependent decision in dogs (*Canis familiaris*). *Journal of Comparative Psychology, 107*, 169–173. https://psycnet.apa.org/doi/10.1037/0735-7036.107.2.169

Diaz-Salvat, C. C., St. Peter, C. C., & Shuler, N. J. (2020). Increased number of responses may account for reduced resurgence following serial training. *Journal of Applied Behavior Analysis, 53*(3), 1542–1558. https://doi.org/10.1002/jaba.686

Doughty, A. H., da Silva, S. P., & Lattal, K. A. (2007). Differential resurgence and response elimination. *Behavioural Processes, 75*(2), 115–128. https://doi.org/10.1016/j.beproc.2007.02.025

Epstein, R. (1983). Resurgence of previously reinforced behavior during extinction. *Behaviour Analysis Letters, 3*(6), 391–397.

Epstein, R. (2015). On the rediscovery of the principle of resurgence. *Revista Mexicana de Análisis de la Conducta, 41*(2), 19–43. https://doi.org/10.5514/rmac.v41.i2.63722

Epstein, R., & Skinner, B. F. (1980). Resurgence of responding after the cessation of response-independent reinforcement. *Proceedings of the National Academy of Sciences of the United States of America, 77*(10), 6251–6253. https://doi.org/10.1073/pnas.77.10.6251

Ferster, C. B., & Skinner, B. F. (1957). Schedules of reinforcement. *Appleton-Century-Crofts*. https://doi.org/10.1037/10627-000

Fisher, W. W., Saini, V., Greer, B. D., Sullivan, W. E., Roane, H. S., Fuhrman, A. M., ... & Kimball, R. T. (2019). Baseline reinforcement rate and resurgence of destructive behavior. *Journal of the Experimental Analysis of Behavior, 111*(1), 75–93. https://doi.org/10.1002/jeab.488

Fisher, W. W., Fuhrman, A. M., Greer, B. D., Mitteer, D. R., & Piazza, C. C. (2020). Mitigating resurgence of destructive behavior using the discriminative stimuli of a multiple schedule. *Journal of the Experimental Analysis of Behavior, 113*(1), 263–277. https://doi.org/10.1002/jeab.552

Fisher, W. W., Greer, B. D., Shahan, T. A., & Norris, H. M. (2023). Basic and applied research on extinction bursts. *Journal of Applied Behavior Analysis, 56*(1), 4–28. https://doi.org/10.1002/jaba.954

Fontes, R. M., Todorov, J. C., & Shahan, T. A. (2018). Punishment of an alternative behavior generates resurgence of a previously extinguished target behavior. *Journal of the Experimental Analysis of Behavior, 110*(2), 171–184. https://doi.org/10.1002/jeab.465

Frye, C. C. J., Rung, J. M., Nall, R. W., Galizio, A., Haynes, J. M., & Odum, A. L. (2018). Continuous nicotine exposure does not affect resurgence of alcohol seeking in rats. *PLoS One, 13*(8), e0202230. https://doi.org/10.1371/journal.pone.0202230

Fuhrman, A. M., Lambert, J. M., & Greer, B. D. (2022). A brief review of expanded-operant treatments for mitigating resurgence. *The Psychological Record, 72*(2), 319–323. https://doi.org/10.1007/s40732-021-00456-z

Galizio, A., Friedel, J. E., & Odum, A. L. (2020). An investigation of resurgence of reinforced behavioral variability in humans. *Journal of the Experimental Analysis of Behavior, 114*(3), 381–393. https://doi.org/10.1002/jeab.637

Gallistel, C. R. (2012). Extinction from a rationalist perspective. *Behavioural Processes, 90*(1), 66–80. https://doi.org/10.1016/j.beproc.2012.02.008

Haney, S. D., Greer, B. D., Mitteer, D. R., & Randall, K. R. (2022). Relapse during the treatment of pediatric feeding disorders. *Journal of Applied Behavior Analysis, 55*(3), 704–726. https://doi.org/10.1002/jaba.913

Herrnstein, R. J. (1970). On the law of effect. *Journal of the Experimental Analysis of Behavior, 13*, 243–266. https://doi.org/10.1901/eab.1970.13-243

Hollard, V., & Davison, M. C. (1971). Preference for qualitatively different reinforcers. *Journal of the Experimental Analysis of Behavior, 16*(3), 375–380. https://doi.org/10.1901/jeab.1971.16-375

Hull, C. L. (1934). The rat's speed-of-locomotion gradient in the approach to food. *Journal of Comparative Psychology, 17*(3), 393–422. https://doi.org/10.1037/h0071299

Jarmolowicz, D. P., & Lattal, K. A. (2014). Resurgence under delayed reinforcement. *The Psychological Record, 64*, 189–193. https://doi.org/10.1007/s40732-014-0040-0

Kestner, K., Redner, R., Watkins, E. E., & Poling, A. (2015). The effects of punishment on resurgence in laboratory rats. *The Psychological Record, 65*, 315–321.

Kestner, K. M., Romano, L. M., St Peter, C. C., & Mesches, G. A. (2018). Resurgence following response cost in a human-operant procedure. *The Psychological Record, 68*(1), 81–87. https://doi.org/10.1007/s40732-018-0270-7

Killeen, P. R. (1994). Mathematical principles of reinforcement. *Behavioral and Brain Sciences, 17*, 105–172. https://psycnet.apa.org/doi/10.1017/S0140525X00033628

Killeen, P. R., & Sitomer, M. T. (2003). MPR. *Behavioural Processes, 62*(1-3), 49–64. https://doi.org/10.1016/s0376-6357(03)00017-2

Kimball, R. T., Greer, B. D., Fuhrman, A. M., & Lambert, J. M. (2023). Relapse and its mitigation: Toward behavioral inoculation. *Journal of Applied Behavior Analysis, 56*(2), 282–301. https://doi.org/10.1002/jaba.971

Kincaid, S. L., Lattal, K. A., & Spence, J. (2015). Super-resurgence: ABA renewal increases resurgence. *Behavioural Processes, 115*, 70–73. https://doi.org/10.1016/j.beproc.2015.02.013

Kuroda, T., Cançado, C. R. X., & Podlesnik, C. A. (2016). Resistance to change and resurgence in humans engaging in a computer task. *Behavioural Processes, 125*, 1–5. https://doi.org/10.1016/j.beproc.2016.01.010

Kuroda, T., Mizutani, Y., Cançado, C. R. X., & Podlesnik, C. A. (2017a). Operant models of relapse in zebrafish (Danio rerio): Resurgence, renewal, and reinstatement. *Behavioural Brain Research, 335*, 215–222. https://doi.org/10.1016/j.bbr.2017.08.023

Kuroda, T., Mizutani, Y., Cançado, C. R. X., & Podlesnik, C. A. (2017b). Reversal learning and resurgence of operant behavior in zebrafish (Danio rerio). *Behavioural Processes, 142*, 79–83. https://doi.org/10.1016/j.beproc.2017.06.004

Lambert, J. M., Bloom, S. E., Samaha, A. L., Dayton, E., & Rodewald, A. M. (2015). Serial alternative response training as intervention for target response resurgence. *Journal of Applied Behavior Analysis, 48*(4), 765–780. https://doi.org/10.1002/jaba.253

Lattal, K. A., & Oliver, A. C. (2020). The control response in assessing resurgence: Useful or compromised tool? *Journal of the Experimental Analysis of Behavior, 113*(1), 77–86. https://doi.org/10.1002/jeab.570

Lattal, K. A., & St. Peter Pipkin, C. (2009). Resurgence of previously reinforced responding: Research and application. *The Behavior Analyst Today, 10*(2), 254–266. https://doi.org/10.1037/h0100669

Lattal, K. A., St. Peter, C., & Escobar, R. (2013). Operant extinction: Elimination and generation of behavior. In G. J. Madden, W. V. Dube, T. D. Hackenberg, G. P. Hanley, & K. A. Lattal (Eds.), *APA handbook of behavior analysis, Vol. 2: Translating principles into practice* (pp. 77–107). American Psychological Association. https://doi.org/10.1037/13938-004

Lattal, K. A., Cançado, C. R., Cook, J. E., Kincaid, S. L., Nighbor, T. D., & Oliver, A. C. (2017). On defining resurgence. *Behavioural Processes, 141*(1), 85–91. https://doi.org/10.1016/j.beproc.2017.04.018

Leitenberg, H., Rawson, R. A., & Mulick, J. A. (1975). Extinction and reinforcement of alternative behavior. *Journal of Comparative and Physiological Psychology, 88*(2), 640.

Lieving, G. A., & Lattal, K. A. (2003). Recency, repeatability, and reinforcer retrenchment: An experimental analysis of resurgence. *Journal of the Experimental Analysis of Behavior, 80*(2), 217–233. https://doi.org/10.1901/jeab.2003.80-217

Mackintosh, N. J. (1974). *The psychology of animal learning*. Academic.

Muething, C., Pavlov, A., Call, N., Ringdahl, J., & Gillespie, S. (2021). Prevalence of resurgence during thinning of multiple schedules of reinforcement following functional communication training. *Journal of Applied Behavior Analysis, 54*(2), 813–823. https://doi.org/10.1002/jaba.791

Neuringer, A., Kornell, N., & Olufs, M. (2001). Stability and variability in extinction. *Journal of Experimental Psychology: Animal Behavior Processes, 27*(1), 79–94. https://doi.org/10.1037/0097-7403.27.1.79

Nevin, J. A. (1974). Response strength in multiple schedules. *Journal of the Experimental Analysis of Behavior, 21*, 389–408. https://doi.org/10.1901/jeab.1974.21-389

Nevin, J. A., & Grace, R. C. (2000). Behavioral momentum and the law of effect. *Behavioral and Brain Sciences, 23*, 90–130. https://doi.org/10.1017/s0140525x00002405

Nevin, J. A., & Shahan, T. A. (2011). Behavioral momentum theory: equations and applications. *Journal of Applied Behavior Analysis, 44*(4), 877–895. https://doi.org/10.1901/jaba.2011.44-877

Nevin, J. A., Mandell, C., & Atak, J. R. (1983). The analysis of behavioral momentum. *Journal of the Experimental Analysis of Behavior, 39*, 49–59. https://doi.org/10.1901/jeab.1983.39-49

Nighbor, T. D., Oliver, A. C., & Lattal, K. A. (2020). Resurgence without overall worsening of alternative reinforcement. *Behavioural Processes, 179*, 104219. https://doi.org/10.1016/j.beproc.2020.104219

Nist, A. N., & Shahan, T. A. (2023). Examining resurgence in rats following expanded-operant treatments. *Journal of the Experimental Analysis of Behavior, 120*(2), 186–203. https://doi.org/10.1002/jeab.870

Oliver, A. C., Nighbor, T. D., & Lattal, K. A. (2018). Reinforcer magnitude and resurgence. *Journal of the Experimental Analysis of Behavior, 110(3)*, 440–450. https://doi.org/10.1002/jeab.481

Page, S., & Neuringer, A. (1985). Variability is an operant. *Journal of Experimental Psychology: Animal Behavior Processes, 11*(3), 429–452. https://doi.org/10.1037/0097-7403.11.3.429

Podlesnik, C. A., & Kelley, M. E. (2015). Translational research on the relapse of operant behavior. *Revista Mexicana de Análisis de la Conducta, 41*(2), 226–251.

Podlesnik, C. A., & Shahan, T. A. (2009). Behavioral momentum and relapse of extinguished operant responding. *Learning & Behavior, 37*, 357-364. 10.3758/LB.37.4.357.

Podlesnik, C. A., & Shahan, T. A. (2010). Extinction, relapse, and behavioral momentum. *Behavioural Processes, 84*(1), 400–411. https://doi.org/10.1016/j.beproc.2010.02.001

Podlesnik, C. A., Jimenez-Gomez, C., & Shahan, T. A. (2006). Resurgence of alcohol seeking produced by discontinuing non-drug reinforcement as an animal model of drug relapse. *Behavioural Pharmacology, 17*, 369–374.

Podlesnik, C. A., Ritchey, C. M., Kuroda, T., & Cowie, S. (2022a). A quantitative analysis of the effects of alternative reinforcement rate and magnitude on resurgence. *Behavioural Processes, 198*, 104641. https://doi.org/10.1016/j.beproc.2022.104641

Podlesnik, C. A., Ritchey, C. M., Waits, J., & Gilroy, S. P. (2022b). A comprehensive systematic review of procedures and analyses used in basic and preclinical studies of resurgence, 1970–2020. *Perspectives on Behavior Science, 46*(1), 137–184. https://doi.org/10.1007/s40614-022-00361-y

Quick, S. L., Pyszczynski, A. D., Colston, K. A., & Shahan, T. A. (2011). Loss of alternative non-drug reinforcement induces relapse of cocaine-seeking in rats: Role of dopamine D1 receptors. *Neuropsychopharmacology, 36*(5), 1015–1020.

Reed, P., & Morgan, T. A. (2007). Resurgence of behavior during extinction depends on previous rate of response. *Learning & Behavior, 35*(2), 106–114. https://doi.org/10.3758/BF03193045

Ritchey, C. M., Kuroda, T., Rung, J. M., & Podlesnik, C. A. (2021). Evaluating extinction, renewal, and resurgence of operant behavior in humans with Amazon Mechanical Turk. *Learning and Motivation, 74*, 101728. https://doi.org/10.1016/j.lmot.2021.101728

Saini, V., Sullivan, W. E., Craig, A. R., DeRosa, N. M., Rimal, A., Derrenbacker, K., & Roane, H. S. (2021). Responding fails to extinguish during human-laboratory experiments of resurgence. *The Psychological Record, 71*, 325–336. https://doi.org/10.1007/s40732-021-00469-8

Shahan, T. A., & Craig, A. R. (2017). Resurgence as choice. *Behavioural Processes, 141*, 100–127. https://doi.org/10.1016/j.beproc.2016.10.006

Shahan, T. A., & Sweeney, M. M. (2011). A mode of resurgence based on behavioral momentum theory. *Journal of the Experimental Analysis of Behavior, 95*, 91–108. https://doi.org/10.1901/jeab.2011.95-91

Shahan, T. A., Craig, A. R., & Sweeney, M. M. (2015). Resurgence of sucrose and cocaine seeking in free-feeding rats. *Behavioural Brain Research, 279*, 47–51. https://doi.org/10.1016/j.bbr.2014.10.048

Shahan, T. A., Browning, K. O., Nist, A. N., & Sutton, G. M. (2020). Resurgence and downshifts in alternative reinforcement rate. *Journal of the Experimental Analysis of Behavior, 114*(2), 163–178. https://doi.org/10.1002/jeab.625

Shahan, T. A., Sutton, G. M., Van Allsburg, J., Avellaneda, M., & Greer, B. D. (2024). Resurgence following higher or lower quality alternative reinforcement. *Journal of the Experimental Analysis of Behavior, 121*(2), 246–258. https://doi.org/10.1002/jeab.904

Silverman, K., Chutuape, M. A., Bigelow, G. E., & Stitzer, M. L. (1999). Voucher-based reinforcement of cocaine abstinence in treatment-resistant methadone patients: Effects of reinforcement magnitude. *Psychopharmacology, 146*, 128–138. https://doi.org/10.1007/s002130051098

Skinner, B. F. (1938). *The behaviour of organisms*. Appleton-Century-Crofts.

Skinner, B. F. (1950). Are theories of learning necessary? *Psychological Review, 57*(4), 193–216. https://doi.org/10.1037/h0054367

Smith, B. M., Smith, G. S., Shahan, T. A., Madden, G. J., & Twohig, M. P. (2017). Effects of differential rates of alternative reinforcement on resurgence of human behavior. *Journal of the Experimental Analysis of Behavior, 107*(1), 191–202. https://doi.org/10.1002/jeab.241

Sweeney, M. M., & Shahan, T. A. (2013). Effects of high, low, and thinning rates of alternative reinforcement on response elimination and resurgence. *Journal of the Experimental Analysis of Behavior, 100*(1), 102–116. https://doi.org/10.1002/jeab.26

Smith, S. W., & Greer, B. D. (2022a). Validating human-operant software: A case example. *Behavior analysis* (Washington, D.C.), 22(4), 389–403. https://doi.org/10.1037/bar0000244

Smith, S. W., & Greer, B. D. (2022b). Phase duration and resurgence. *Journal of the experimental analysis of behavior*, 117(1), 91–104. https://doi.org/10.1002/jeab.725

Sweeney, M. M., & Shahan, T. A. (2016). Resurgence of target responding does not exceed increases in inactive responding in a forced-choice alternative reinforcement procedure in humans. *Behavioural Processes, 124*, 80–92. https://doi.org/10.1016/j.beproc.2015.12.007

Tiger, J. H., Hanley, G. P., & Bruzek, J. (2008). Functional communication training: a review and practical guide. *Behavior Analysis in Practice, 1*(1), 16–23. https://doi.org/10.1007/BF03391716

Todd, T. P. (2013). Mechanisms of renewal after the extinction of instrumental behavior. *Journal of Experimental Psychology: Animal Behavior Processes, 39*, 193–207. https://doi.org/10.1037/a0032236

Trask, S., Schepers, S. T., & Bouton, M. E. (2015). Context change explains resurgence after extinction of operant behavior. *Mexican Journal of Behavior Analysis, 41*, 187–210.

Trask, S., & Bouton, M. E. (2016). Discriminative properties of the reinforcer can be used to attenuate the renewal of extinguished operant behavior. *Learning & Behavior, 44*(2), 151–161. https://doi.org/10.3758/s13420-015-0195-9.

Volkert, V. M., Lerman, D. C., Call, N. A., & Trosclair-Lasserre, N. (2009). An evaluation of resurgence during treatment with functional communication training. *Journal of Applied Behavior Analysis, 42*(1), 145–160. https://doi.org/10.1901/jaba.2009

Walter, K. M., & Dickson, C. A. (2023). Response effort and resurgence. *Journal of the Experimental Analysis of Behavior, 119*(2), 373–391. https://doi.org/10.1002/jeab.835

Wathen, S. N., & Podlesnik, C. A. (2018). Laboratory models of treatment relapse and mitigation techniques. *Behavior Analysis: Research and Practice, 18*(4), 362–387. https://doi.org/10.1037/bar0000119

Wilson, A. N., Glassford, T. S., & Koerkenmeier, S. M. (2016). Effects of Response Effort on Resurgence. *Behavior Analysis in Practice, 9*(2), 174–178. https://doi.org/10.1007/s40617-016-0122-3

Winterbauer, N. E., & Bouton, M. E. (2010). Mechanisms of resurgence of an extinguished instrumental behavior. *Journal of Experimental Psychology: Animal Behavior Processes, 36*(3), 343–353. https://doi.org/10.1037/a0017365

Winterbauer, N. E., & Bouton, M. E. (2012). Effects of thinning the rate at which the alternative behavior is reinforced on resurgence of an extinguished instrumental response. *Journal of Experimental Psychology: Animal Behavior Processes, 38*(3), 279. https://doi.org/10.1037/a0028853

Chapter 2
Applied Research on Mitigating Resurgence

Halle M. Norris, Daniel R. Mitteer, Casey Irwin Helvey, and Brian D. Greer

As the previous chapter noted, *resurgence* is a form of relapse in which target responding re-emerges following a worsening of conditions for an alternative response (Epstein, 1985; Lattal et al., 2017; Lattal & Wacker, 2015; see also Greer & Shahan, 2019, and Shahan & Craig, 2017, for related definitions). In clinical settings, resurgence of socially maintained destructive behavior, such as self-injurious behavior or aggression, occurs regularly during treatment (Briggs et al., 2018; Falligant et al., 2022a; Kranak & Falligant, 2021; Mitteer et al., 2022; Muething et al., 2021). Consider a common treatment for destructive behavior known as

Grants 2R01HD079113, 2R01HD093734, 1R01HD109266, and 1R01HD108617 from the National Institute of Child Health and Human Development provided partial support for this work.
The authors have no conflicts of interest to declare.
Daniel Mitteer is now at the Marcus Autism Center and Emory University. Halle Norris is now at Children's Mercy Hospital.

H. M. Norris
Children's Specialized Hospital–Rutgers University Center for Autism Research, Education, and Services (CSH–RUCARES), Somerset, NJ, USA

D. R. Mitteer · C. Irwin Helvey (✉)
Children's Specialized Hospital–Rutgers University Center for Autism Research, Education, and Services (CSH–RUCARES), Somerset, NJ, USA

Rutgers Robert Wood Johnson Medical School, New Brunswick, NJ, USA
e-mail: cih18@rutgers.edu

B. D. Greer
Children's Specialized Hospital–Rutgers University Center for Autism Research, Education, and Services (CSH–RUCARES), Somerset, NJ, USA

Rutgers Robert Wood Johnson Medical School, New Brunswick, NJ, USA

Rutgers Brain Health Institute, Piscataway, NJ, USA

M. P. Kranak (ed.), *Behavioral Treatments for Individuals with Autism*, Autism and Child Psychopathology Series,
https://doi.org/10.1007/978-3-031-91965-7_2

functional communication training (FCT; Tiger et al., 2008). FCT is a differential-reinforcement procedure that involves providing reinforcement for an appropriate alternative response, called a functional communication response (FCR; Carr & Durand, 1985), and often includes an extinction contingency for destructive behavior. For example, when destructive behavior is maintained by access to tangibles, FCT might involve teaching an individual to exchange a card to access a preferred tangible item while the behavior analyst withholds that same tangible item following instances of destructive behavior. FCT is typically implemented with an initially dense reinforcement schedule to teach the FCR and rapidly decrease destructive behavior. Once reliable treatment effects are observed, the schedule of reinforcement is thinned to make treatment implementation more practical. It is during this critical time that resurgence is likely to occur, with researchers finding at least one instance of resurgence in 76–91% of applications of FCT schedule thinning (Briggs et al., 2018; Falligant et al., 2022a; Kranak & Falligant, 2021; Mitteer et al., 2022; Muething et al., 2021).

In other applied settings, unplanned decreases in reinforcer availability can occur due to treatment-integrity errors. For example, resurgence might happen if an FCR goes unreinforced (e.g., while a caregiver is attending to another child) or if technological errors occur (e.g., the Internet connection becomes unavailable). Unfortunately, resurgence of destructive behavior can pose serious injury risks (e.g., tissue damage, broken bones). Even if destructive behavior resurges at a lower intensity, increased destructive behavior may result in individuals inadvertently reinforcing it (e.g., Mitteer et al., 2018), decreasing the likelihood that treatment effects will maintain. Resurgence is such a pressing concern that those seeking certification as board-certified behavior analysts will soon be required to demonstrate competency in planning for and mitigating potential treatment relapse like resurgence (Behavior Analysis Certification Board [BACB], 2020).

Although there has been a recent uptick of applied research on resurgence (Kestner & Peterson, 2017; Perrin et al., 2022), much of the work that has been done includes translational and basic studies (Podlesnik et al., 2023). The preceding chapter provided a comprehensive overview of the methods and procedures that have been used to evaluate resurgence in the basic literature. In general, similar arrangements (e.g., three-phase designs, dependent variables) have been used in the translational and applied literature. According to a recent literature review by Perrin et al. (2022), most of the applied research on resurgence has been done with children under the age of 18 who were diagnosed with autism spectrum disorder. Perrin et al. also found that the existing research has primarily focused on the following areas: (a) schedules of reinforcement for target and alternative responses (e.g., Fisher et al., 2018, 2019), (b) phase duration (e.g., Greer et al., 2020), (c) schedule thinning (e.g., Briggs et al., 2018; Volkert et al., 2009), (d) stimulus control (e.g., Fuhrman et al., 2016), and (e) teaching multiple alternative responses (i.e., expanding the operant class; e.g., Lambert et al., 2017). Notably, many of the specific questions within these lines of research have been informed by quantitative models of resurgence, including behavioral momentum theory (e.g., Fisher et al., 2018; Nevin & Shahan, 2011) and resurgence as choice (e.g., Greer & Shahan, 2019; Shahan &

Craig, 2017; see Chap. 1 for additional details). Although a comprehensive science of resurgence mitigation is still developing, understanding the extant data and relevant theories can guide behavior analysts toward thinking critically about resurgence and developing modifications to improve commonly prescribed treatments.

"Prescribed Fires"

Kimball et al. (2023) describe the effect of minimizing the impact of treatment challenges on the relapse of destructive behavior as *behavioral inoculation*. They distinguish the term *behavioral inoculation* from the actual procedures used by behavior analysts to achieve this outcome. In the context of resurgence, resurgence-mitigation procedures refer to the combination of strategies and technologies that behavior analysts employ throughout assessment and treatment to produce *behavioral inoculation*. Currently, behavioral inoculation is an aspiration, and our science is not yet at the point that we can prevent resurgence. Reducing resurgence during one portion of treatment may mean increased destructive behavior in another part of assessment or treatment.

Our clinical-research group has become accustomed to viewing resurgence within a "prescribed fire" metaphor. In wildland-fire science, prescribed fires are intentional, contained ignitions aimed at bolstering ecosystem resilience and minimizing the impact of wildfires (i.e., accidental ignitions; Hiers et al., 2020). In behavior analysis, we may be unable to stop resurgence from occurring completely, but we may be able to better control when it will occur such that behavior resurges in a safe, well-resourced environment similar to how wildland fire scientists reduce more dangerous wildfires using prescribed fires in tightly controlled locations. This makes resurgence-mitigation procedures crucial by arranging for "prescribed" resurgence in well-controlled clinical settings to avoid significant relapse later outside of the behavior analyst's care (e.g., at home, school).

Resurgence-Mitigation Procedures

The following section will outline and analyze resurgence-mitigation strategies that have been demonstrated as efficacious or promising in clinical literature. It is important to note that some resurgence-mitigation procedures have more empirical support than others, and this list is only meant to describe strategies that have been evaluated with humans, in either an applied or clinical setting. The focus of this chapter is on mitigation strategies that have been evaluated clinically and shown some success. However, promising translational research that has not yet been evaluated clinically is described later in this chapter. We have chosen to organize the discussion of mitigation strategies based on when in time they are implemented within the treatment progression. That is, descriptions of procedures that behavior analysts could implement in baseline (i.e., Phase 1) will come first, followed by procedures implemented in treatment (i.e., Phase 2), and finally procedures implemented during treatment challenges (i.e., Phase 3).

Baseline: Phase 1

Recall that in baseline (i.e., Phase 1), target behavior is reinforced according to some schedule of reinforcement. In clinical settings, this target behavior is often dangerous (e.g., aggression, self-injurious behavior, pica), whereas in a translational evaluation, it may be arbitrary (e.g., button presses, answering math questions). The following sections will describe manipulations to the independent variable that can be made in baseline to potentially mitigate resurgence in future treatment challenges.

Reinforcement Schedules in Baseline

The impact that the schedule of reinforcement in baseline (i.e., Phase 1) has on the magnitude of resurgence has been studied by various research teams. This phenomenon has been evaluated in many settings, including but not limited to nonhuman animal laboratories, human-operant experiments, and within clinical settings involving treatment of destructive behavior. Multiple quantitative theories (e.g., behavioral momentum theory; resurgence as choice) predict, and research supports, that higher rates of reinforcement for the target behavior in baseline produce more resurgence in subsequent treatment challenges.

Fisher et al. (2019) compared high and low rates of reinforcement in baseline with seven individuals who engaged in destructive behavior. In Experiment 1, they compared a dense variable-interval (VI) 2-s schedule of reinforcement to a leaner (e.g., VI 90-s) schedule of reinforcement. Experiment 2 replicated this but with a dense schedule more common during FCT (i.e., fixed-ratio [FR] 1). Across both experiments, programming a denser schedule of reinforcement exacerbated resurgence during a treatment challenge involving periods of extinction (e.g., what might occur when reinforcers are unavailable, broken, or disrupted in some way). This suggests that programming a leaner schedule of reinforcement during baseline may help minimize resurgence later on in treatment. However, considering the "prescribed fire" metaphor again, behavior analysts must consider whether they can safely manage high rates of destructive behavior engendered by the lean reinforcement schedules during baseline and, if so, whether that is preferred to managing potential resurgence later on in treatment.

Duration of Baseline

The duration of exposure to reinforcement for the target behavior has also been shown to have an effect on resurgence of target behavior during future treatment challenges. This can be referred as baseline duration, whether that is within a typical resurgence sequence or conceptualized as time prior to contacting treatment. For example, clinicians could view the age in which an individual began treatment for destructive behavior as an indicator of duration of baseline, if we are assuming that prior to treatment the client was likely contacting reinforcement for their destructive behavior. This can be better understood with reference to learning history, as a longer baseline phase would constitute more history of a target behavior contacting reinforcement. Bruzek et al. (2009) evaluated this phenomenon with caregivers of infants and their responses to simulated infant crying. Their results suggest that responses with a longer history of reinforcement are more likely to show resurgence than responses with shorter exposures to reinforcement contingencies. Although more translational in nature, Smith and Greer (2022) also replicated these effects with human participants through an experiment conducted on Amazon's Mechanical Turk platform.

Treatment: Phase 2

Phase 2 can be referred to generally as "Treatment." This phase often involves the introduction and reinforcement of an alternative response, like an FCR, and extinction for the target response, such as destructive behavior.

Inclusion or Exclusion of Extinction

As described above, Phase 2 often includes the target behavior being placed on extinction. However, more recently, researchers and practitioners have been evaluating the effects of treatments without the use of extinction. Implementing extinction for a target behavior may not be feasible in some settings, due to safety, resources, or other variables. Due to this, much research has focused on the efficacy of treatments without extinction and their effects on resurgence. Brown et al. (2020) evaluated this both clinically and translationally. In Experiment 1, two individuals with destructive behavior experienced repeated exposure to resurgence evaluations with and without extinction during differential reinforcement of alternative behavior (DRA). Because treatments with and without extinction can produce highly disparate rates of reinforcement, the researchers ensured similar rates of reinforcement across their two treatment conditions by delivering noncontingent reinforcement (NCR) during the DRA-with-extinction condition. Despite this, the majority of reinforcer deliveries in the DRA-with-extinction evaluation were delivered contingent on an alternative response, rather than noncontingently. When considering differences in baseline responding, they observed higher levels of target responding during the resurgence test (i.e., Phase 3) in the DRA-without-extinction condition versus in the DRA-with-extinction-and-NCR condition. Additional research is necessary to better understand how to mitigate resurgence when arranging treatments without extinction.

Discriminative Stimuli

Discrimination training during treatment (i.e., Phase 2) has shown promise in research thus far with regard to mitigating resurgence (Fisher et al., 2020; Fuhrman et al., 2016). In fact, it has been described as the most robust single-mitigation strategy in applied research to date (Fisher et al., 2020). The use of discriminative stimuli in FCT (e.g., multiple schedules) is common and can be adapted easily to fit the preferences of the implementers and client (e.g., modality of discriminative stimuli; see Norris et al., in press). In FCT with multiple schedules, discriminative stimuli (e.g., colored cards) signal to the participant when the FCR will and will not produce reinforcement (i.e., reinforcement and extinction components). Fuhrman et al. (2016) compared traditional FCT and FCT with multiple schedules in three-phase arrangements sequentially for two participants. Both participants engaged in a higher proportion of baseline responding in the extinction challenge for traditional FCT compared to FCT with a multiple schedule.

Fisher et al. (2020) replicated and extended Fuhrman et al. (2016) by comparing traditional FCT with and without discriminative stimuli. Fisher et al. conducted a multielement design where one of the contexts contained discriminative stimuli to signal the reinforcement and extinction components. Across four participants, lower proportion of baseline responding was observed in the context in which the discriminative stimulus was present to signal the extinction component.

The literature on the use of discriminative stimuli and its effects on resurgence suggest that these stimuli gain stimulus control over FCRs therefore leading to less resurgence when these discriminative stimuli are present to signal availability or unavailability of reinforcement than when these stimuli are not present. Further, some researchers compare the use of discriminative stimuli to the generalization-decrement hypothesis (Nevin et al., 2017), in that treatment challenges (i.e., Phase 3) may be more like treatment sessions (i.e., Phase 2) than baseline (i.e., Phase 1) due to the inclusion of discriminative stimuli signaling reinforcement or extinction during treatment but not during baseline.

Expanding the Operant Class

For a variety of reasons, it is possible that certain FCRs may be more difficult for a novel listener to be able to reinforce immediately if they are unfamiliar with the client, treatment, or reinforcer. Unfortunately, a delay or failure of the implementer reinforcing the FCR may produce resurgence. Behavior analysts may consider broadening a client's FCR repertoire by systematically teaching multiple appropriate FCRs for the same reinforcer. For example, if a client approaches a distant cousin at a family reunion and emits the FCR, "help" to gain help in finding a different preferred video on an iPad, the distant cousin is not likely to understand or deliver that reinforcer correctly. However, if the client has been systematically taught to emit multiple topographically different FCRs (e.g., "help," "new video," "Elmo," "change") and to scroll through those FCRs when contacting extinction, then resurgence may be less likely to occur (Lambert et al., 2017). However, clients are unlikely to scroll through multiple FCRs when contacting extinction without prior teaching.

Lag schedules have been used in research to systematically teach and maintain response variability across FCR topographies. A lag schedule requires that a response be different in a specified way (e.g., topography) from a specified number of previous responses to be reinforced (Cooper et al., 2020). For example, Falcomata et al. (2018) implemented a lag-5 schedule of reinforcement to teach and maintain variability across five topographically different FCRs. Adami et al. (2017) specifically evaluated lag schedules in the context of FCT. Both studies demonstrated success in establishing variability in responding across the FCR topographies.

Similarly, some researchers have evaluated serial training in order to promote response variability when contacting extinction. Serial training involves teaching and then subsequently extinguishing recently taught FCRs in a sequential manner, until all targeted responses have been taught, reinforced, and extinguished, except for the final topography. Results of serial training have been promising in the effects on future response variability during periods of extinction. Although the research on the effects of expanding the operant class and teaching response variability has yielded mixed results on resurgence (Adami et al., 2017; Lambert et al., 2017), behavior analysts may still consider implementing these procedures into a treatment package. Adaptive response variability may be useful when initial FCRs contact extinction such that, at the very least, it may delay the re-emergence of destructive behavior and give the implementer time to correct fidelity errors and reinforce an appropriate response (Adami et al., 2017; Falcomata et al., 2018).

Treatment Challenges: Phase 3

Most resurgence-mitigation research has focused on strategies to implement in Phase 1 or 2 (i.e., baseline or treatment) to avoid worsened outcomes in Phase 3. Phase 3 represents a challenge to treatment, such as prolonged periods of extinction or other worsening conditions (e.g., decreased rate, quality, or immediacy of reinforcement; increased response effort for alternative behavior). As the term "phase" implies, these might be planned treatment challenges. For example, Wacker et al. (2013) programmed repeated extinction tests throughout treatment and Rose and Beaulieu (2019) specifically evaluated "denial probes" in which a reinforcer was unavailable for an entire appointment. In other cases, these treatment challenges are unplanned. Nevertheless, the goal of most resurgence-mitigation research is to determine how to offset a large increase in dangerous destructive behavior during these particular times. Returning to our prescribed-fire metaphor, the bulk of research is designed at controlling the occurrence of resurgence during baseline and treatment (i.e., prescribed fires) in the hopes that high-magnitude resurgence will be less likely to occur during treatment challenges (i.e., wildfires).

With that said, just because wildfire scientists have compelling preventative strategies to offset wildfires does not mean they have stopped developing innovative methods of putting out wildfires when they occur. Similarly, behavior-analytic researchers have begun to investigate how best to support clients during treatment challenges (irrespective of previous mitigation strategies during Phases 1 and 2). A subset of studies has evaluated strategies that may be effective when implemented during the treatment challenges. Some research has suggested that programming noncontingent reinforcement or fixed-time deliveries of reinforcement during treatment challenges may mitigate resurgence (Bouton & Trask, 2016; Marsteller & St. Peter, 2014). In practice, this may include delivering the functional reinforcer on a response-independent schedule or providing continuous, noncontingent access to the functional reinforcer during treatment challenges. For caregivers, this may be a natural modification to make as they may already be programming NCR-like arrangements when they know something difficult may occur in their child's environment (e.g., bringing extra toys and anticipating increased screen-time when bringing the client to a doctor's office).

Research also suggests that the use of competing stimuli during the extinction component could aid in reaching terminal schedules of reinforcement quickly and with minimal increases in destructive behavior. Competing stimuli or activities during the extinction component has also been shown to prevent resurgence of destructive behavior during schedule thinning (e.g., Fuhrman et al., 2018). Miller et al. (2021) showed that for two participants, the addition of competing stimuli during the extinction component allowed for rapid schedule thinning to occur with less resurgence of destructive behavior when compared to a condition with no competing stimuli.

Promising Translational Research

To this point, we have described various approaches to mitigating resurgence in applied contexts with humans that have produced varying degrees of success. In this section, we describe two approaches to resurgence mitigation that have shown promise in pre-clinical evaluations conducted with nonhuman animals or with humans in translational or human-operant preparations designed to mimic the assessment, treatment, and potential resurgence of problem behavior. We also describe in this section findings from retrospective studies that analyzed cohorts of patients whose problem behavior was treated using routine clinical procedures but for whom important information was uncovered regarding the variables associated with the resurgence of problem behavior as it naturally occurs. As we describe below, the collective findings across these types of studies suggest future targets for prospectively designed clinical trials and single-case applied research on resurgence mitigation.

Size of the Decrease in Reinforcer Availability

Basic, translational, and applied researchers have recently begun to turn their attention to one simple predictor of resurgence and resurgence magnitude—size of the decrease in reinforcer availability—as a potential target for mitigating resurgence in applied contexts. Guided by the findings of Shahan, Browning, Nist et al. (2020b) conducted with nonhuman animals, Shahan and Greer (2021) reanalyzed the data from two then-recent retrospective evaluations of resurgence (Mitteer et al., 2022; Muething et al., 2021) conducted across large, independent cohorts of patients whose problem behavior was treated using functional communication training (FCT; Carr & Durand, 1985) and for whom reinforcement schedule thinning was accomplished using multiple schedules (e.g., Fisher et al., 1998; Greer et al., 2016; Hanley et al., 2001). Shahan and Greer's findings replicated those of Shahan, Browning, Nist et al. by showing that the magnitude of resurgence increased as a function of the size of the decrease in functional reinforcer availability, meaning that when behavior analysts programmed larger schedule-thinning steps, resurgence tended to be greater. Furthermore, both investigations showed that responding increased exponentially as a function of the size of the decrease in reinforcer availability, meaning that large schedule-thinning steps tended to produce more resurgence. An independent investigation conducted by Falligant, Hagopian, et al. (2022b) replicated the findings reported by Shahan and Greer, and these researchers detected a similar exponential function relating resurgence magnitude to the size of the decrease in alternative reinforcement.

These research findings are promising, as two independent clinics replicated the findings of a highly controlled basic study on resurgence conducted with rats in a retrospective evaluation that examined similar transitions. However, the retrospective clinical studies reanalyzed by Shahan and Greer (2021) and by Falligant, Hagopian et al. (2022b) did not control the types of transitions programmed across patients. Therefore, schedule-thinning steps were highly disparate within and across patients and clinics, as were the schedule-thinning sequences used. Therefore, Greer et al. (2024) attempted to correct these limitations by enrolling participants in a prospective clinical evaluation that controlled the size and sequence of schedule-thinning steps within and across participants while using multiple schedules. When differently sized schedule-thinning steps were quasirandomly sequenced in Experiment 2, Greer et al. showed that resurgence tended to be greatest with the largest decreases in reinforcer availability. However, when these same schedule-thinning steps were arranged from smallest to largest in Experiments 1 and 2, little resurgence occurred, suggesting that the order in which schedule-thinning steps occur may moderate the degree to which resurgence magnitude is controlled by the size of the decrease in reinforcer availability.

The implications of this line of research are likely to be important for future clinical practice. For example, one promising finding across studies is that resurgence tends to be minimal when schedule-thinning steps are kept small (e.g., a 20% or smaller decrease in reinforcer availability; Greer et al., 2024). Whether a schedule-thinning progression comprised of only small steps mitigates resurgence throughout the schedule-thinning process is an important question for future research, and our team is currently conducting such a study to help address this question.

A second promising finding is that the order of schedule-thinning steps may itself be an important consideration when conducting reinforcement schedule thinning (Greer et al., 2024). Whether larger schedule-thinning steps programmed later in the process of reinforcement schedule thinning are less prone to producing high-magnitude resurgence is another important question for future research, which we also plan to evaluate.

On/Off Cycling of Alternative Reinforcement

Another line of research that has shown promise as a potentially useful approach to mitigating socially significant resurgence is to expose target responding to extinction early and often when initiating treatment with alternative reinforcement (e.g., FCT). Studies that have investigated this approach to resurgence mitigation have often cycled between treatment sessions that arrange reinforcement for an alternative response, followed by sessions that suspend alternative reinforcement, while extinction remains in place for target responding across sessions. So-called on/off cycles in treatment, as compared to treatments that do not suspend reinforcement for the alternative response, have tended to show better resurgence mitigation in nonhuman animals (Schepers & Bouton, 2015; Shahan, Browning, & Nall, 2020a; Trask et al., 2018).

Smith and Greer (2023) recently extended this line of research to humans in an Internet-based, human-operant task. Participants were recruited through Amazon's Mechanical Turk, where workers select tasks (e.g., surveys, brief studies) to complete for money. Participants enrolled in this study experienced a series of addition problems on either a star or square that moved around one side of the screen. New addition problems replaced previously answered addition problems throughout the experiment. All sessions lasted 2 min, and each session was separated by a 5-s blackout.

In Phase 1, participants earned money according to a VI 15-s schedule by correctly answering addition problems on a star that moved randomly around the left side of the screen for five sessions. In Phase 2, the star remained on the left side of the screen, and a second addition problem appeared and moved randomly around the right side of the screen for 11 sessions. Answering star questions no longer produced reinforcement following Phase 1, and the reinforcement schedule arranged for answering square questions correctly in Phase 2 differed across the three experimental groups. Two control groups experienced a consistent reinforcement schedule for answering square questions correctly, with one group experiencing a dense VI 5-s schedule of alternative reinforcement and the other group experiencing a relatively lean VI 15-s schedule of alternative reinforcement. The third group served as a test group, and participants randomized to this group experienced a VI 5-s schedule of alternative reinforcement on even-numbered sessions in Phase 2 and extinction for both the target and alternative response on odd-numbered sessions. Phase 3 included six sessions with all responses remaining available but with reinforcement suspended for both the target and alternative response. across all sessions.

Relative to the two control groups, the on/off cycling group in Smith and Greer (2023) showed greater suppression of target responding and better discrimination between the target and alternative response in Phase 2. The test group also showed less target responding across Phases 2 and 3 than did the control groups, suggesting that cycling between periods with and without alternative reinforcement may produce favorable outcomes both during and following intervention. However, as is always the case, promising initial findings such as these must be replicated, ideally by independent researchers, before behavior analysts consider applying the approach under consideration. Our research team is currently working to safely extend this line of research to the clinical context, and although initial outcomes are encouraging (for a recent laboratory demonstration, see Shahan et al., 2024), additional data and time are needed to more fully understand the potential benefits and drawbacks of using this approach to mitigate socially significant resurgence.

Discussion and Other Considerations

In this chapter, we provided an overview of applied mitigation research related to resurgence, or the recurrence of target behavior following a worsening in reinforcement conditions. Several strategies (e.g., use of treatment signals, programming alternative reinforcement or activities) have empirical support, and other techniques (e.g., on/off cycling) show promising outcomes that may prove helpful in applied work following translation. Yet, the domain of applied resurgence mitigation is still in its infancy and there are several areas of future research that will be compelling to investigate.

Implementer Behavior

When examining forms of treatment relapse like resurgence, behavior analysts often focus on the behavioral outcomes of the direct recipients of treatment services (e.g., children with destructive behavior). However, there are two primary reasons why behavior analyst should expand their focus to include key stakeholders, like caregivers, teachers, and other implementers. First, considering stakeholders during treatment development and care transition aligns with the paradigm of family-centered care (Brown et al., 2022), which may increase the social validity of treatment goals, procedures, and outcomes. Thus, there is great practical relevance to expanding an evaluation of treatment relapse to include the relevant behavior of key stakeholders and determine how best to support them as part of family-centered care.

Second, it is important to consider that many of the mitigation strategies mentioned in this chapter rely on the implementers delivering the treatment strategies with high procedural fidelity (i.e., as the treatments are intended to be implemented; Gresham et al., 2000). For example, Fisher et al. (2020) found that presenting the treatment signal associated with extinction mitigated resurgence of destructive behavior during prolonged periods of extinction. However, would this still be the case if the implementers had implemented extinction of FCRs or destructive behavior poorly or had they inadvertently obscured the treatment signal during this critical time?

Unfortunately, researchers have found that many variables including those affecting the resurgence of client behavior may also affect implementer behavior. In studies of caregivers roleplaying FCT procedures with confederates, a worsening of reinforcement conditions for caregivers (e.g., increased confederate destructive behavior following treatment implementation) disrupted their procedural fidelity (Mitteer et al., 2018; Williams et al., 2023), resulting in critical errors such as delivering functional reinforcement following destructive behavior. Additional variables like contextual changes may also disrupt procedural fidelity. In an experiment on teacher behavior, Berdeaux et al. (2022) taught teachers to implement three different function-based treatments with confederates who displayed escape-maintained challenging behavior. When the experimenters added distractor confederates to the classroom, this change disrupted procedural fidelity of at least one treatment for all teachers.

Most recently, Yassa et al. (2024) taught trainees to implement FCT with multiple schedules within a similar confederate arrangement; then, the experimenters assessed the disruption of implementer behavior during a "training-challenge sequence" that programmed periods in which the trainees implemented the treatment with (a) a behavioral-protocol change, (b) a novel confederate with different behavioral functions and discriminative stimuli, and (c) a confederate who displayed relapsed destructive behavior and persistent FCRs during periods of signaled extinction. Yassa et al. found that the training-challenge sequence disrupted implementer fidelity at least once for all participants and in 62% of the training challenges. Some of these errors involved delivering the functional reinforcer incorrectly and failing to ensure that treatment signals remained visible during treatment.

Addressing Both Client and Implementer Behavior to Mitigate Resurgence

Taken together, research on implementer behavior indicates that those responsible for delivering treatment strategies designed to mitigate resurgence may occasionally deviate from the prescribed interventions, especially when the implementation context differs from the initial training arrangement. This suggests two important lines of future research. One is determining the effects of different types of implementer errors on client behavior and assessing the durability of prescribed mitigation strategies. An example of this research direction can be found in Mitteer et al. (2021) in which the experimenters emulated the frequency and types of errors caregivers made in Mitteer et al. (2018) when delivering a version of FCT with children with autism. Although conducted in the context of a translational human-operant experiment to avoid worsening actual challenging behavior, the authors found that matching experimenter behavior to the caregiver errors in Mitteer et al. (2018) led to high levels of relapsed target behavior for all children and extinction of alternative behavior for the majority of children. Researchers might take a similar approach following outcomes like those in Yassa et al. (2024) wherein they program equivalent procedural-fidelity errors during FCT with discriminative stimuli within a translational arrangement to determine how disruptive those errors might be for client performance.

If these errors are shown to have a large impact on client performance, it would suggest that researchers ought to examine strategies to bolster procedural fidelity (and mitigate relapse of undesirable implementer behavior). Consider refinements like treatment signals and competing activities, which appear to mitigate resurgence of client destructive behavior. Researchers might be able to take these promising approaches and apply them to implementer behavior, such as arranging reminders of training procedures and the importance of certain treatment components for long-term success (i.e., incorporating treatment signals) or coaching caregivers to seek alternative activities (e.g., listening to music, completing other caregiving responsibilities) to attenuate discomfort or stress associated with treatment adherence not producing immediate treatment effects. Ultimately, researchers may need to address resurgence in relation to the client and the implementer to promote long-term effects of behavioral interventions.

Generality and Effectiveness Research

Research often progresses from initial efficacy studies in the laboratory toward effectiveness evaluations in the community, where the former represent tightly controlled applications of an independent variable by experts with small-scope dependent variables, and the latter address larger-scale applications of a treatment by typical implementers and broader dependent variables (Hoagwood et al., 1995). As might be evident from our chapter describing translational and initial applied work on resurgence mitigation, the field of behavior analysis finds itself still in the early research stages akin to efficacy research. That is, researchers have been focused on translating findings from basic laboratory studies to human participants (e.g., Smith & Greer, 2022; Williams et al., 2023) or conducting initial pilot work on applied resurgence mitigation (e.g., Fisher et al., 2020; Fuhrman et al., 2016). These types of studies are critical for assessing mitigation effects while minimizing the relevance of threats to internal validity (e.g., history, diffusion of treatment) that might be more pervasive outside of tightly controlled settings with highly trained implementers.

With that said, it will be important to assess the generality of promising mitigation strategies in less rigorous environments and by those with less specialized training in resurgence mitigation (e.g., master's level practitioners in behavior-analytic clinics or who conduct home-based or school-based services). Additionally, an aspect of effectiveness research is that it might assess changes in impactful measures outside of typical dependent variables (e.g., changes in the rate of destructive behavior). Resurgence-mitigation research that examines effectiveness might, for example, evaluate the extent to which the strategies reduce clinical readmissions, emergency-department visits, or the use of restraint and seclusion—not just keeping destructive behavior low during changes in reinforcement conditions. Although more research will be needed to determine well-established interventions for mitigating resurgence, we encourage researchers to consider the generality of their techniques following their efficacy evaluations.

Conclusion

Although still in its infancy, applied research on resurgence mitigation holds promise for improving the clinical care of the clients and families we serve. Researchers have identified strategies that can effectively reduce resurgence of destructive behavior (e.g., Fisher et al., 2020; Fuhrman et al., 2016). Equally important, investigators have conducted the necessary work to rule out potential strategies that end up being less impactful (e.g., Fuhrman et al., 2022; Irwin Helvey et al., 2023), which further guides research endeavors and resources away from less compelling independent variables and instead toward those with favorable findings. As researchers continue to develop helpful strategies, we encourage them to examine promising strategies within the context of client-implementer interactions and their generality within effectiveness research.

References

Adami, S., Falcomata, T. S., Muething, C. S., & Hoffman, K. (2017). An evaluation of lag schedules of reinforcement during functional communication training: Effects on varied mand responding and challenging behavior. *Behavior Analysis in Practice, 10*(3), 209–213. https://doi.org/10.1007/s40617-017-0179-7

Behavior Analyst Certification Board. (2020). *Ethics code for behavior analysts*. https://bacb.com/wp-content/ethics-code-for-behavior-analysts/.

Berdeaux, K. L., Lerman, D. C., & Williams, S. D. (2022). Effects of environmental distractions on teachers' procedural integrity with three function-based treatments. *Journal of Applied Behavior Analysis, 55*(3), 832–850. https://doi.org/10.1002/jaba.918

Bouton, M. E., & Trask, S. (2016). Role of the discriminative properties of the reinforcer in resurgence. *Learning & Behavior, 44*, 137–150. https://doi.org/10.3758/s13420-015-0197-7

Briggs, A. M., Fisher, W. W., Greer, B. D., & Kimball, R. T. (2018). Prevalence of resurgence of destructive behavior when thinning reinforcement schedules during functional communication training. *Journal of Applied Behavior Analysis, 51*(3), 620–633. https://doi.org/10.1002/jaba.472

Brown, K. R., Greer, B. D., Craig, A. R., Sullivan, W. E., Fisher, W. W., & Roane, H. S. (2020). Resurgence following differential reinforcement of alternative behavior implemented with and without extinction. *Journal of the Experimental Analysis of Behavior, 113*(2), 449–467. https://doi.org/10.1002/jeab.588

Brown, K. R., Hurd, A. M., Randall, K. R., Szabo, T., & Mitteer, D. R. (2022). A family-centered care approach to behavior-analytic assessment and intervention. In *Behavior analysis in practice, SI: Compassion in applied behavior analysis* (pp. 1–17). https://doi.org/10.1007/s40617-022-00756-y

Bruzek, J. L., Thompson, R. H., & Peters, L. C. (2009). Resurgence of infant caregiving responses. *Journal of the Experimental Analysis of Behavior, 92*(3), 327–343. https://doi.org/10.1901/jeab.2009-92-327

Carr, E. G., & Durand, V. M. (1985). Reducing behavior problems through functional communication training. *Journal of Applied Behavior Analysis, 18*(2), 111–126. https://doi.org/10.1901/jaba.1985.18-111

Cooper, J. O., Heron, T. E., & Heward, W. L. (2020). *Applied behavior analysis*. Pearson.

Epstein, R. (1985). Extinction-induced resurgence: Preliminary investigations and possible applications. *The Psychological Record, 35*, 143–153. https://doi.org/10.1007/bf03394918

Falcomata, T. S., Muething, C. S., Silbaugh, B. C., Adami, S., Hoffman, K., Shpall, C., & Ringdahl, J. E. (2018). Lag schedules and functional communication training: Persistence of Mands and relapse of problem behavior. *Behavior Modification, 42*(3), 314–334. https://doi.org/10.1177/0145445517741475

Falligant, J. M., Chin, M. D., & Kurtz, P. F. (2022a). Renewal and resurgence of severe problem behavior in an intensive outpatient setting: Prevalence, magnitude, and implications for practice. *Behavioral Interventions, 37*(3), 909–924. https://doi.org/10.1002/bin.1878

Falligant, J. M., Hagopian, L. P., Kranak, M. P., & Kurtz, P. F. (2022b). Quantifying increases in problem behavior following downshifts in reinforcement: A retrospective analysis and replication. *Journal of the Experimental Analysis of Behavior, 118*(1), 148–155. https://doi.org/10.1002/jeab.769

Fisher, W. W., Kuhn, D. E., & Thompson, R. H. (1998). Establishing discriminative control of responding using functional and alternative reinforcers during functional communication training. *Journal of Applied Behavior Analysis, 31*(4), 543–560. https://doi.org/10.1901/jaba.1998.31-543

Fisher, W. W., Greer, B. D., Fuhrman, A. M., Saini, V., & Simmons, C. A. (2018). Minimizing resurgence of destructive behavior using behavioral momentum theory. *Journal of Applied Behavior Analysis, 51*(4), 831–853. https://doi.org/10.1002/jaba.499

Fisher, W. W., Saini, V., Greer, B. D., Sullivan, W. E., Roane, H. S., Fuhrman, A. M., Craig, A. R., & Kimball, R. T. (2019). Baseline reinforcement rate and resurgence of destructive behavior. *Journal of the Experimental Analysis of Behavior, 111*(1), 75–93. https://doi.org/10.1002/jeab.488

Fisher, W. W., Fuhrman, A. M., Greer, B. D., Mitteer, D. R., & Piazza, C. C. (2020). Mitigating resurgence of destructive behavior using the discriminative stimuli of a multiple schedule. *Journal of the Experimental Analysis of Behavior, 113*(1), 263–277. https://doi.org/10.1002/jeab.552

Fuhrman, A. M., Fisher, W. W., & Greer, B. D. (2016). A preliminary investigation on improving functional communication training by mitigating resurgence of destructive behavior. *Journal of Applied Behavior Analysis, 49*(4), 884–899. https://doi.org/10.1002/jaba.338

Fuhrman, A. M., Greer, B. D., Zangrillo, A. N., & Fisher, W. W. (2018). Evaluating competing activities to enhance functional communication training during reinforcement schedule thinning. *Journal of Applied Behavior Analysis, 51*(4), 931–942. https://doi.org/10.1002/jaba.486

Fuhrman, A. M., Lambert, J. M., & Greer, B. D. (2022). A brief review of expanded-operant treatments for mitigating resurgence. *The Psychological Record, 72*(2), 319–323. https://doi.org/10.1007/s40732-021-00456-z

Greer, B. D., & Shahan, T. A. (2019). Resurgence as choice: Implications for promoting durable behavior change. *Journal of Applied Behavior Analysis, 52*(3), 816–846. https://doi.org/10.1002/jaba.573

Greer, B. D., Fisher, W. W., Saini, V., Owen, T. M., & Jones, J. K. (2016). Functional communication training during reinforcement schedule thinning: An analysis of 25 applications. *Journal of Applied Behavior Analysis, 49*(1), 105–121. https://doi.org/10.1002/jaba.265

Greer, B. D., Fisher, W. W., Retzlaff, B. J., & Fuhrman, A. M. (2020). A preliminary evaluation of treatment duration on the resurgence of destructive behavior. *Journal of the Experimental Analysis of Behavior, 113*(1), 251–262. https://doi.org/10.1002/jeab.567

Greer, B. D., Shahan, T. A., Irwin Helvey, C., Fisher, W. W., Mitteer, D. R., & Fuhrman, A. M. (2024). Resurgence of destructive behavior following decreases in alternative reinforcement: A prospective analysis. *Journal of Applied Behavior Analysis, 57*(3), 599–614. https://doi.org/10.1002/jaba.1083

Gresham, F. M., MacMillan, D. L., Beebe-Frankenberger, M. E., & Bocian, K. M. (2000). Treatment integrity in learning disabilities intervention research: Do we really know how treatments are implemented? *Learning Disabilities Research & Practice, 15*(4), 198–205. https://doi.org/10.1207/SLDRP1504_4

Hanley, G. P., Iwata, B. A., & Thompson, R. H. (2001). Reinforcement schedule thinning following treatment with functional communication training. *Journal of Applied Behavior Analysis, 34*(1), 17–38. https://doi.org/10.1901/jaba.2001.34-17

Hiers, J. K., O'Brien, J. J., Varner, J. M., Butler, B. W., Dickinson, M., Furman, J., Gallagher, M., Godwin, D., Goodrick, S. L., Hood, S. M., Hudak, A., Kobziar, L. N., Linn, R., Loudermilk, E. L., McCaffrey, S., Robertson, K., Rowell, E. M., Skowronski, N., Watts, A. C., & Yedinak, K. M. (2020). Prescribed fire science: The case for a refined research agenda. *Fire Ecology, 16*(11), 1–15. https://doi.org/10.1186/s42408-020-0070-8

Hoagwood, K., Hibbs, E., Brent, D., & Jensen, P. (1995). Introduction to the special section: Efficacy and effectiveness in studies of child and adolescent psychotherapy. *Journal of Consulting and Clinical Psychology, 63*(5), 683–687. https://psycnet.apa.org/doi/10.1037/0022-006X.63.5.683

Irwin Helvey, C. M., Fisher, W. W., Greer, B. D., Fuhrman, A. M., & Mitteer, D. R. (2023). Resurgence of destructive behavior following differential rates of alternative reinforcement. *Journal of Applied Behavior Analysis, 56*(4), 804–815. https://doi.org/10.1002/jaba.1010

Kestner, K. M., & Peterson, S. (2017). A review of resurgence literature with human participants. *Behavior Analysis: Research & Practice, 17*(1), 1–17. https://doi.org/10.1037/bar0000039

Kimball, R. T., Greer, B. D., Fuhrman, A. M., & Lambert, J. M. (2023). Relapse and its mitigation: Toward behavioral inoculation. *Journal of Applied Behavior Analysis, 56*(2), 282–301. https://doi.org/10.1002/jaba.971

Kranak, M. P., & Falligant, J. M. (2021). Further investigation of resurgence following schedule thinning: Extension to an inpatient setting. *Behavioral Interventions, 36*(4), 1003–1012. https://doi.org/10.1002/bin.1831

Lambert, J. M., Bloom, S. E., Samaha, A. L., & Dayton, E. (2017). Serial functional communication training: Extending serial DRA to mands and problem behavior. *Behavioral Interventions, 32*(4), 311–325. https://doi.org/10.1002/bin.1493

Lattal, K. A., & Wacker, D. (2015). Some dimensions of recurrent operant behavior. *Mexican Journal of Behavior Analysis, 41*(2), 1–13. https://www.redalyc.org/pdf/593/59341195001.pdf

Lattal, K. A., Cançado, C. R., Cook, J. E., Kincaid, S. L., Nighbor, T. D., & Oliver, A. C. (2017). On defining resurgence. *Behavioural Processes, 141*(1), 85–91. https://doi.org/10.1016/j.beproc.2017.04.018

Marsteller, T. M., & St. Peter, C. C. (2014). Effects of fixed-time reinforcement schedules on resurgence of problem behavior. *Journal of Applied Behavior Analysis, 47*(3), 455–469. https://doi.org/10.1002/jaba.134

Miller, S. A., Fisher, W. W., Greer, B. D., Saini, V., Keevy, M., & D. (2021). Procedures for determining and then modifying the extinction component of multiple schedules for destructive behavior. *Journal of Applied Behavior Analysis, 55*(2), 463–480. https://doi.org/10.1002/jaba.896

Mitteer, D. R., Greer, B. D., Fisher, W. W., Briggs, A. M., & Wacker, D. P. (2018). A laboratory model for evaluating relapse of undesirable caregiver behavior. *Journal of the Experimental Analysis of Behavior, 110*(2), 252–266. https://doi.org/10.1002/jeab.462

Mitteer, D. R., Greer, B. D., Randall, K. R., Kimball, R. T., & Smith, S. W. (2021). Empirically deriving omission and commission errors for relapse tests: A demonstration of reverse translation. *Behavior Analysis: Research and Practice, 21*(4), 351–363. https://doi.org/10.1037/bar0000218

Mitteer, D. R., Greer, B. D., Randall, K. R., & Haney, S. D. (2022). On the scope and characteristics of relapse when treating severe destructive behavior. *Journal of Applied Behavior Analysis, 55*(3), 688–703. https://doi.org/10.1002/jaba.912

Muething, C., Pavlov, A., Call, N., Ringdahl, J., & Gillespie, S. (2021). Prevalence of resurgence during thinning of multiple schedules of reinforcement following functional communication training. *Journal of Applied Behavior Analysis, 54*(2), 813–823. https://doi.org/10.1002/jaba.791

Nevin, J. A., & Shahan, T. A. (2011). Behavioral momentum theory: Equations and applications. *Journal of Applied Behavior Analysis, 44*(4), 877–895. https://doi.org/10.1901/jaba.2011.44-877

Nevin, J. A., Craig, A. R., Cunningham, P. J., Podlesnik, C. A., Shahan, T. A., & Sweeney, M. M. (2017). Quantitative models of persistence and relapse from the perspective of behavioral momentum theory: Fits and misfits. *Behavioral Processes, 141*(1), 92–99. https://doi.org/10.1016/j.beproc.2017.04.016

Norris, H. M., Mitteer, D. R., Hurd, A. M., & Brown, K. R. (in press). Integrating client and implementer preferences during functional communication training with discriminative stimuli. *Behavior Analysis in Practice.*

Perrin, J., Morris, C., & Kestner, K. (2022). Resurgence of clinically relevant behavior: A systematic review. *Education and Treatment of Children, 45*(1), 85–104. https://doi.org/10.1007/s43494-021-00054-2

Podlesnik, C. A., Ritchey, C. M., Waits, J., & Gilroy, S. P. (2023). A comprehensive systematic review of procedures and analyses used in basic and preclinical studies of resurgence, 1970–2020. *Perspectives on Behavior Science, 46*(1), 137–184. https://doi.org/10.1007/s40614-022-00361-y

Rose, J. C., & Beaulieu, L. (2019). Assessing the generality and durability of interview-informed functional analyses and treatment. *Journal of Applied Behavior Analysis, 52*(1), 271–285. https://doi.org/10.1002/jaba.504

Schepers, S. T., & Bouton, M. E. (2015). Effects of reinforcer distribution during response elimination on resurgence of an instrumental behavior. *Journal of Experimental Psychology. Animal Learning and Cognition, 41*(2), 179–192. https://doi.org/10.1037/xan0000061

Shahan, T. A., & Craig, A. R. (2017). Resurgence as choice. *Behavioural Processes, 141*(1), 100–127. https://doi.org/10.1016/j.beproc.2016.10.006

Shahan, T. A., & Greer, B. D. (2021). Destructive behavior increases as a function of reductions in alternative reinforcement during schedule thinning: A retrospective quantitative analysis. *Journal of the Experimental Analysis of Behavior, 116*(2), 243–248. https://doi.org/10.1002/jeab.708

Shahan, T. A., Browning, K. O., & Nall, R. W. (2020a). Resurgence as choice in context: Treatment duration and on/off alternative reinforcement. *Journal of the Experimental Analysis of Behavior, 113*(1), 57–76. https://doi.org/10.1002/jeab.563

Shahan, T. A., Browning, K. O., Nist, A. N., & Sutton, G. M. (2020b). Resurgence and downshifts in alternative reinforcement rate. *Journal of the Experimental Analysis of Behavior, 114*(2), 163–178. https://doi.org10.1002/jeab.625

Shahan, T. A., Sutton, G. M., & Avellaneda, M. (2024). Resurgence mitigation across extended extinction following four and eight cycles of on/off alternative reinforcement. *Behavioural Processes, 220*, 105082. https://doi.org/10.1016/j.beproc.2024.105082

Smith, S. W., & Greer, B. D. (2022). Phase duration and resurgence. *Journal of the Experimental Analysis of Behavior, 117*(1), 91–104. https://doi.org/10.1002/jeab.725

Smith, S., & Greer, B. D. (2023). Translational evaluation of on/off alternative reinforcement cycling. *Journal of the Experimental Analysis of Behavior, 120*(3), 429–439. https://doi.org/10.1002/jeab.879

Tiger, J. H., Hanley, G. P., & Bruzek, J. (2008). Functional communication training: A review and practical guide. *Behavior Analysis in Practice, 1*(1), 16–23. https://doi.org/10.1007/BF03391716

Trask, S., Keim, C. L., & Bouton, M. E. (2018). Factors that encourage generalization from extinction to test reduce resurgence of an extinguished operant response. *Journal of the Experimental Analysis of Behavior, 110*(1), 11–23. https://doi.org/10.1002/jeab.446

Volkert, V. M., Lerman, D. C., Call, N. A., & Trosclair-Lasserre, N. (2009). An evaluation of resurgence during treatment with functional communication training. *Journal of Applied Behavior Analysis, 42*(1), 145–160. https://doi.org/10.1901/jaba.2009.42-145

Wacker, D. P., Harding, J. W., Berg, W. K., Lee, J. F., Schieltz, K. M., Padilla, Y. C., Nevin, J. A., & Shahan, T. A. (2013). An evaluation of persistence of treatment effects during long-term treatment of destructive behavior. *Journal of the Experimental Analysis of Behavior, 96*(2), 261–282. https://doi.org/10.1901/jeab.2011.96-261

Williams, C. L., Montague, K. L., Bernstein, A. M., Call, N. A., & Slocum, S. K. (2023). Expanding a laboratory model for evaluating relapse of caregiver nonadherence. *Journal of the Experimental Analysis of Behavior, 120*(3), 363–375. https://doi.org/10.1002/jeab.873

Yassa, R., Mitteer, D. R., Greer, B. D., Angley, S. M., McCabe, L. H., & Elwasli, O. M. (2024). Teaching trainees to implement functional communication training with multiple schedules: An evaluation of training effects and durability. *Journal of Applied Behavior Analysis, 57*(4), 999–1015. https://doi.org/10.1002/jaba.2915

Chapter 3
Basic Research on Renewal

Ryan T. Kimball, Andrew R. Craig, and William E. Sullivan

Imagine, for a moment, that you are a clinician working with learners who engage in severe challenging behavior (e.g., aggression, self-injury) at a clinic-based service setting. One of your clients, Johnny, was recently outplaced by his school to the day treatment program at your clinic to decrease his aggression, which occurs when teachers give him difficult academic instructions. You then crafted a behavior intervention plan (BIP) based on the results of a functional behavioral assessment. The plan included important components like differentially reinforcing appropriate requests for breaks from, and help with, difficult academic instructions; withholding reinforcement for aggression (i.e., extinction); and gradually increasing the number of instructions Johnny must complete before he can earn a break (i.e., demand fading). Fortunately, your treatment produced robust changes in Johnny's behavior, and you have not observed any aggression for several weeks. After training Johnny's teacher to implement the BIP in the clinic with flawless treatment integrity, you discharged Johnny from services, and he returned to the classroom. However, within a day of Johnny's return to the classroom, you received notice that despite the teacher doing precisely what they were supposed to do according to the BIP, Johnny's aggression returned at high levels. Unfortunately, recent applied research on the prevalence of treatment relapse suggests situations like the one described above are likely common for clinicians (e.g., Mitteer et al., 2022; Muething et al., 2020).

The re-emergence of Johnny's aggression when he returned to the classroom setting despite the teacher following the BIP is called *renewal*, which is defined as the

R. T. Kimball (✉)
University of Saint Joseph, West Hartford, CT, USA
e-mail: rkimball@usj.edu

A. R. Craig · W. E. Sullivan
SUNY Upstate Medical University, Syracuse, NY, USA

M. P. Kranak (ed.), *Behavioral Treatments for Individuals with Autism*, Autism and Child Psychopathology Series,
https://doi.org/10.1007/978-3-031-91965-7_3

return of a previously eliminated target response (e.g., aggression) following a change in context that was in place during treatment, in the absence of any changes in contingencies (Kimball & Kranak, 2022; Podlesnik et al., 2017). Basic researchers often study renewal in an arrangement that mimics the conditions that the client, Johnny, experienced in the example described above. As an illustration, consider Experiment 1 from Kelley et al. (2015). First, pigeons' key pecking in an operant chamber resulted in reinforcement (i.e., access to food) in Context A. In Context A, the center key light flashed between white and red every 0.1 s. The conditions in Context A are analogous to a history of reinforcement for Johnny's aggression in a non-treatment setting (e.g., a school classroom). Next, experimenters extinguished key pecking in Context B, wherein the center key light flashed between white and red every 0.5 s. Context B conditions were analogous to treatment for Johnny's aggression in a different, therapeutic setting (e.g., a clinic). Finally, the experimenters observed a re-emergence of key pecking when the pigeons returned to Context A in the renewal test, despite that key pecking remained on extinction. The renewal of key pecking following the context change is analogous to the re-emergence of Johnny's aggression during the return to the classroom setting.

Our contemporary understanding of renewal as it occurs in applied settings has roots in basic research with nonhuman animals: if one considers the introduction sections of recently published applied studies on renewal, they will find that the impetus for the research often stems from the basic research laboratory findings (e.g., Haney et al., 2021). Investigating renewal in the basic laboratory is advantageous for several reasons (Podlesnik & Kelley, 2015). For example, researching renewal in the basic laboratory with nonhuman animals permits researchers to control subjects' experimental history and isolate the role of context change on the return of previously eliminated target responding. These goals may be challenging to do with the renewal of socially significant behavior in some applied settings with more dynamic environments (e.g., schools and in-home services). Additionally, basic research on renewal avoids potential risks of studying renewal of challenging behavior in applied settings, such as client and staff injuries. Thus, the basic laboratory is often the ideal arena for research that lays the groundwork for future applied and translational research on important topics like relapse (including renewal) mitigation (e.g., Bernal-Gamboa et al., 2022; Kuroda et al., 2021).

This chapter discusses research on renewal from the basic laboratory. Although basic research on renewal is relevant to many socially significant behaviors such as drug abuse, gambling, and overeating (Bouton & Todd, 2014), we wrote the chapter intending to highlight content most relevant to clinicians working with individuals who engage in severe challenging behavior. The basic processes that undergird relapse of each of these socially significant behaviors (and other behaviors not listed), however, are the same. Further, although the origins of contemporary basic research on operant renewal were primarily influenced by studies focused on the return of previously extinguished Pavlovian responses (e.g., Archer et al., 1979; Bouton & King, 1983), we mainly consider basic research concerning operant behavior. First, we review approaches to studying renewal as an operant model of treatment relapse. Next, we discuss what researchers mean by "context," environmental variables that impact renewal, and renewal-mitigation procedures. We then provide a critical analysis of Context Theory and the basic research on which the theory is based. Finally, we offer directions for future research.

Renewal as an Operant Model of Treatment Relapse

Treatment relapse of challenging behavior may occur for a number of reasons, but basic researchers often study renewal as an operant model of relapse that occurs due to a change in the treatment context (Kelley et al., 2015). Moreover, because applied research suggests that clinicians should strive to program and test for the generality of behavior change by conducting treatment in multiple settings (i.e., familiar and novel contexts), renewal is an ideal model for studying relapse that may occur during planned and unplanned context changes (Falcomata & Wacker, 2013). Researchers frequently use three variations of a well-established three-phase design to study renewal: ABA, ABC, and AAB. Each procedural variation for studying renewal resembles unique context changes that may occur during the treatment of challenging behavior (Kimball & Kranak, 2022). As a result, basic researchers often refer to the relapse effects observed with the ABA, ABC, and AAB procedural variations as different *types* of renewal (e.g., Todd, 2013).

With ABA renewal, the target response (e.g., lever pressing for rats) produces reinforcement and is acquired in Context A during Phase 1. During Phase 2, the target response no longer produces reinforcement and is eliminated via extinction in Context B. In Phase 3, researchers return the subject to Context A to test for the re-emergence of the target response in the face of continued extinction (e.g., Bouton et al., 2011). Phase 3 is the renewal test. Investigating ABA renewal in the basic laboratory is beneficial because it allows researchers to study a unique sequence of conditions in which treatment occurs in a distinct context (i.e., Context B) and relapse occurs following a transition to a familiar context associated with a history of reinforcement for the target response. Clinicians may encounter ABA renewal when treatment occurs in a clinic, and relapse is observed when returning to the home environment (Neely et al., 2024).

The preparation for studying ABC renewal is very similar to the ABA renewal preparation except that experimenters test for an increase in the recently eliminated target response in a novel context that the subject has not yet encountered (i.e., Context C) instead of a familiar context. Studying the re-emergence of target responding during a transition to a novel context is significant because it demonstrates that renewal may occur even in an environment unrelated to a history of reinforcement for the target response. For example, Bouton et al. (2011, Experiment 3) reinforced rats' lever pressing in Context A on a variable interval (VI) 30-s schedule and then extinguished that target response in Context B. Distinct contexts were programmed using visual and olfactory cues. Next, experimenters observed a renewal of lever pressing during a transition to Context C for 15 of 16 rats. Clinicians may observe ABC renewal under various circumstances, such as when a new behavior technician works with the client after treatment has exclusively been conducted with one interventionist (Neely et al., 2024).

The preparation for studying AAB renewal diverges from ABA and ABC preparations because treatment (i.e., extinction) occurs in the context already associated with reinforcement for the target response (Context A) instead of a different context (Context B). As an illustration, Bouton et al. (2011, Experiment 1) reinforced rats' lever pressing in Context A and then withdrew reinforcement for lever pressing in the same context until responding extinguished. Finally, the experimenters detected a renewal of lever pressing for 16 of 16 rats during a transition to a novel Context B. Similar to ABC renewal, AAB renewal demonstrates that merely removing the organism from the treatment context where extinction occurred can result in the re-emergence of an extinguished target response. The AAB renewal preparation simulates the sequence of treatment conditions that clients may experience during the in-home treatment of challenging behavior (Kimball & Kranak, 2022). Clinicians can imagine a situation in which there is a history of reinforcement for challenging behavior in the client's home. Then, a treatment that includes extinction for challenging behavior also occurs in the home. After robust treatment outcomes are obtained and the clinician trains the caregiver to implement the treatment with fidelity, the caregiver may feel confident enough to take their child on community outings to novel contexts the child has not been to before (e.g., a new grocery store). This transition to a novel context may allow AAB renewal to occur despite the caregiver properly implementing the treatment during the context change.

Some basic research suggests that the magnitude of operant ABA renewal tends to be greater than ABC and AAB renewal (e.g., Bernal-Gamboa et al., 2017; Bouton et al., 2011; Todd et al., 2012), suggesting that the strength of renewal effects may be more significant when returning to a familiar context associated with a history of reinforcement for the target response relative to transitioning to an unfamiliar context. These data may imply that clinicians should take extra care when conducting generalization training in contexts where challenging behavior has historically been reinforced. Still, other studies have failed to find such differences between renewal types across operant and Pavlovian conditioning paradigms (e.g., Muñiz-Moreno & Loy, 2023; Todd, 2013), so further research on this matter is warranted.

What Is a Context?

Outcomes from the basic laboratory emphasize the important role of context change in determining the maintenance of behavior change. Researchers broadly define context as any environmental stimulus conditions that influence behavior (Podlesnik et al., 2017). Readers should note that this definition is likely intentionally broad to encompass the diverse range of stimuli that can comprise a context. Understanding the variables contributing to a context may help clinicians and researchers anticipate which environmental manipulations will constitute a change in that context. It may also help them anticipate situations where renewal is likely to occur and plan their treatment and/or research protocols accordingly. Here, we will provide an overview of the methods that researchers have used to manipulate context during basic laboratory research on renewal.

Physical Environment

The lion's share of laboratory studies on renewal have manipulated the physical contexts used during the acquisition of the target response, extinction, and renewal testing. Nakajima et al. (2000) provided an early example of renewal in the context of operant behavior, and they manipulated visual, auditory, and tactile cues in two sets of operant chambers for rats to create their contexts. In one context, the chamber floor was covered with a black acrylic plate, a ball chain was suspended from the chamber ceiling, and a light positioned above the lever flashed throughout the session. In the other, the stainless-steel grid floor was exposed, the chain was absent, a white acrylic plate bisected the chamber to reduce floor space, and a tone was presented throughout the session. During baseline, rats earned food pellets by pressing the lever. During treatment and the renewal test, lever pressing was placed on extinction. Nakajima et al. included three groups of rats: AAA, AAB, and ABA. The letters in these group names indicated the contexts in place across phases, and which of the two contexts described above was Context A and Context B was counterbalanced across rats. During baseline, rats in each group lever pressed at elevated rates. When food reinforcement was suspended during treatment, lever pressing decreased across sessions for rats in each group. During the renewal test, lever pressing initially increased for rats in the ABA group, thus demonstrating renewal of food-motivated operant behavior. Rates of lever pressing for rats in the AAA and AAB groups remained near zero. In the interest of clarity, the specific manipulations of the physical context used across laboratories tend to differ, and the extent to which AAB context manipulations are sufficient to produce renewal might depend on the specific methods researchers use to arrange those physical contexts.

Social Variables

Browning and Shahan (2018) extended the study of renewal to contexts produced by social variables. They used operant chambers for rats that were bisected by a sheet of ¼-inch hardware cloth, splitting the chambers into two compartments. The front compartment included a lever and dipper aperture, and the back compartment was used to introduce a second rat with which the rats whose behavior was being studied could interact in a limited capacity through the hardware-cloth divider. During baseline, two groups of rats pressed levers for sucrose, and experimental rats were alone in the operant chambers. In treatment, lever pressing was extinguished. For rats in the AAA group, no other stimulus change was arranged. However, a second rat was placed in the back compartment for rats in the ABA group. Finally, during the renewal test, the second rat was removed for the ABA group to test for renewal, and no stimulus change was arranged for rats in the AAA group. Renewed lever pressing occurred for the ABA group but not the AAA group.

It was possible that the presence of a second rat during extinction of lever pressing presented a source of alternative, social reinforcement in Browning and Shahan's (2018) Experiment 1. Inasmuch, it was possible that removing the second rat in the renewal test essentially resulted in the suspension of alternative reinforcement, thereby resulting in a *resurgence* (i.e., a different type of relapse; see Chap. 1, Mauzy et al., this volume) of lever pressing. They followed up on this possibility in their Experiment 2 by reversing A and B context assignments. That is, for the ABA group, Context A was associated with the presence of the second rat, and Context B with its absence. Again, lever pressing increased for rats in the ABA group during the renewal test and did not change between phases for rats in the AAA group. Thus, the presence of a social stimulus, like another rat in an operant chamber, may contribute to the conditioning context, and changing the availability of that stimulus following extinction may result in renewal. Continued basic research on renewal during changes in social stimuli seems warranted given its parallel to renewal that occurs due to changes in treatment implementers in clinical practice (see Muething et al., 2020).

Interoceptive Manipulations

The stimuli so far reviewed that may contribute to contexts have been rather concrete: both the physical environment and social stimuli are directly observable components of the organism's environment. Interoceptive stimuli, those within the bounds of the organism's skin, also have been shown to contribute to contexts that, if changed following extinction, may result in renewed behavior. For example, Bouton et al. (1990) evaluated the extent to which drug states could serve as contextual stimuli in the context of fear conditioning with rats. During baseline, rats experienced a single session of fear conditioning. They were placed in operant chambers and foot shocks were delivered to associate the chamber with shock. Next, rats were injected with a benzodiazepine tranquilizer on each day of treatment. Half of the rats were placed in the operant chambers 30 min following injection, and these rats experienced extinction of the chamber-shock relation in that no shocks were delivered. The other half of the rats were handled before being placed back in their home cages on each day of treatment. Finally, rats experienced two renewal test sessions conducted on separate days. During both test sessions, rats were placed in the operant chambers. Prior to one session, rats were injected with the drug, and they were injected with saline prior to the other (order counterbalanced across rats).

Rats who underwent extinction training under the drug's influence exhibited substantially more freezing when tested following saline injection than following drug injection. Importantly, freezing did not differ between saline and drug tests for rats that did not experience extinction training during treatment, suggesting that differences between groups that did experience extinction training are not attributable to any potential motoric effects produced by drug intoxication. Thus, removing drug intoxication during the test resulted in renewal of freezing.

Additionally, Schepers and Bouton (2017) demonstrated that hunger states (i.e., satiety vs. food deprivation) may also serve as contexts that exert control over response suppression. They trained rats to press a lever for sucrose reward during baseline under conditions of satiety. That is, rats had free access to food outside of sessions. Next, lever pressing was extinguished in treatment under conditions of food deprivation—rats had 1 hour of access to food following sessions. Finally, during the renewal test, rats experienced two different kinds of test conditions in a counterbalanced order over days. In the sated condition, they had free access to food for 23 hours prior to sessions. In the deprived condition, they experienced food deprivation for 23 hours prior to sessions. During the renewal test, lever pressing renewed when rats were tested under conditions of satiety, but lever pressing remained low during conditions of food deprivation.

Time

Adding to the list of comparatively abstract stimuli that may contribute to contexts, temporal variables have been shown to impact renewal. For example, Bouton and García-Gutiérrez (2006) studied acquisition, extinction, and renewal of a Pavlovian approach response in two groups of rats. During baseline, rats experienced conditioning trials wherein the presentation of a tone (i.e., a conditioned stimulus or CS) terminated with the delivery of a food pellet (i.e., the unconditioned stimulus or US). The Pavlovian approach response was nose poking into the food aperture. Half of these trials were separated by a 4-min intertrial interval (ITI), and the other half were separated by a 16-min ITI. Next, during treatment, rats experienced a single extinction training session containing eight extinction trials and four test trials. The extinction trials entailed presentation of the CS in the absence of the US. Half of the rats experienced a 4-min ITI, and the other half experienced a 16-min ITI. Following extinction trials, a 16-min ITI was arranged, after which test trials began. These trials were identical to extinction trials, but they were separated by 8-min ITIs. If time served as a context in this setting, Bouton and García-Gutiérrez hypothesized that introduction of the 16-min ITI following extinction trials would serve as a context change for rats that experienced a 4-min ITI between extinction trials but not for rats that experienced a 16-min ITI between extinction trials.

By the end of the 48 conditioning trials, rats reliably nose poked into the food receptacle when the CS was presented. During treatment, nose poking in the presence of the CS was reduced to low levels in both groups. Consistent with Bouton and García-Gutiérrez's (2006) hypothesis, presentation of the 16-min ITI did not affect nose poking during the CS for rats that also experienced a 16-min ITI during extinction. For rats that experienced the 4-min ITI during extinction, however, nose poking in the presence of the CS significantly increased relative to terminal performance during extinction, demonstrating renewal.

Variables That Impact Renewal

Basic research indicates that several variables may impact the likelihood and magnitude of renewal, such as baseline and treatment reinforcement rates, baseline response rates, baseline and treatment durations, the types of interventions used during treatment to decrease target responding (e.g., extinction, differential reinforcement), and the similarity between treatment and non-treatment settings. The following section summarizes basic research findings on these variables.

Rate of Reinforcement

Many basic investigations and a small collection of applied studies indicate that baseline reinforcement rates for target responding affect the persistence of behavior during treatment (e.g., Lerman et al., 1996; Nevin & Wacker, 2013; Pipkin & Vollmer, 2009). In addition, applied research suggests that clinicians should pay close attention to the reinforcement schedules they program for alternative behaviors during treatment, ideally progressing from a dense schedule at the onset of treatment and then thinning to a leaner schedule later in treatment that may be more feasible to implement in the natural environment (Briggs et al., 2023; Kranak & Brown, 2024). Given the importance of considering reinforcement rates during the treatment of severe challenging behavior, clinicians should know how baseline and treatment reinforcement rates may influence renewal.

Baseline

To our knowledge, only two basic research studies have expressly examined the effects of baseline reinforcement rate on renewal, and the results of both studies suggest that higher rates of baseline reinforcement produce higher magnitudes of renewal (Berry et al., 2014; Podlesnik & Shahan, 2009). First, consider Experiment 3 from Podlesnik and Shahan (2009). In baseline, pigeons' pecks to a key produced food reinforcement on a VI 120-s schedule in two components of a multiple schedule in Context A, which was signaled by steady illumination of the house light in the operant chamber. In addition, experimenters also delivered response-independent food reinforcers on a variable time (VT) 20-s schedule in one component. Next, experimenters exposed pigeons' key pecks to a phase of extinction in a different context (Context B, signaled by a flashing house light) in which responding resulted in no programmed consequences. Finally, extinction continued for key pecking, and the experimenters returned the pigeons to Context A. Results indicated that higher magnitudes of renewal occurred in the multiple schedule component that previously included additional response-independent reinforcer deliveries. It is worth highlighting that Podlesnik and Shahan manipulated baseline reinforcement rates by providing additional response-independent reinforcers on a VT schedule in the dense component.

Alternatively, Berry et al. (2014) compared the effects of dense and lean baseline reinforcement schedules on renewal with pigeons but manipulated reinforcement rates by programming two distinct schedules of response-dependent reinforcement in a multiple schedule. During baseline in Context A of Experiment 1, key pecking produced food reinforcement on a VI 30-s schedule in one multiple schedule component (dense) and a VI 120-s schedule in the other component (lean). Next, experimenters extinguished key pecking in both multiple schedule components in Context B. Contexts A and B were signaled by steady and flashing key lights during multiple schedule components, respectively. Finally, experimenters tested for renewal in Context A while extinction remained in place. Results of Experiment 1 replicated the findings from Podlesnik and Shahan in that ABA renewal was greater in the multiple schedule component that included dense baseline reinforcement rates relative to the component associated with lean baseline reinforcement rates. Berry and colleagues found similar results in a second experiment with ABC renewal wherein contexts were signaled by different operant chambers with different physical characteristics. Although clinicians treating severe challenging behavior do not often manipulate baseline reinforcement rates (Kimball et al., 2023a; St. Peter Pipkin & Vollmer, 2009), the findings from Podlesnik and Shahan and Berry et al. potentially imply that challenging behaviors with higher reinforcement rates before treatment may be susceptible to higher renewal magnitudes later.

Treatment

As far as we know, Kimball et al. (2023b) is the only study that has evaluated the effects of reinforcement rates in Context B on the magnitude of renewal. College students served as participants, and they engaged with a computer task that involved pressed moving response keys. Kimball, Salvetti et al. compared the effects of dense and lean differential reinforcement of alternative behavior (DRA) schedules on ABA renewal in a within-subjects design. The experimenters programmed different contexts by changing the background color of the computer screen. During baseline in Context A, target responding produced reinforcement (i.e., points and animated bursts of confetti) on a VI 3-s schedule in the dense arrangement and a VI 12-s schedule in the lean arrangement. Following baseline in Context A, experimenters placed target responding on extinction in Context B and differentially reinforced participants' responses on an alternative response key on a VI 3-s schedule in the dense arrangement and a VI 12-s schedule in the lean arrangement. In the ABA renewal test, the same extinction and DRA contingencies remained in place in Context A, and experimenters found higher renewal magnitudes in the lean arrangement relative to the dense arrangement. The experimenters hypothesized that the DRA and extinction procedures produced a suppressive effect on renewed target responding and that these effects depended on the rate of reinforcement for the alternative response. If these results generalize, clinicians may consider that higher magnitudes of renewal may be more likely in applied settings if the reinforcement schedule for the alternative responses (e.g., FCR) is relatively lean. Still, these results should be interpreted cautiously because the experimenters manipulated both baseline and DRA reinforcement parameters.

Baseline Response Rate

The extent to which target response rate during baseline affects the magnitude of renewal is an underexplored research question. We are unaware of published studies that have expressly manipulated target response rate in baseline as an independent variable. Nevertheless, Podlesnik et al. (2017) reanalyzed the findings from Bouton et al. (2011) and Podlesnik and Shahan (2009), and the retrospective analysis suggested that higher target response rates during baseline were correlated with higher magnitudes of ABA renewal in rats and pigeons. Be that as it may, the retrospective findings for Podlesnik and Shahan's data are challenging to interpret because the researchers manipulated reinforcement rates for the target response in baseline, and the data showed that higher baseline reinforcement rates preceded higher magnitudes of renewal. Said differently, it is difficult to know if the target response rate or reinforcement rate contributed to the higher magnitudes of renewal. Fortunately, further consideration of the results from Berry et al. (2014) seemingly clarifies that baseline reinforcement rate might be a better predictor of renewal magnitude. Recall that both Berry et al. and Podlesnik and Shahan found that dense baseline reinforcement rates produced higher magnitudes of renewal than lean reinforcement rates. However, Berry et al. observed higher target response rates in the dense condition, which contrasts with the results from Podlesnik and Shahan, who observed higher target response rates in the lean condition.

Considering that both studies found that dense baseline reinforcement rates produced higher magnitudes of renewal than lean reinforcement rates despite differences in the conditions that produced the highest baseline response rate, we cannot confidently say that baseline response rate affects renewal magnitude. At present, research suggests that clinicians should not consider baseline response rate as an indicator of the potential future magnitude of renewal. Down the line, future studies that examine the role of baseline response rate on the magnitude of renewal should include control procedures to account for baseline reinforcement rates and vice versa (see Craig et al., 2019, for further discussion).

Duration of Baseline in Context A and Treatment with Extinction

Renewal occurs during transitions to familiar environments associated with a history of reinforcement for the target response (ABA renewal) and transitions to novel environments unassociated with extinction for the target response (ABC and AAB renewal). Therefore, from a conceptual standpoint, it seems reasonable to expect that longer reinforcement histories for the target response in Context A may produce higher magnitudes of renewal and that more prolonged exposure to extinction during treatment may result in weakened renewal effects. Nevertheless, basic research on renewal demonstrates that it is not actually that simple.

Duration of Baseline in Context A

Several studies have investigated the effects of different baseline durations in Context A on the magnitude of renewal with rats. Todd et al. (2012) compared the effects of 4 versus 12 sessions of baseline reinforcement for the target response in Context A on both ABA and ABC renewal. The experimenters programmed different contexts using visual and olfactory stimuli. Results showed that the magnitude of ABA and ABC renewal was greater following 12 baseline sessions in Context A relative to 4 sessions. However, as noted by others (e.g., Craig et al., 2019), the experiment's results are confounded by the fact that rats that experienced 12 sessions in baseline exhibited much higher response rates in baseline than rats that experienced 4 baseline sessions. Therefore, it does not appear possible to determine if the extended exposure to baseline was truly the catalyst that produced the increased magnitude of renewal. The ambiguous results from Todd et al. are a common theme of research in this area. For example, Madrigal et al. (2018) also sought to compare the effects of 4 versus 12 sessions of baseline reinforcement for the target response on the magnitude of ABA renewal with rats. The results implied that 12 baseline sessions resulted in greater ABA renewal than 4 baseline sessions; however, Madrigal et al.'s findings were confounded by differences in baseline response rates between groups as well as the number of scheduled and obtained reinforcers during baseline (see also Nieto et al., 2023; Experiment 2 on ABC renewal). These collective findings illustrate the complexity of comparing durations of exposure to baseline reinforcement in Context A on renewal magnitude and suggest that more research is vital. For now, clinicians should look to other baseline variables (e.g., reinforcement rate) as potential indicators of future renewal magnitude.

Duration of Treatment with Extinction

Little is known about the effects of treatment duration with extinction in Context B (ABA and ABC renewal) or Context A (AAB renewal) on the magnitude of renewal. Bouton et al. (2011) found that tripling the number of extinction sessions (i.e., 12 versus 4 sessions) failed to mitigate the magnitude of AAB renewal with rats. Nieto et al. (2023), who manipulated context using visual and physical stimuli, found that conducting 36 extinction sessions in Context B mitigated the magnitude of ABC renewal relative to conducting 4 extinction sessions. However, the researchers found that these renewal mitigation effects were wiped out when they doubled the number of baseline reinforcement sessions for the target response. Clearly, additional research is needed in this area to clarify the conditions under which the duration of exposure to extinction during treatment affects renewal. Future research should also endeavor to compare the effects of different treatment durations with extinction on ABA renewal. The findings of the few studies on this variable suggest that clinicians should not expect extended treatment durations to affect the magnitude of renewal.

Additional Treatment Procedures Beyond Extinction

Although basic researchers have primarily studied operant renewal when the target behavior is decreased and suppressed via extinction alone (e.g., Bouton et al., 2011), researchers have also studied renewal following treatments that include alternative reinforcement such as DRA, noncontingent reinforcement (NCR), differential reinforcement of other behavior (DRO), and punishment. Measuring renewal during the availability of alternative reinforcement is particularly relevant to clinicians, given that treatments to reduce challenging behavior rarely entail extinction alone (Kimball et al., 2020). Clinicians almost always craft treatment packages with at least some alternative reinforcement (e.g., FCT; Tiger et al., 2008). Therefore, from a translational point of view, basic research that includes extinction plus alternative reinforcement during treatment and renewal tests may have more ecological validity with respect to interventions aimed at decreasing severe challenging behavior in clinical settings.

DRA

Researchers have demonstrated that ABA renewal occurs despite the availability of DRA during renewal tests (Kimball et al., 2023b; Ritchey et al., 2022). In other words, basic research shows that target responding will still renew during a context change from a therapeutic setting to a familiar environment even though contingencies for target and alternative responding heavily favor engaging in the alternative response. For example, Ritchey et al. (2022, Experiment 5) examined ABA renewal during DRA with adult human participants who engaged with a computer task on

Amazon Mechanical Turk (MTurk). Target responding produced reinforcement during baseline in Context A on a VI 2-s schedule. Next, experimenters differentially reinforced an alternative response on a VI 2-s schedule, and the target response resulted in no programmed consequences (i.e., extinction) in Context B. Contexts A and B were signaled by visual stimuli on the background computer screen. Then, during the renewal test in Context A, experimenters observed a renewal of target responding despite no change in the contingencies for target and alternative responding. Still, despite an increase in the target response rate in the renewal test, alternative response rates remained relatively high. Results such as these imply that clinicians should potentially prepare for renewal during context changes even if they have recently eliminated challenging behavior with a DRA-based BIP.

DRO

Like DRA, basic research also suggests renewal occurs despite DRO contingencies that promote the inhibition of target responding (e.g., Kearns & Weiss, 2007; Rey et al., 2020). As an illustration, Nakajima et al. (2002, Experiment 1) reinforced rats' lever pressing on a VI 30-s schedule in Context A. Next, experimenters placed lever pressing on extinction and introduced a resetting DRO 30-s schedule in Context B. Contexts A and B were signaled with a combination of visual, auditory, and tactile stimuli. Then, Nakajima et al. observed ABA renewal of lever pressing in a return to Context A despite the continuation of the DRO contingency (see also Finch et al., 2022 for ABC renewal). Bernal-Gamboa and Nieto (2018) found similar results with ABC renewal in rats, but the authors also compared renewal during DRO versus extinction alone. Notably, the experimenters found zero differences in the magnitude of renewal between the rats that experienced the renewal test with extinction and the group of rats with the DRO contingency programmed during the test. The findings from these reviewed studies suggest clinicians should potentially be wary of renewal even if a DRO-based intervention has successfully suppressed challenging behavior.

NCR

Beyond differential reinforcement procedures, a few basic research studies have also demonstrated that renewal occurs despite the delivery of response-independent reinforcers during treatment and the renewal test (i.e., NCR). For instance, Nakajima et al. (2002, Experiment 2) first reinforced rats' lever pressing in Context A. Next, experimenters reduced targeting responding to low levels in Context B by extinguishing lever pressing and introducing a variable time (VT) 30-s schedule of reinforcement. Finally, the experimenters observed ABA renewal of lever pressing when they returned the rats to Context A and continued presenting noncontingent reinforcers according to the VT 30-s schedule (see also Kearns & Weiss, 2007). Finch et al. (2023) found similar results with ABA and ABC renewal with college students who engaged with a computer task. The results of basic research on renewal during NCR suggest that clinicians should keep renewal on their radar during context changes despite NCR-based interventions that introduce abolishing operations (Langthorne & McGill, 2009) for challenging behavior.

Delay to Reinforcement

To our knowledge, Morfín et al. (2021) is the only study that has examined the impact of delay to reinforcement on renewal. Researchers first reinforced rats' lever pressing on a VI 30-s schedule in baseline in Context A. Next, the researchers assigned the rats to two groups. One group of rats experienced extinction for lever pressing in Context B and the other group experienced a delay-to-reinforcement contingency in which lever pressing was reinforced on a VI 18-s schedule, but once lever pressing met the VI contingency, the delivery of that reinforcer was delayed by 12 s. Contexts were signaled by visual, olfactory, and tactile stimuli. Next, the researchers compared ABA renewal between groups when the rats returned to Context A, but lever pressing was placed on extinction for both groups. The results showed that the delay-to-reinforcement group exhibited less ABA renewal than the group of rats that experienced extinction in Context B. The results from Morfín et al. should be interpreted with caution because the renewal test was confounded by the delay-to-reinforcement group not only experiencing a context change during the test but a removal of reinforcement, too. Nevertheless, if these findings generalize, they might have implications for reducing challenging behavior when programming extinction is not feasible or ethically palatable (see Briggs et al., 2019, for further discussion).

Punishment

Basic researchers have found that renewal occurs during context changes following the elimination of target responding in Context B with punishment. As an illustration, Bouton and Schepers (2015) examined both ABA and ABC renewal of rats' lever pressing following exposure to punishment of the target response, and contexts were signaled by olfactory, visual, and tactile stimuli. In Context A, lever pressing produced reinforcement on a VI 30-s schedule. Next, in Context B, lever pressing continued to produce reinforcement on the VI 30-s schedule, but lever pressing also resulted in intermittent punishment via shock delivered on a VI 90-s schedule. Then, experimenters observed renewal when rats returned to Context A (Experiment 1) or transitioned rats to a novel Context C (Experiment 2) while extinction was programmed for lever pressing and punishment was removed.

In related experiments, Broomer and Bouton (2023) and Kuroda et al. (2020) compared ABA renewal following Context B conditions in which target responding was eliminated via punishment or extinction. While Broomer and Bouton did not detect any differences in the magnitude of renewal following punishment versus extinction with rats, Kuroda et al. found that the magnitude of renewal was greater following punishment plus extinction in Context B relative to extinction alone with zebrafish. Notwithstanding these differences in findings, the collective results of these reviewed studies on renewal following punishment suggest that learning during punishment may be context-specific (Bouton & Schepers, 2015). However, all of these studies share the same procedural confound in the renewal test that arguably clouds the interpretation of the results, at least from an applied perspective. Specifically, each study removed the punishment contingency during the renewal test that was in effect in Context B. The removal of the punishment contingency presents interpretation challenges because renewal is the relapse of responding *produced by a context change*. When context changes coincide with contingency changes, it is difficult to isolate the variable(s) responsible for behavior change. Thus, when punishment is removed in the renewal test, the magnitude of relapse may be influenced by the context change, withdrawing punishment, or both. What's more, when punishment is required to produce socially significant decreases in challenging behavior in clinical practice (see Hurd et al., 2024, for discussion), clinicians are encouraged to program punishment across all settings to increase the likelihood of stimulus generalization (Lerman & Vorndran, 2002). Future basic research studies might consider retaining the punishment contingency during renewal tests so that results may shed more light on what renewal may look like in applied settings when punishment is present.

Similarity Between Treatment and Non-Treatment Contexts

Although only a single study has evaluated the impact of context similarity on operant renewal, we believe it is worth considering, given that a handful of applied studies (e.g., Haney et al., 2021) have used context similarity as a renewal-mitigation procedure for socially significant behavior. In a series of experiments with rats, Todd et al. (2012) used a mixture of different contextual manipulations, including the type of operant chamber (i.e., two different models of Med Associates chambers), visual stimuli, and olfactory stimuli to compare the magnitude of ABC renewal when Contexts B and C were relatively similar (Experiments 1 and 3) versus when Contexts A and C were relatively similar (Experiments 2 and 3). Though the precise details of how the experimenters constructed the various contextual arrangements are beyond the scope of this chapter, Todd et al. found that the magnitude of ABC renewal was larger when the extinction context (Context B) was relatively distinct from the testing context (Context C). In other words, the magnitude of renewal was larger if the acquisition context (Context A) was relatively similar to the novel testing context (Context C). Contrastingly, the experimenters observed smaller magnitudes of renewal if Context B was relatively similar to Context C. Todd et al. found similar results with ABA renewal when they made Context B more or less distinct from Context A. These collective findings appear to imply that clinicians might consider making efforts to increase the similarity between treatment settings (e.g., clinic therapy room) and both novel (e.g., new school classroom) and familiar settings (e.g., home) in practice.

Renewal-Mitigation Procedures

A long-standing goal of applied behavior analysis has been to increase the longevity and durability of behavioral treatments (Baer et al., 1968). One role that basic research has played in meeting that goal is testing and refining relapse mitigation procedures in controlled settings before measuring the effects of the procedures on socially significant behavior in applied settings. An effective relapse-mitigation procedure reduces the potentially damaging impact of relapse by reducing the magnitude and persistence of relapse effects during treatment challenges (Kimball et al., 2023a). In the case of renewal, basic research has identified a few mitigation techniques specifically tailored to lessen the impact of relapse during treatment context changes. Although applied researchers have examined additional renewal-mitigation procedures with challenging behavior (see Chap. 4, Grunewald et al., this volume), we reserve our discussion to procedures with demonstrated efficacy in the basic lab.

Extinction Cues

Several studies have demonstrated that distinct environmental cues (i.e., stimuli) historically paired with extinction for the target response can be presented during context changes to reduce the magnitude of operant ABA, ABC, and AAB renewal (e.g., Bernal-Gamboa et al., 2022; Gámez & Bernal-Gamboa, 2019; Nieto et al., 2020). The presentation of extinction cues signals that extinction is still in effect despite transitions to familiar contexts that have previously included reinforcement for the target response (ABA renewal) or novel contexts without established reinforcement histories for the target response (ABC or AAB renewal). Willcocks and McNally (2014, Experiment 1) provided an early example of how extinction cues may be used to mitigate ABA renewal. In Context A, rats' nose pokes produced beer on an FR 1 schedule, and then experimenters placed that response on extinction in Context B until responding decreased to low levels. Contexts A and B were signaled with olfactory and tactile cues. During each extinction session in Context B, the experimenters presented a periodic audible tone that lasted 1 min and repeated every 6 min. Next, in a test for ABA renewal, experimenters returned the rats to Context A with extinction still in place. Half of the rats experienced continued presentation of the periodic audible tone in the test, and half did not. Notably, Willcocks and McNally found that target response rates were significantly lower for the rats that experienced the extinction cue in the ABA renewal test than for those that did not experience the extinction cue during the test.

Multiple Context Training

Another renewal-mitigation procedure with demonstrated efficacy is called multiple context training. Multiple context training involves exposing the target response to extinction in multiple stimulus contexts before testing for renewal instead of exposing the target response to extinction in only a single context. While this procedure has been chiefly tested with Pavlovian responses (see Bustamante et al., 2024, for a review), a few studies on the renewal of operant behavior have shown promising mitigation effects (e.g., Bernal-Gamboa et al., 2020). Consider the results from Bernal-Gamboa et al. (2017), which demonstrated that multiple context training can mitigate both operant ABA and ABC renewal. In Experiment 1, experimenters reinforced rats' lever pressing with food on a VI 30-s schedule in Context A. Next, half of the rats experienced extinction for lever pressing in Context B for one session a day across 3 days. The other half of the rats experienced extinction in three different contexts (B, C, and D) across 3 days, such that each of the three extinction sessions occurred in a novel and distinct context. The experimenters programmed the various contexts using visual and tactile stimuli. Finally, the experimenters tested for renewal with all rats in a novel context (Context E), akin to a test for ABC renewal. Results showed that the rats that experienced multiple context training exhibited a reduced magnitude of ABC renewal relative to those that only experienced extinction in a single context. The experimenters repeated those same procedures with two more groups of rats and found that multiple context training did not mitigate ABA renewal. However, in Experiment 2, the experimenters found that multiple context training did mitigate ABA renewal after extinction occurred in three distinct contexts but across 12 sessions instead of only 3. Additional research is needed to determine more precisely the conditions under which multiple-context training influences renewal produced by different kinds of context changes (i.e., ABA, ABC, and AAB renewal).

Conceptual Analyses of Renewal

So far in this chapter, we have described various manipulations that have been used in laboratory settings to understand renewal of Pavlovian and operant behavior. The effects of these manipulations have been shown to be robust and have been replicated across species in a variety of preparations (for review, see Podlesnik et al., 2017). These manipulations demonstrate *that* previously eliminated behavior may renew when the context changes. They do not, however, clearly demonstrate *why* context change causes renewal. Although there have been various conceptual analyses of renewal that attempt to answer this "why" question (Podlesnik & Shahan, 2009, 2010; Shahan et al., 2020), the most widely applied analysis is offered by Bouton and colleagues' Context Theory (Bouton, 2002, 2004; Trask et al., 2015).

According to Context Theory, the different phases of a renewal preparation generate different types of learning, and those types of learning come under the control of the contexts in which they occurred. Specifically, during Phase 1 (e.g., Context A), when an operant response produces a reinforcer or a US is presented following a CS, organisms develop excitatory response-reinforcer or CS-US associations. Simply put, with excitatory learning that occurs with operant behavior, the organism associates the context in which reinforcers are delivered for target responding with reinforcement. Therefore, when the organism encounters that context, target responding increases because that context has historically been a predictor of forthcoming reinforcement (Todd, 2013). The associations developed following excitatory learning come under the control of the Phase-1 context, but also tend to generalize readily to other contexts. During Phase 2, an operant response is placed on extinction and no longer produces a specific outcome, or a CS may be presented repeatedly without also presenting the US. Under these contingencies, the organism learns an inhibitory response-no-reinforcer or CS-no-US association, and this inhibitory learning comes under the control of the Phase-2 context (e.g., Context B). Said differently, inhibitory learning is learning not to respond, and the organism associates the extinction context with "no reinforcer" (Bouton, 1993, 1994, 2014; Nelson et al., 2011). Unlike the context-general excitatory learning generated in Phase 1, the inhibitory learning generated in Phase 2 is context-specific. When the context subsequently is changed in Phase 3 (whether a familiar context, as in ABA renewal, or a new context, as in AAB and ABC renewal), the inhibitory learning generated during Phase 2 fails to generalize to Phase 3. The excitatory learning generated during Phase 1, however, does generalize, thus resulting in renewal.

The basic arguments put forward by Context Theory have received general support in that the manipulation of variables that should affect the degree to which excitatory and inhibitory learning generalize between contexts has been shown to impact renewal in expected ways. For example, in ABA renewal, the Phase-3 transition back to the same context that previously was associated with renewal during Phase 1 should result in substantial generalization of excitatory learning to that context and thus substantial renewal of extinguished behavior. In ABC and ABB renewal, however, one may expect less generalization of excitatory learning because the Phase-3 context differs from the Phase-1 context. This line of reasoning has been supported in that ABA renewal tends to be greater than ABC or AAB renewal (Bouton et al., 2011). Moreover, one would expect Phase-3 contexts that are more similar to Phase-2 contexts to promote stronger generalization of inhibitory learning, and thus less renewal, than Phase-3 contexts that are less like Phase-2 contexts. As described above, this argument, too, has found empirical support (e.g., Todd et al., 2012).

A Note on the Relation Between Context Control and Stimulus Control

In the above section, we referred to "contextual control" of excitatory and inhibitory learning. Readers familiar with the concept of "stimulus control" may wonder about the extent to which these concepts are related. As Podlesnik et al. (2017) reviewed, stimulus control usually refers to control over a behavior that is exerted by a specific, discrete stimulus derived from that stimulus' unique relation to a specific outcome. For example, an educator may reinforce their students' requests for breaks from demands only when a green "go" signal is presented in the classroom (see Saini et al., 2016). As the material in this chapter has illustrated, the concept of "context" often is more loosely defined and may encompass several (or all) discrete stimuli in an individual's environment. Discrete stimuli and contexts may result in equivalent control over excitatory learning, inhibitory learning, and behavior, but the controlling stimuli are more (in the case of stimulus control) or less (in the case of context control) specific.

Directions for Future Research and Conclusion

Trends in the recently published basic research suggest at least two distinct avenues for future research essential for understanding renewal during the treatment of challenging behavior in applied settings. First, the results of a collection of studies (e.g., Keevy et al., 2022; Kincaid et al., 2015) suggest that future basic research is warranted to more conclusively determine how the magnitude of renewal is affected by the co-occurrence of other forms of relapse (King et al., 2024). While many basic studies have investigated renewal in isolation (e.g., Bouton et al., 2011), some researchers have suggested that relapse types may co-occur in applied settings on some occasions due to the dynamic nature of stimulus and reinforcement conditions in clinical practice (Sweeney & Shahan, 2015). For instance, after successfully reducing challenging behavior in a clinic setting with a DRA-based treatment like FCT (Context B), renewal may be observed when the learner returns to the non-treatment setting (e.g., school classroom; Context A). When renewal occurs, it is plausible that other treatment challenges may co-occur, such as treatment integrity errors of omission in which the treatment implementer fails to reinforce the alternative response (e.g., FCR; Mitteer et al., 2018). The omission of reinforcement for the alternative response could result in a different type of relapse called *resurgence*, which is the re-emergence of a previously eliminated target response when a more recently reinforced alternative response contacts worsening reinforcement conditions, such as temporary extinction (Lattal et al., 2017). Some basic studies have found that the magnitude of relapse was greater during tests that included both a context change (renewal) and the elimination of alternative reinforcement (resurgence) relative to the magnitude of relapse when either type of treatment challenge occurred in isolation. For example, Podlesnik et al. (2019, Experiment 2) reinforced rats' target responding (left lever press) in baseline in Context A. Next, researchers placed the target response on extinction and simultaneously differentially reinforced an alternative response (right lever press) in Context B. Contexts A and B were signaled with visual stimuli. Then, during the combined relapse test, researchers alternated between conditions in which the alternative response was placed on extinction in Context B (i.e., resurgence alone) and the alternative response was placed on extinction plus the rats returned to Context A (i.e., resurgence and renewal) in a counterbalanced order. Results showed that for most subjects, the combined effects of context change and suspending reinforcement produced higher magnitudes of relapse relative to suspending reinforcement alone (see also King & Hayes, 2016; Ritchey et al., 2022). Still, other studies have failed to demonstrate these effects (e.g., Sweeney & Shahan, 2015).

After conducting a systematic literature review, King et al. (2024) recently noted that only 2 of the 27 reviewed experiments included the proper control procedures to fairly compare the combined and isolated effects of renewal and resurgence. Accordingly, basic researchers should consider addressing this shortage of studies with more well-controlled experiments, given the high prevalence of these relapse phenomena in clinical practice (Briggs et al., 2018; Muething et al., 2020). Future studies should also expand this line of research by investigating the combined effects of renewal and other forms of relapse, such as reinstatement (Kranak & Falligant, 2023) and spontaneous recovery (Thrailkill et al., 2018).

A second clear direction for future basic research is continuing to investigate what researchers have dubbed the "nonsequential" renewal arrangement (Sullivan et al., 2018). Traditionally, basic research on ABA and ABC renewal employs a standard three-phase arrangement in which each phase is sequentially introduced. Phase 1 establishes a reinforcement history for the target response in Context A, and Phase 2 introduces a contingency to decrease and suppress target responding in Context B. Lastly, Phase 3 tests for renewal by presenting the same contingency for target responding from Phase 2, but in either a familiar or a novel context. In spite of how often researchers have used this approach, some researchers have noted that it fails to account for a critical aspect of how ABA services are often provided during the treatment of challenging behavior. Besides those receiving service in inpatient settings, many learners receive treatment for their challenging behavior in a clinical setting (e.g., outpatient clinic) during part of the day, and then return to the non-treatment setting later in the day (e.g., home). Said another way, learners typically experience repeated exposure to the setting historically associated with a history of reinforcement for challenging behavior (i.e., Context A) while undergoing treatment in the clinical setting (i.e., Context B). Thus, from a translational point of view, the traditional sequential three-phase arrangement for studying renewal may lack ecological validity with respect to outpatient treatments because sequentially exposing behavior to Context A exclusively and then Context B exclusively may not map onto the events that transpire in clinical practice. To address this potential issue, a few studies have compared renewal following the traditional sequential three-phase arrangement and a nonsequential renewal arrangement in which subjects are intermittently exposed to reinforcement for the target response in Context A while experiencing treatment in Context B (Craig et al., 2019, 2020; Sullivan et al., 2018).

Consider Craig et al. (2019) as an example. During baseline in Context A, experimenters reinforced rats' lever pressing on a VI 30-s schedule. Next, experimenters assigned rats to either the Sequential or the Nonsequential groups for treatment in Context B. The Sequential group experienced one daily session of extinction for the target response in Context B until the phase was complete. In contrast, rats in the Nonsequential group experienced two sessions per day: one session in which target responding was placed on extinction in Context B and another in which target responding was reinforced on a VI 30-s schedule in Context A. Contexts A and B were signaled with different auditory, olfactory, visual, and tactile stimuli. In Phase 3, the experimenters exposed all rats to the same type of renewal test in Context A, where target responding produced no consequences (i.e., extinction). Craig et al. observed more renewal on average for the Nonsequential group relative to the Sequential group. Sarno and Kestner (2024) recently replicated these findings but also found that olfactory extinction cues did not mitigate ABA renewal in a nonsequential renewal arrangement. Undoubtedly, the findings from Craig et al. and Sarno and Kestner suggest that continued exploration of renewal in nonsequential arrangements is warranted to evaluate the generality of the phenomenon and further test the effects of renewal-mitigation procedures found to be effective with sequential arrangements (e.g., multiple context training).

In summary, clinicians and applied researchers should consider basic research on renewal as a resource to better understand when, how, and why context changes in clinical practice result in treatment relapse. Years of basic research on renewal have served as an invaluable bedrock of knowledge for applied and translational researchers to identify (a) the conditions in which renewal occurs, (b) the variables that impact renewal, and (c) procedures to mitigate the magnitude of renewal. If clinicians wish to increase the longevity and durability of their treatments, engagement with basic research on renewal (i.e., the general source of their methods) is imperative (Sidman, 2011).

References

Archer, T., Sjödén, P. O., Nilsson, L. G., & Carter, N. (1979). Role of exteroceptive background context in taste-aversion conditioning and extinction. *Animal Learning & Behavior, 7*, 17–22. https://doi.org/10.3758/BF03209650

Baer, D. M., Wolf, M. M., & Risley, T. R. (1968). Some current dimensions of applied behavior analysis. *Journal of Applied Behavior Analysis, 1*(1), 91–97. https://doi.org/10.1901/jaba.1968.1-91

Bernal-Gamboa, R., Nieto, J., & Gámez, A. M. (2020). Conducting extinction in multiple contexts attenuates relapse of operant behavior in humans. *Behavioural Processes, 181*, 104261. https://doi.org/10.1016/j.beproc.2020.104261

Bernal-Gamboa, R., & Nieto, J. (2018). Evidencia de renovación instrumental ABC previamente eliminada con los procedimientos de extinción y omisión. *Revista Argentina de Ciencias del Comportamiento, 10*(2), 11–18.

Bernal-Gamboa, R., Nieto, J., & Uengoer, M. (2017). Effects of extinction in multiple contexts on renewal of instrumental responses. *Behavioural Processes, 142*, 64–69. https://doi.org/10.1016/j.beproc.2017.06.003

Bernal-Gamboa, R., Nieto, J., & Uengoer, M. (2017). Effects of extinction in multiple contexts on renewal of instrumental responses. *Behavioural Processes, 142*, 64–69. https://doi.org/gbz5xb

Bernal-Gamboa, R., Mason, T. A., Nieto, J., & Gámez, A. M. (2022). An analysis of extinction-cue features in the reduction of operant behavior relapse. *The Psychological Record, 72*(1), 65–73. https://doi.org/10.1007/s40732-021-00472-z

Berry, M. S., Sweeney, M. M., & Odum, A. L. (2014). Effects of baseline reinforcement rate on operant ABA and ABC renewal. *Behavioural Processes, 108*, 87–93. https://doi.org/10.1016/j.beproc.2014.09.009

Bouton, M. E. (1993). Context, time, and memory retrieval in the interference paradigms of Pavlovian learning. *Psychological Bulletin, 114*(1), 80. https://psycnet.apa.org/doi/10.1037/0033-2909.114.1.80

Bouton, M. E. (1994). Conditioning, remembering, and forgetting. *Journal of Experimental Psychology: Animal Behavior Processes, 20*(3), 219. https://psycnet.apa.org/doi/10.1037/0097-7403.20.3.219

Bouton, M. E. (2002). Context, ambiguity, and unlearning: Sources of relapse after behavioral extinction. *Biological Psychiatry, 52*, 976–986. https://doi.org/10.1016/S0006-3223(02)01546-9

Bouton, M. E. (2004). Context and behavioral processes in extinction. *Learning & Memory, 11*(5), 485–494. https://doi.org/10.1101/lm.78804

Bouton, M. E. (2014). Why behavior change is difficult to sustain. *Preventive Medicine, 68*, 29–36. https://doi.org/10.1016/j.ypmed.2014.06.010

Bouton, M. E., & García-Gutiérrez, A. (2006). Intertrial interval as a contextual stimulus. *Behavioural Processes, 71*, 307–317. https://doi.org/10.1016/j.beproc.2005.12.003

Bouton, M. E., & King, D. A. (1983). Contextual control of the extinction of conditioned fear: Tests for the associative value of the context. *Journal of Experimental Psychology: Animal Behavior Processes, 9*(3), 248. https://psycnet.apa.org/doi/10.1037/0097-7403.9.3.248

Bouton, M. E., & Schepers, S. T. (2015). Renewal after the punishment of free operant behavior. *Journal of Experimental Psychology: Animal Learning and Cognition, 41*(1), 81. https://psycnet.apa.org/doi/10.1037/xan0000051

Bouton, M. E., & Todd, T. P. (2014). A fundamental role for context in instrumental learning and extinction. *Behavioural Processes, 104*, 13–19. https://doi.org/10.1016/j.beproc.2014.02.012

Bouton, M. E., Kenney, F. A., & Rosengard, C. (1990). State-dependent fear extinction with two benzodiazepine tranquilizers. *Behavioral Neuroscience, 104*, 44–55. https://doi.org/10.1037/0735-7044.104.1.44

Bouton, M. E., Todd, T. P., Vurbic, D., & Winterbauer, N. E. (2011). Renewal after the extinction of free operant behavior. *Learning & Behavior, 39*(1), 57–67. https://doi.org/10.3758/s13420-011-0018-6

Briggs, A. M., Fisher, W. W., Greer, B. D., & Kimball, R. T. (2018). Prevalence of resurgence of destructive behavior when thinning reinforcement schedules during functional communication training. *Journal of Applied Behavior Analysis, 51*(3), 620–633. https://doi.org/10.1002/jaba.472

Briggs, A. M., Dozier, C. L., Lessor, A. N., Kamana, B. U., & Jess, R. L. (2019). Further investigation of differential reinforcement of alternative behavior without extinction for escape-maintained destructive behavior. *Journal of Applied Behavior Analysis, 52*(4), 956–973. https://doi.org/10.1002/jaba.648

Briggs, A. M., Mitteer, D. R., Bergmann, S., & Greer, B. D. (2023). Reinforcer thinning: General approaches and considerations for maintaining skills and mitigating relapse. In *Handbook of applied behavior analysis: Integrating research into practice* (pp. 105–122). Springer International Publishing. https://doi.org/10.1007/978-3-031-19964-6_6

Broomer, M. C., & Bouton, M. E. (2023). A comparison of renewal, spontaneous recovery, and reacquisition after punishment and extinction. *Learning & Behavior, 51*(3), 262–273. https://doi.org/10.3758/s13420-022-00552-2

Browning, K. O., & Shahan, T. A. (2018). Renewal of extinguished operant behavior following changes in social context. *Journal of the Experimental Analysis of Behavior, 110*, 430–439. https://doi.org/10.1002/jeab.472

Bustamante, J., Soto, M., Miguez, G., Quezada-Scholz, V. E., Angulo, R., & Laborda, M. A. (2024). Extinction in multiple contexts reduces the return of extinguished responses: A multilevel meta-analysis. *Learning & Behavior, 52*(3), 209–223. https://doi.org/10.3758/s13420-023-00609-w

Craig, A. R., Sullivan, W. E., & Roane, H. S. (2019). Further evaluation of a nonsequential approach to studying operant renewal. *Journal of the Experimental Analysis of Behavior, 112*(2), 210–223. https://doi.org/10.1002/jeab.546

Craig, A. R., Sullivan, W. E., Browning, K. O., DeRosa, N. M., & Roane, H. S. (2020). Re-exposure to reinforcement in Context A during treatment in Context B reduces ABC renewal. *Journal of the Experimental Analysis of Behavior, 113*(1), 141–152. https://doi.org/10.1002/jeab.569

Falcomata, T. S., & Wacker, D. P. (2013). On the use of strategies for programming generalization during functional communication training: A review of the literature. *Journal of Developmental and Physical Disabilities, 25*, 5–15. https://doi.org/10.1007/s10882-012-9311-3

Finch, K. R., Williams, C. L., & Kestner, K. M. (2022). ABA and ABC renewal during ongoing omission training. *The Psychological Record, 72*(4), 675–695. https://doi.org/10.1007/s40732-022-00524-y

Finch, K. R., Kestner, K. M., & Amanieh, H. (2023). ABA and ABC renewal during an ongoing fixed-time schedule. *The Psychological Record, 73*(1), 105–117. https://doi.org/10.1007/s40732-022-00513-1

Gámez, A. M., & Bernal-Gamboa, R. (2019). The reoccurrence of voluntary behavior in humans is reduced by retrieval cues from extinction. *Acta Psychologica, 200*, 102945. https://doi.org/10.1016/j.actpsy.2019.102945

Haney, S. D., Piazza, C. C., Peterson, K. M., & Greer, B. D. (2021). An evaluation of a renewal-mitigation procedure for inappropriate mealtime behavior. *Journal of Applied Behavior Analysis, 54*(3), 903–927. https://doi.org/10.1002/jaba.815

Hurd, A. M., Brown, K. R., & Randall, K. R. (2024). Stimulus avoidance assessment: A systematic literature review. *Perspectives on Behavior Science, 47*, 139–166. https://doi.org/10.1007/s40614-024-00398-1

Kearns, D. N., & Weiss, S. J. (2007). Contextual renewal of cocaine seeking in rats and its attenuation by the conditioned effects of an alternative reinforcer. *Drug and Alcohol Dependence, 90*(2–3), 193–202. https://doi.org/10.1016/j.drugalcdep.2007.03.006

Keevy, M., Bai, J. Y., Ritchey, C. M., & Podlesnik, C. A. (2022). Examining combinations of stimulus and contingency changes with children diagnosed with autism spectrum disorder and pigeons. *Learning and Motivation, 78*, 101806. https://doi.org/10.1016/j.lmot.2022.101806

Kelley, M. E., Liddon, C. J., Ribeiro, A., Greif, A. E., & Podlesnik, C. A. (2015). Basic and translational evaluation of renewal of operant responding. *Journal of Applied Behavior Analysis, 48*(2), 390–401. https://doi.org/10.1002/jaba.209

Kimball, R. T., & Kranak, M. P. (2022). Six things clinicians should know about renewal. *Education and Treatment of Children, 45*(4), 395–410. https://doi.org/10.1007/s43494-022-00078-2

Kimball, R. T., Greer, B. D., Randall, K. R., & Briggs, A. M. (2020). Investigations of operant ABA renewal during differential reinforcement. *Journal of the Experimental Analysis of Behavior, 113*(1), 187–205. https://doi.org/10.1002/jeab.577

Kimball, R. T., Greer, B. D., Fuhrman, A. M., & Lambert, J. M. (2023a). Relapse and its mitigation: Toward behavioral inoculation. *Journal of Applied Behavior Analysis, 56*(2), 282–301. https://doi.org/10.1002/jaba.971

Kimball, R. T., Salvetti, E. L., Day, L. E., Karis, R., Silveira, J., Jr., & Kranak, M. P. (2023b). Operant ABA renewal during dense and lean schedules of differential reinforcement. *Journal of the Experimental Analysis of Behavior, 119*(3), 529–538. https://doi.org/10.1002/jeab.840

Kincaid, S. L., Lattal, K. A., & Spence, J. (2015). Super-resurgence: ABA renewal increases resurgence. *Behavioural Processes, 115*, 70–73. https://doi.org/10.1016/j.beproc.2015.02.013

King, J. E., & Hayes, L. J. (2016). The role of discriminative stimuli on response patterns in resurgence. *The Psychological Record, 66*, 325–335. https://doi.org/10.1007/s40732-016-0175-2

King, H., Martone, L., Laureano, B., & Falligant, J. M. (2024). A systematic review of enhanced resurgence paradigms. *Journal of the Experimental Analysis of Behavior, 121*(2), 266–278. https://doi.org/10.1002/jeab.902

Kranak, M. P., & Brown, K. R. (2024). Updated recommendations for reinforcement schedule thinning following functional communication training. *Behavior Analysis in Practice, 17*(1), 87–106. https://doi.org/10.1007/s40617-023-00863-4

Kranak, M. P., & Falligant, J. M. (2023). Treatment integrity, commission errors, and reinstatement: A primer. *Education and Treatment of Children, 46*(3), 249–262. https://doi.org/10.1007/s43494-023-00104-x

Kuroda, T., Gilroy, S. P., Cançado, C. R., & Podlesnik, C. A. (2020). Effects of punishing target response during extinction on resurgence and renewal in zebrafish (Danio rerio). *Behavioural Processes, 178*, 104191. https://doi.org/10.1016/j.beproc.2020.104191

Kuroda, T., Ritchey, C. M., Cançado, C. R., & Podlesnik, C. A. (2021). Punishment in training contexts decreases operant renewal in zebrafish (Danio rerio). *Learning and Motivation, 74*, 101712. https://doi.org/10.1016/j.lmot.2021.101712

Langthorne, P., & McGill, P. (2009). A tutorial on the concept of the motivating operation and its importance to application. *Behavior Analysis in Practice, 2*, 22–31. https://doi.org/10.1007/BF03391745

Lattal, K. A., Cançado, C. R., Cook, J. E., Kincaid, S. L., Nighbor, T. D., & Oliver, A. C. (2017). On defining resurgence. *Behavioural Processes, 141*, 85–91. https://doi.org/10.1016/j.beproc.2017.04.018

Lerman, D. C., & Vorndran, C. M. (2002). On the status of knowledge for using punishment: Implications for treating behavior disorders. *Journal of Applied Behavior Analysis, 35*(4), 431–464. https://doi.org/10.1901/jaba.2002.35-431

Lerman, D. C., Iwata, B. A., Shore, B. A., & Kahng, S. (1996). Responding maintained by intermittent reinforcement: Implications for the use of extinction with problem behavior in clinical settings. *Journal of Applied Behavior Analysis, 29*(2), 153–171. https://doi.org/10.1901/jaba.1996.29-153

Madrigal, K., Hernández, C., & Flores, C. (2018). Effects of the number of acquisition sessions and scheduled reinforcers on ABA renewal. *Learning and Motivation, 63*, 162–168. https://doi.org/10.1016/j.lmot.2018.07.002

Mitteer, D. R., Greer, B. D., Fisher, W. W., Briggs, A. M., & Wacker, D. P. (2018). A laboratory model for evaluating relapse of undesirable caregiver behavior. *Journal of the Experimental Analysis of Behavior, 110*(2), 252–266. https://doi.org/10.1002/jeab.462

Mitteer, D. R., Greer, B. D., Randall, K. R., & Haney, S. D. (2022). On the scope and characteristics of relapse when treating severe destructive behavior. *Journal of Applied Behavior Analysis, 55*(3), 688–703. https://doi.org/10.1002/jaba.912

Morfín, L. R. M., Flores, C., & Madrigal, K. D. (2021). Effects of delay of reinforcement on ABA renewal. *Behavioural Processes, 189*, 104440. https://doi.org/10.1016/j.beproc.2021.104440

Muething, C., Call, N., Pavlov, A., Ringdahl, J., Gillespie, S., Clark, S., & Mevers, J. L. (2020). Prevalence of renewal of problem behavior during context changes. *Journal of Applied Behavior Analysis, 53*(3), 1485–1493. https://doi.org/10.1002/jaba.672

Muñiz-Moreno, J., & Loy, I. (2023). ABA, AAB and ABC renewal with Pavlovian conditioning of tentacle lowering procedure in the snail Cornu aspersum. *Behavioural Processes, 209*, 104889. https://doi.org/10.1016/j.beproc.2023.104889

Nakajima, S., Tanaka, S., Urushihara, K., & Imada, H. (2000). Renewal of extinguished lever-press responses upon return to the training context. *Learning and Motivation, 31*(4), 416–431. https://doi.org/10.1006/lmot.2000.1064

Nakajima, S., Urushihara, K., & Masaki, T. (2002). Renewal of operant performance formerly eliminated by omission or noncontingency training upon return to the acquisition context. *Learning and Motivation, 33*(4), 510–525. https://doi.org/10.1016/S0023-9690(02)00009-7

Neely, J. A., Liddon, C. J., Kimball, R. T., Fuhrman, A. M., & Valentino, A. L. (2024). Understanding and reacting to relapse: Considerations for practitioners. *Behavior Analysis in Practice*. Advanced online publication. https://doi.org/10.1007/s40617-024-00997-z

Nelson, J. B., Sanjuan, M. D. C., Vadillo-Ruiz, S., Pérez, J., & León, S. P. (2011). Experimental renewal in human participants. *Journal of Experimental Psychology: Animal Behavior Processes, 37*(1), 58–70. https://psycnet.apa.org/doi/10.1037/a0020519

Nevin, J. A., & Wacker, D. P. (2013). Response strength and persistence. In G. J. Madden et al. (Eds.), *APA handbooks in psychology: APA handbook of behavior analysis, vol. 2: Translating principles into practice* (pp. 109–128). American Psychological Association. https://doi.org/10.1037/13938-005

Nieto, J., Mason, T. A., Bernal-Gamboa, R., & Uengoer, M. (2020). The impacts of acquisition and extinction cues on ABC renewal of voluntary behaviors. *Learning & Memory, 27*(3), 114–118. https://doi.org/10.1101/lm.050831.119

Nieto, J., Mason, T. A., García-Salazar, J., Bernal-Gamboa, R., & Gámez, A. M. (2023). The impact of prolonging extinction on the ABC "super renewal" of instrumental responses in rats. *Behavioural Processes, 209*, 104891. https://doi.org/10.1016/j.beproc.2023.104891

St. Peter Pipkin, C., & Vollmer, T. R. (2009). Applied implications of reinforcement history effects. *Journal of Applied Behavior Analysis, 42*(1), 83–103. https://doi.org/10.1901/jaba.2009.42-83

Podlesnik, C. A., & Kelley, M. E. (2015). Translational research on the relapse of operant behavior. *Revista Mexicana de Análisis de la Conducta, 41*(2), 226–251. https://psycnet.apa.org/doi/10.5514/rmac.v41.i2.63774

Podlesnik, C. A., & Shahan, T. A. (2009). Behavioral momentum and relapse of extinguished operant responding. *Learning & Behavior, 37*, 357–364. https://doi.org/10.3758/LB.37.4.357

Podlesnik, C. A., & Shahan, T. A. (2010). Extinction, relapse, and behavioral momentum. *Behavioural Processes, 84*, 400–411. https://doi.org/10.1016/j.beproc.2010.02.001

Podlesnik, C. A., Kelley, M. E., Jimenez-Gomez, C., & Bouton, M. E. (2017). Renewed behavior produced by context change and its implications for treatment maintenance: A review. *Journal of Applied Behavior Analysis, 50*(3), 675–697. https://doi.org/10.1002/jaba.400

Podlesnik, C. A., Kuroda, T., Jimenez-Gomez, C., Abreu-Rodrigues, J., Cançado, C. R., Blackman, A. L., Silverman, K., Villegas-Barker, J., Galbato, M., & Teixeira, I. S. C. (2019). Resurgence is greater following a return to the training context than remaining in the extinction context. *Journal of the Experimental Analysis of Behavior, 111*(3), 416–435. https://doi.org/10.1002/jeab.505

Rey, C. N., Thrailkill, E. A., Goldberg, K. L., & Bouton, M. E. (2020). Relapse of operant behavior after response elimination with an extinction or an omission contingency. *Journal of the Experimental Analysis of Behavior, 113*(1), 124–140. https://doi.org/10.1002/jeab.568

Ritchey, C. M., Kuroda, T., & Podlesnik, C. A. (2022). Evaluating effects of context changes on resurgence in humans. *Behavioural Processes, 194*, 104563. https://doi.org/10.1016/j.beproc.2021.104563

Saini, V., Miller, S. A., & Fisher, W. W. (2016). Multiple schedules in practical application: Research trends and implications for future investigation. *Journal of Applied Behavior Analysis, 49*(2), 421–444. https://doi.org/10.1002/jaba.300

Sarno, B. G., & Kestner, K. M. (2024). A replication of a nonsequential renewal model and a failure to attenuate nonsequential renewal with extinction cues. *The Psychological Record, 74*(3), 237–250. https://doi.org/10.1007/s40732-024-00608-x

Schepers, S. T., & Bouton, M. E. (2017). Hunger as a context: food seeking that is inhibited during hunger can renew in the context of satiety. *Psychological Science, 28*(11), 1640–1648. https://doi.org/10.1177/0956797617719084

Shahan, T. A., Browning, K. O., & Nall, R. W. (2020). Resurgence as choice in context: Treatment duration and on/off alternative reinforcement. *Journal of the Experimental Analysis of Behavior, 113*, 57–76. https://doi.org/10.1002/jeab.563

Sidman, M. (2011). Can an understanding of basic research facilitate the effectiveness of clinicians? Reflections and personal perspectives. *Journal of Applied Behavior Analysis, 44*(4), 973–991. https://doi.org/10.1901/jaba.2011.44-973

Sullivan, W. E., Saini, V., & Roane, H. S. (2018). A nonsequential approach to the study of operant renewal: A reverse translation. *Journal of the Experimental Analysis of Behavior, 110*(1), 74–86. https://doi.org/10.1002/jeab.456

Sweeney, M. M., & Shahan, T. A. (2015). Renewal, resurgence, and alternative reinforcement context. *Behavioural Processes, 116*, 43–49. https://doi.org/10.1016/j.beproc.2015.04.015

Thrailkill, E. A., Kimball, R. T., Kelley, M. E., Craig, A. R., & Podlesnik, C. A. (2018). Greater reinforcement rate during training increases spontaneous recovery. *Journal of the Experimental Analysis of Behavior, 109*(1), 238–252. https://doi.org/10.1002/jeab.307

Tiger, J. H., Hanley, G. P., & Bruzek, J. (2008). Functional communication training: A review and practical guide. *Behavior Analysis in Practice, 1*(1), 16–23. https://doi.org/10.1007/BF03391716

Todd, T. P. (2013). Mechanisms of renewal after the extinction of instrumental behavior. *Journal of Experimental Psychology: Animal Behavior Processes, 39*(3), 193. https://psycnet.apa.org/doi/10.1037/a0032236

Todd, T. P., Winterbauer, N. E., & Bouton, M. E. (2012). Effects of the amount of acquisition and contextual generalization on the renewal of instrumental behavior after extinction. *Learning & Behavior, 40*(2), 145–157. https://doi.org/10.3758/s13420-011-0051-5

Trask, S., Schepers, S. T., & Bouton, M. E. (2015). Context change explains resurgence after the extinction of operant behavior. *Mexican Journal of Behavior Analysis, 41*, 187–210.

Willcocks, A. L., & McNally, G. P. (2014). An extinction retrieval cue attenuates renewal but not reacquisition of alcohol seeking. *Behavioral Neuroscience, 128*(1), 83–91. https://doi.org/10.1037/a0035595

Chapter 4
Renewal in Clinical Practice: Implications and Mitigation Strategies

Kayla Grunewald, Hunter C. King, Shane H. Phillips, Caleb Spink, John Michael Falligant, and Michael P. Kranak

Relapse, or the recurrence of previously reinforced but currently eliminated behavior is a common impediment to the successful treatment of problem behavior (Kimball et al., 2023). Common forms of relapse, such as resurgence and reinstatement, are based upon changes in reinforcement conditions for alternative and target responses, respectively (see Chap. 2, Norris et al., this volume and Chap. 6, Stephens et al., this volume). Relapse is typically evaluated in basic and translational studies using a three-phase arrangement (see Wathen & Podlesnik, 2018). This three-phase arrangement mirrors the general course of treatment for problem behavior (see Chap. 1, Mauzy et al., this volume; Chap. 3, Kimball et al., this volume; and Kranak & Falligant, 2023). Along with resurgence and reinstatement, there is a third distinct type of relapse, also commonly evaluated in a three-phase arrangement, relevant to the treatment of problem behavior: *renewal*.

Renewal, unlike other forms of relapse, occurs as a function of changes in stimulus conditions, or contexts. A *context change* refers to an alteration of cues that could influence an organism's behavior—these include a wide variety of

K. Grunewald · H. C. King
Oakland University, Rochester, MI, USA

S. H. Phillips · J. M. Falligant
Auburn University, Auburn, AL, USA

C. Spink
Kennedy Krieger Institute, Baltimore, MD, USA

M. P. Kranak (✉)
Oakland University and Oakland University Center for Autism, Rochester, MI, USA
e-mail: kranak@oakland.edu

M. P. Kranak (ed.), *Behavioral Treatments for Individuals with Autism*, Autism and Child Psychopathology Series,
https://doi.org/10.1007/978-3-031-91965-7_4

exteroceptive (e.g., location, apparatus, people, reinforcers) and interoceptive (e.g., deprivation and drug states, stress) stimuli (see Bouton, 2019). Specifically related to problem behavior, the most common types of context changes are those related to a change in either (a) the intervention agent or (b) the location in which treatment is being implemented (Kimball & Kranak, 2022). However, more subtle stimuli (e.g., items in a room, clothing, furniture, presence/absence of other individuals) could also constitute a context, and their alteration could be a context change that influences behavior (Randall et al., 2024). The critical feature of renewal is that, following a context change, the contingencies for problem and appropriate behavior remain unchanged, and yet problem behavior reemerges (Saini & Mitteer, 2020).

Renewal is typically assessed using a three-phase procedure consisting of conditioning, extinction, and testing phases. For clarity, the contexts associated with these phases are labeled as "A," "B," and "C," respectively (Bouton et al., 2011). For example, in an ABC arrangement, an experimenter conditions a response in context "A," extinguishes the response in context "B," and tests for renewal in context "C." In this scenario, each phase occurs in a distinct context. Conversely, if the renewal test is conducted in the same context as the conditioning phase, this is referred to as an ABA arrangement. We provide clinical examples of these arrangements in several vignettes at the end of this chapter.

Additive Relapse

The corpus of literature on renewal points to a context change, in the absence of contingencies changes, as a necessary condition in understanding behavioral mechanisms of renewal (Podlesnik et al., 2017). However, to complicate matters, simultaneous changes in context (i.e., renewal) and contingencies (i.e., resurgence) are likely quite prevalent in community settings, raising questions as to whether relapse following said changes would result in a magnitude of relapse beyond either change in isolation (Kimball et al., 2025). This effect is referred to as additive relapse (see King et al., 2024 for a review), which is measured by comparing the magnitude of relapse amid a context change in isolation, a contingency change in isolation, and a simultaneous change in context and contingencies. Additive relapse has been a focus among a small, yet growing number of investigations with important implications for increasing client's readiness for the dynamic environmental conditions anticipated following treatment (Kimball et al., 2023).

To illustrate additive relapse, consider a child who engages in high rates of challenging behavior at home when they are unable to access a preferred toy. During treatment, the child is taught to emit a functional communication response (FCR) that results in access to the reinforcer that previously maintained challenging behavior (i.e., the toy). The child met all treatment goals and treatment was successfully generalized to caregivers. Upon returning home, a context previously associated with reinforcement for challenging behavior, caregivers necessarily allocate time to household chores. During this time, the child emits the FCR for a preferred toy, but it went unnoticed by caregivers. After several unsuccessful attempts to access caregivers' attention, the child proceeded to engage in challenging behavior, but at a magnitude far greater than that observed prior to treatment. Here, additive relapse might occur because two conditions were met: (a) the child was re-exposed to a familiar environment (i.e., home) associated with high rates of reinforcement for challenging behavior and (b) a reduction in alternative reinforcement occurred because the caregivers forgot to reinforce their child's FCR.

Research on additive relapse almost exclusively stems from basic experiments with nonhuman animals (Bolívar et al., 2017; Kincaid et al., 2015; Podlesnik & Fleet, 2014) and translational studies with typically developing humans in well-controlled laboratory settings (Alessandri & Cancado, 2020; King & Hayes, 2016; Williams & St. Peter, 2020). In a notable exception with a clinically relevant sample, Kimball et al. (2018) evaluated whether a simultaneous change in context and contingencies modulated relapse to a greater extent, relative to a contingency change alone, in three children with autism spectrum disorder and one typically developing child. All procedures occurred in an early intervention program, and target and alternative responses consisted of analogue responses (i.e., stacking rings; placing ball into one of two plastic bins; sorting colored blocks in buckets of corresponding colors) for each child. A standard three-phase relapse arrangement was conducted, where target responses were reinforced on a fixed-ratio (FR) 1 schedule in Phase 1, then placed on extinction in Phase 2 while the alternative response was reinforced on a FR 1 schedule. Phase 3 represented the relapse test and consisted of two conditions. The first condition tested for resurgence by discontinuing reinforcer deliveries for both the alternative and target response. The second condition evaluated the combined effects of renewal and resurgence by providing materials only for the target response and ceasing reinforcer deliveries. The second condition was designed to resemble a scenario in which a caregiver inadvertently forgets to provide their child with materials needed to emit the FCR (context change), thus eliminating opportunities for the FCR to produce reinforcement (contingency change). Across all participants, a greater magnitude of relapse was observed in the second condition (renewal + resurgence) compared to resurgence alone in the first condition. Although the effects of renewal were not isolated in a separate comparison condition, a necessary condition for evaluating additive relapse, Kimball et al.'s (2018) findings shed light on the potential exigent treatment challenges caregivers likely experience in natural settings.

Given the limited research on additive relapse, especially in applied studies, a dearth of empirical guidance exists for how to effectively mitigate this form of relapse in practice. Although yet to be subjected to the phenomenon of additive relapse specifically, practical guidance might be gleaned from studies evaluating relapse mitigation strategies for resurgence (see Chap. 2, Norris et al., this volume and Kranak & Falligant, 2021) and renewal (see below) in isolation. For instance, extinction cues have been shown to mitigate renewal and resurgence in separate experimental arrangements (Nieto et al., 2020). This procedure involves the repeated pairing of an extinction-correlated stimulus (S-delta materials; colored stimulus) with the unavailability of reinforcement for problem behavior in the clinic, then presenting the S-delta when treatment is generalized to a different setting (e.g., home or school). Here, renewal of challenging behavior is mitigated by using the same S-delta to signal the unavailability of reinforcement for problem behavior in multiple settings, thus increasing the similarity of stimulus conditions between those settings. Additionally, prior investigations support the use of other strategies for mitigating relapse amid contextual and contingency changes, such as (a) extended extinction, where the duration of the extinction component in a multiple schedule is systematically increased across schedule thinning steps to reduce the likelihood challenging behavior will reemerge during generalization programming (see Briggs et al., 2023, for a review), (b) dosage of treatment, where longer exposures to treatment can increase the discriminability of contingencies for the FCR and challenging behavior, thus reducing the likelihood of relapse when alternative reinforcement is reduced (Fisher et al., 2018) or when treatment is generalized to a new context (Wacker et al., 2011), and (c) multiple context training, where the number of environmental conditions that control behavior is systematically increased by implementing the same contingencies in multiple settings (Balooch & Neumann, 2011; Haney et al., 2021).

Renewal of Undesirable Caregiver Behavior

While renewal is often investigated in the context of the reemergence of undesirable client behavior, undesirable caregiver behavior can also reemerge under similar conditions. In practice, treatment is typically implemented in a clinic setting by trained therapists until a predetermined treatment goal is achieved. At this juncture, practitioners often program for generalization by training caregivers to implement treatment in the clinic to high levels of treatment integrity. Indeed, a wealth of research supports caregivers' capacity to precisely implement a variety of behavioral interventions (King et al., 2023; LaBrot et al., 2022; Nuta et al., 2021; Preas & Mathews, 2021); however, near perfect treatment integrity is quite difficult to maintain when transferring treatment from the clinic to a setting (e.g., home) previously associated with reinforcement for challenging behavior. This transition represents an important context change during which challenging behavior may reemerge, which in turn increases the possibility of commission and omission errors on behalf of the caregiver. Given the clear implications of this dynamic for improving the chances of maintaining long-term treatment efficacy, scholars have begun to investigate the conditions under which renewal of undesirable caregiver behavior occurs.

A translational study by Mitteer et al. (2018) evaluated caregivers' propensity for treatment integrity errors in situations emulating common issues believed to affect caregivers' treatment adherence in naturalistic settings. In their study, confederates served as children who wore colored shirts to facilitate discrimination between three treatment phases. The primary outcome variable was undesirable caregiver behavior, defined as delivering a programmed reinforcer within 2 s of the confederate's challenging behavior and failing to deliver the programmed reinforcer within 2 s of the confederate's FCR. Phase 1 was conducted in a home-like context where the caregiver's delivery of reinforcers terminated the confederate's challenging behavior. In Phase 2, caregivers implemented functional communication training (FCT) in a clinic context where delivering the reinforcer for challenging behavior or the FCR terminated both responses. In Phase 3, treatment was reimplemented in the home-like context, during which caregiver behavior had no effect on confederate's challenging behavior or FCRs. In other words, caregiver's treatment adherence was placed on extinction. Study findings indicated three of four caregivers exhibited treatment integrity errors in the form of omission (i.e., failing to reinforcer FCRs) and commission errors (i.e., delivering the reinforcer for challenging behavior) when treatment was reimplemented in the training context (Phase 1).

Findings from Mitteer et al. (2018) align with prior research indicating caregiver integrity errors are often maintained via the transient reduction of children's challenging behavior (i.e., negative reinforcement; Stocco & Thompson, 2015; Patterson, 1982)—a contingency presumably established in specific contexts (e.g., homes) prior to caregiver's understanding of operant functions of behavior. Thus, escalations in challenging behavior in certain environmental contexts may result in the reemergence of strategies (i.e., contingent reinforcement) that historically reduced or mitigated challenging behavior in those contexts. This underscores the importance of individualized caregiver and stakeholder training to enhance their capacity to maintain high levels of treatment integrity amid contextual changes, which could entail systemically decreasing feedback contingent on high levels of treatment integrity in contexts that increasingly resemble the physical characteristics of home or other naturalistic settings (Durand & Carr, 1991; Falcomata et al., 2010; Hanley et al., 2021; Neely et al., 2020).

Applied Relevance

It is understandable that renewal is a common phenomenon when considering the goals of generalizing treatment implementation across settings and intervention agents following success in initial treatment settings (Kimball & Kranak, 2022; Wacker et al., 2011). As changes in context are constant, common, and unavoidable in daily life, renewal becomes even more important to consider and mitigate during the course of behavioral treatment, where renewal is commonplace. For example, Muething et al. (2020) conducted a retrospective consecutive controlled case series (CCCS; Hagopian, 2020) and found that renewal occurred in nearly 70% of applications of functional communication training (FCT) in an outpatient setting. Falligant et al. (2021) replicated Muething et al. (2020) and similarly found renewal occurred in nearly 60% of applications of FCT in an inpatient setting. Others have documented similar prevalence estimates for renewal across service settings (Haney et al., 2022; Mitteer et al., 2022). Consider a few additional examples illustrating the applied relevance of renewal. Haney et al. (2022) found that out of 19 participants, 25 different treatment packages, and 38 overall transitions (opportunities where renewal might occur), renewal occurred in 63% of the participants, across 52% of treatment packages, and in 47% of the possible transitions to which participants were exposed. Collectively, renewal has been shown to occur across a range of topographies of problem behavior, different diagnoses, and all functional classes including both socially and automatically maintained problem behavior (Falligant et al., 2022, 2024; Muething et al., 2022).

Mitigation Strategies

Multiple Context Training

Multiple context training entails implementing treatment (e.g., FCT) in systematic fashion across a variety of contexts. Doing so prepares individuals to undergo treatment, or rather, for treatment to be implemented in environments other than initial treatment settings (Kimball & Kranak, 2022). During multiple context training, contexts are systematically varied so individuals come to associate treatment contingencies with contexts *other than* initial treatment contexts (Bernal-Gamboa et al., 2020; Kimball et al., 2023). Said another way, multiple context training exposes individuals to different and distinct contexts (e.g., new therapists, new treatment rooms, community-based settings) while maintaining the same contingencies that were present during treatment. From this perspective, multiple context training could be interpreted simply as implementing treatment across (a) a variety of intervention agents and (b) in many different settings other than the initial treatment location, all in a systematic manner.

As mentioned in the preceding chapter, there is a wealth of nonhuman data supporting multiple context training as a strategy for mitigating renewal (see Bustamante et al., 2024). Data obtained from large-scale retrospective analyses of renewal also support multiple context training in this capacity (Falligant et al., 2021, 2022, 2024; Muething et al., 2020). Thus, although there is a comparative shortage of research explicitly on multiple context training in applied settings (Kimball et al., 2023), what data we do have suggest multiple context training is a viable strategy for mitigating renewal. This is also supported by related work in generalization training more broadly (Falcomata & Wacker, 2013; Neely et al., 2018; Stokes & Baer, 1977). Further, given that renewal is a stimulus control phenomenon and that multiple context training is rooted in principles of stimulus control, it follows that multiple context training could be considered as the most promising strategy for mitigating renewal (Bouton, 2004). This is a perspective that our clinical and translational research group has come to adopt in recent years.

A reasonable question one might have at this point is, "How many different contexts are necessary to mitigate renewal?" Currently, the best data-based answer to that question is, "more is better" (Falligant et al., 2021, 2022). The current standard for conducting multiple context training emphasizes conducting *many sessions* across *few contexts*. However, results from both basic studies and retrospective applied analyses, stimulus control principles, and Context Theory suggest that multiple context training should entail conducting fewer sessions across as many contexts as possible (Bouton & Broomer, 2023; Falligant et al., 2021, 2022; Nieto et al., 2023).

Consider a hypothetical example where a clinician is able to conduct five sessions of multiple context training. Following the current standard, the clinician conducts three sessions (sessions 1–3) with the client's mom as the intervention agent, and an additional two sessions (sessions 4 and 5) in a commons area of the clinic rather than the treatment room. Here, the client would have been exposed to only two contexts (beyond the initial context) containing treatment contingencies. Contrast this with an alternative approach. Following a novel approach—one we recommend to readers—the clinician conducts one session with the client's mom (session 1), one session in a new treatment room (session 2), one session in a playground area (session 3), one session at a local store (session 4), and one session with a new therapist (session 5). Here, the client would have been exposed to five different contexts, each containing the same contingencies present in the initial treatment setting.

Programming Common Stimuli

In studies of renewal, behavioral changes established in one context (i.e., clinic, familiar therapists) sometimes do not generalize to other contexts (e.g., homes, schools, novel therapists), suggesting renewal might be more likely when treatment occurs in environments distinct from those to which clients are transitioned following treatment. Studies of stimulus control indicate treatment effects generalized to novel contexts to the extent those new contexts resemble the physical characteristics of the treatment context (Lazareva, 2012; Swartzentruber, 1993). Therefore, efforts should be made to modify the clinic to resemble generalization setting(s) (i.e., *programming common stimuli*).

During this procedure, clients are exposed to familiar stimuli (e.g., people, places, objects) while treatment contingencies remain in effect. Exposing clients to familiar stimuli during treatment allows those stimuli to be paired with treatment contingencies (e.g., reinforcement for appropriate behavior and extinction for challenging behavior) to establish their stimulus control over behavior. Consequently, when treatment is generalized from the clinic to a different setting in which those stimuli are present, challenging behavior is less likely to reemerge (Piazza et al.,

1996; Falcomata & Wacker, 2013). Two common approaches for mitigating renewal effects by programming common stimuli include the integration of familiar people and physical stimuli during treatment.

Haney et al. (2021) evaluated both approaches in an outpatient clinic with children who engaged in inappropriate mealtime behavior (IMB). All study procedures were conducted using an ABA renewal preparation. Renewal mitigation strategies included the introduction of caregivers as interventionists for four children and the introduction of caregivers and familiar stimuli associated with the client's home for two children (i.e., Jade and Julian). In Context A, trained therapists contingently reinforced IMB by the removal of nonpreferred food. Context B served as the mitigation condition, where caregivers of all children were trained to implement a function-based extinction treatment. For two children, the treatment room was also modified to emulate the kitchen in their household. Specifically, a video projector displayed a picture onto the treatment room wall depicting the view from Jade's mealtime chair at home (i.e., dining table, table centerpiece, clock, refrigerator) and Julian's kitchen (e.g., table with blue cloth, blue bowls, bookshelf, candles, paintings). Familiar physical items were also placed in their respective treatment rooms. When treatment was reimplemented in Context A, challenging behavior either did not reoccur or occurred at comparatively lower rates relative to control conditions in which mitigation strategies were absent.

The effects of programming common stimuli on the maintenance of treatment outcomes are widely documented in the behavioral literature (Arnold-Saritepe et al., 2023; Falcomata & Wacker, 2013; Stokes & Baer, 1977). This procedure is strongly correlated with renewal given its focus on increasing the similarity of the clinic context and contexts historically associated with reinforcement for challenging behavior. Therefore, practitioners are strongly encouraged to consider the likelihood of encountering renewal amid clinically necessary context changes and how stimuli can be incorporated into treatment to promote the maintenance of desirable behavioral in familiar and novel contexts.

Contingency-Correlated Stimuli

Renewal may be mitigated by programming contextual stimuli that are correlated with operant extinction for challenging or alternative behavior (Podlesnik et al., 2017). These approaches have been used in several applied investigations of renewal to transfer treatment across different caregivers and environments (e.g., Greer et al., 2019). For example, Fisher et al. (2015) used extinction cues to rapidly transfer treatment effects across settings with three children who engaged in aggression, property destruction, and elopement. First, a functional analysis (FA) was conducted for each participant. Once the function of problem behavior was identified, participants were taught how to emit a functional communication response (FCR) that produced the same functional reinforcer that maintained challenging behavior. Next, therapists established a multiple schedule to signal periods of time in which the FCR would (S^D) or would not (S^Δ) be reinforced. In this arrangement, a therapist wore a yellow wristband during the S^D component and removed it from the participant's sight during the S^Δ component. This meant that if the participants emitted the FCR (e.g., "attention please") while the therapist was wearing the yellow wristband, the therapist would provide attention. Otherwise, there were no consequences for the FCR when the therapist was not wearing the yellow wristband. All participants engaged in high rates of the FCR during the S^D component of the multiple schedule and much lower rates during the S^Δ component, indicating stimulus control of the FCR by the yellow bracelet. Importantly, participants engaged in low levels of challenging behavior when the schedule-correlated stimulus was used.

Stimuli correlated with the availability or unavailability of reinforcement for problem and/or alternative behavior may promote generalization of desirable changes during context changes. Thus, clinicians might consider adding a variety of cues to signal when reinforcement is and is not available. This can readily be accomplished by using a variety of signaled schedules. For example, Bland et al. (2016) further demonstrated the effectiveness of schedule-correlated stimuli in a unique translational study with pigeons that evaluated persistence of target (problem) behavior when reinforcement for an alternative behavior was either signaled or not. To do this, pigeons pecked either a target key or alternative key that produced a reinforcer. Alternative reinforcement was signaled by a change in light near the key. A variety of disruptors were also added that allowed persistence of behaviors to be assessed. Results showed that when alternative reinforcement was signaled, the target behavior was less resistant to change than when alternative reinforcement was not signaled. Additionally, the alternative response was more resistant to change when alternative reinforcement was signaled. These findings support the use of signaling the availability/unavailability of reinforcement in a clinical setting. Signaling the availability of reinforcement for an FCR may rapidly decrease problem behavior while increasing the persistence of the FCR. Along these lines, programming common stimuli is a recommended strategy for promoting generalization and mitigating renewal (Stokes & Baer, 1977). Identifying extinction cues and incorporating them into multiple different contexts can assist with treatment generalization and maintenance.

Vignette 1

Aurora was an 8-year-old female diagnosed with autism spectrum disorder. Teachers at her school (Context A) reported that she frequently demonstrated physical aggression towards her classmates and paraeducators as well as property destruction when presented with prompts to do independent tasks such as classwork. She was referred to a board-certified behavior analyst (BCBA) to assess and treat her challenging behavior. At the clinic (Context B), the BCBA conducted an FA and determined the function of Aurora's challenging behavior to be accessible to social attention. Her behavioral treatment consisted of differential reinforcement of an alternative behavior (DRA) and extinction. During functional communication training (FCT) Aurora was taught how to use a response card to request attention from her peers and school staff. Once Aurora presented her card, she had access to a short positive interaction with her staff or peer—challenging behavior did not receive programmed consequences (i.e., staff did not attend to challenging behavior). Following FCT and extinction, Aurora's challenging behavior quickly reduced to near-zero levels and appropriate communication responses increased. Subsequently, the BCBA trained her school staff to implement her behavioral treatment with high levels of procedural fidelity. However, Aurora's BCBA noted that, upon her return to her classroom (Context A), Aurora reverted to engaging in high levels of challenging behavior and infrequently used the FCR when presented with independent work. This is a classic example of ABA renewal.

Aurora's challenging behavior was acquired and reinforced in Context A. When she began treatment in Context B, her challenging behavior was placed on extinction and an appropriate alternative behavior was reinforced. When she returned to Context A, her challenging behavior relapsed. To remedy this, the BCBA implemented schedule-correlated stimuli in the classroom. In the clinic setting, the BCBA placed a red card on Aurora's desk to signal when reinforcement was not available for the FCR and a green card to signal the availability of reinforcement for the FCR. Signaling the availability of reinforcement for the alternative response resulted in clinically significant reductions in challenging behavior in the clinic. The BCBA then trained school staff to embed the schedule-correlated stimuli within the classroom setting. Once school staff began using the schedule-correlated stimuli in the classroom, Aurora's challenging behavior remained at near-zero levels while appropriate FCRs occurred frequently. The BCBA and school staff then successfully faded the schedule-correlated stimuli, and Aurora was able to appropriately and independently request for attention with minimal challenging behavior.

Vignette 2

In a very similar example, imagine that Aurora's challenging behavior was established in the classroom (Context A). This time though, the BCBA conducted their functional analysis and treatment evaluation (e.g., FCT plus extinction) in the classroom, with the teacher implementing the intervention with guidance from the BCBA. Aurora's challenging behavior decreased to near-zero levels and appropriate FCRs increased. Once the mastery criterion was met, the BCBA did a maintenance and generalization check at the clinic where she received ABA services (Context B) during situations where she was prompted to do low-preferred tasks such as independent math work and sitting independently at her assigned center. Aurora reverted to engaging in high levels of challenging behavior and infrequently requested attention when presented with low-preferred tasks. This is an example of AAB renewal. Aurora's challenging behavior was acquired in Context A, subsequently extinguished in Context A, and then reemerged in Context B when Aurora began emitting problem behavior at the clinic.

In both examples, it is likely that Aurora would have higher magnitude renewal (i.e., higher rate and intensity challenging behavior) in the ABA example than the AAB example. Both ABA and AAB renewal can result in the reemergence of challenging behavior which can cause stress on the family and client as well as inhibit progress in the academic, functional, and/or social domains. Indeed, research has shown that ABA renewal generally produces a greater magnitude of renewal than AAB (e.g., Bouton et al., 2011). In ABA renewal, challenging behavior is maintained by a history of reinforcement and S^Ds in the environment. For example, Aurora's parents may have inadvertently reinforced her challenging behavior for years. Her parents are robust S^Ds that signal the availability of reinforcement for challenging behavior. Although the behavior may be extinguished in a novel setting (Context B), when returning to Context A, the individual is again exposed to S^Ds correlated with a rich reinforcement history which can result in greater renewal.

Vignette 3

Charlie (pseudonym), a 9-year-old male diagnosed with autism spectrum disorder, was referred to the assessment and treatment of severe behavior. Charlie reportedly began engaging in physical aggression and property destruction approximately 2 years ago, which primarily occurred at home with his caregivers. Shortly following Charlie's admission, a functional analysis (FA) was conducted to confirm the maintaining variables for his challenging behavior. The FA consisted of four test conditions (attention, demand, tangible, no-interaction) and one toy-play control condition. Initially, FA conditions were implemented by trained staff; however, due to low rates of challenging behavior, both caregivers were trained to implement FA conditions. This modification was effective as high rates of challenging behavior were observed which consistently occurred in the attention condition relative to the control condition. Therefore, the team concluded Charlie's challenging behavior was attention maintained, but only with caregivers.

In light of caregivers' stimulus control over Charlie's behavior, caregivers served as interventions throughout Charlie's attention treatment evaluation. First, functional communication training was conducted to establish a vocal functional communication response (FCR) for attention: "Attention, please." Following Charlie's acquisition of the FCR, treatment commenced, which included differential reinforcement of alternative behavior (DRA) for the FCR, extinction for challenging behavior, and noncontingent access (NCA) to a moderately preferred item identified form a stimulus preference assessment.

A multiple schedule (i.e., a red/green stimulus board) was used to signal the availability and unavailability of alternative reinforcement. During initial treatment sessions, emitting the FCR was reinforced on a continuous schedule that resulted in 10 s of access to caregiver attention. Following low and stable rates of challenging behavior across consecutive sessions, schedule thinning commenced. The team collectively agreed on terminal schedule criterion of 10 min. During schedule thinning, the inter-reinforcement interval was systematically increased by 1-min increments, and progressing through each thinning step required a 90% or greater reduction in challenging behavior from baseline rates for three consecutive sessions. Charlie successfully tolerated increasingly longer periods of extinction and attained his terminal schedule goal of 10 min.

The team then initiated generalization training commensurate with Charlie's tendency to primarily engage in challenging behavior in the home. Caregivers reported their home office as a particularly relevant context as issues tended to arise when their attention was allocated to work-related tasks on their computer. Therefore, the following day, caregivers brought several items (i.e., laptop, small lamp, books) from their home office to the clinic. The treatment room was modified via the inclusion of a small desk with a laptop and two chairs for both caregivers, as well as a smaller table with a lamp and several books. At the onset of the session, caregivers presented the red side of the stimulus board and informed Charlie their attention would be unavailable for a little while. All other treatment procedures remained the same (i.e., DRA, extinction, NCA). As expected, Charlie engaged in challenging behavior given the treatment room now resembled a salient aspect of the home context historically associated with reinforcement for challenging behavior. However, after several sessions rapid treatment gains were observed in the "home-like" context, indicating treatment could now be generalized to the actual home. Caregivers and Charlie responded well to this transition, evidenced by caregivers' continued adherence to treatment procedures in light of minor and infrequent instances of challenging behavior. Therapists provided bi-weekly consultation for three weeks before concluding all treatment goals were met and treatment could be terminated.

Acknowledgments Chapter preparation was partially supported by grants 1R21HD113881-01, 1R21HD112724-01A1, and 1R21HD113794-01A1 from the National Institute of Child Health and Human Development (NICHD), as well as a NARSAD Young Investigator Grant from the Brain and Behavior Research Foundation (BBRF). The content is solely the responsibility of the authors and does not necessarily reflect the official views of the NICHD or BBRF.

Kayla Grunewald is now at Journey Therapy Center.

References

Alessandri, J., & Cançado, C. R. X. (2020). Context affects resurgence of negatively reinforced human behavior. *Behavioural Processes, 170*, 104018. https://doi.org/10.1016/j.beproc.2019.104018

Arnold-Saritepe, A. M., Phillips, K. J., Taylor, S. A., Gomes-Ng, S., Lo, M., & Daly, S. (2023). Generalization and maintenance. In J. L. Matson (Ed.), *Handbook of applied behavior analysis for children with autism: Clinical guide to assessment and treatment* (pp. 415–433). Springer Nature Switzerland AG. https://doi.org/10.1007/978-3-031-27587-6_21

Balooch, S. B., & Neumann, D. L. (2011). Effects of multiple contexts and context similarity on the renewal of extinguished conditioned behaviour in an ABA design with humans. *Learning and Motivation, 42*(1), 53–63. https://doi.org/10.1016/j.lmot.2010.08.008

Bernal-Gamboa, R., Nieto, J., & Gámez, A. M. (2020). Conducting extinction in multiple contexts attenuates relapse of operant behavior in humans. *Behavioural Processes, 181*, 10426. https://doi.org/10.1016/j.beproc.2020.104261

Bland, V. J., Bai, J. Y., Fullerton, J. A., & Podlesnik, C. A. (2016). Signaled alternative reinforcement and the persistence of operant behavior. *Journal of the Experimental Analysis of Behavior, 106*(1), 22–33. https://doi.org/10.1002/jeab.212

Bolívar, H. A., Cox, D. J., Barlow, M. A., & Dallery, J. (2017). Evaluating resurgence procedures in a human operant laboratory. *Behavioural Processes, 140*, 150–160. https://doi.org/10.1016/j.beproc.2017.05.004

Bouton, M. E. (2004). Context and behavioral processes in extinction. *Learning & Memory, 11*(5), 485–494. https://doi.org/10.1101/lm.78804

Bouton, M. E. (2019). Extinction of instrumental (operant) learning: Interference, varieties of context, and mechanisms of contextual control. *Psychopharmacology, 236*(1), 7–19.

Bouton, M. E., & Broomer, M. C. (2023). Learning to stop responding. *Behavioural Processes, 206*, 104830. https://doi.org/10.1016/j.beproc.2023.104830

Bouton, M. E., Todd, T. P., Vurbic, D., & Winterbauer, N. E. (2011). Renewal after the extinction of free operant behavior. *Learning & Behavior, 39*(1), 57–67. https://doi.org/10.3758/s13420-011-0018-6

Briggs, A. M., Mitteer, D. R., Bergmann, S., & Greer, B. D. (2023). Reinforcer thinning: General approaches and considerations for maintaining skills and mitigating relapse. In *Handbook of applied behavior analysis: Integrating research into practice* (pp. 105–122). Springer International Publishing.

Bustamante, J., Soto, M., Miguez, G., Quezada-Scholz, V. E., Angulo, R., & Laborda, M. A. (2024). Extinction in multiple contexts reduces the return of extinguished responses: A multilevel meta-analysis. *Learning & Behavior, 52*(3), 209–223. https://doi.org/10.3758/s13420-023-00609-w

Durand, V. M., & Carr, E. G. (1991). Functional communication training to reduce challenging behavior: Maintenance and application in new settings. *Journal of Applied Behavior Analysis, 24*(2), 251–264. https://doi.org/10.1901/jaba.1991.24-251

Falcomata, T. S., Roane, H. S., Feeney, B. J., & Stephenson, K. M. (2010). Assessment and treatment of elopement maintained by access to stereotypy. *Journal of Applied Behavior Analysis, 43*(3), 513–517. https://doi.org/10.1901/jaba.2010.43-513

Falcomata, T. S., & Wacker, D. P. (2013). On the use of strategies for programming generalization during functional communication training: A review of the literature. *Journal of Developmental and Physical Disabilities, 25*, 5–15. https://doi.org/10.1007/s10882-012-9311-3

Falligant, J. M., Kranak, M. P., McNulty, M. K., Schmidt, J. D., Hausman, N. L., & Rooker, G. W. (2021). Prevalence of renewal of problem behavior: Replication and extension to an inpatient setting. *Journal of Applied Behavior Analysis, 54*(1), 367–373. https://doi.org/10.1002/jaba.740

Falligant, J. M., Chin, M. D., & Kurtz, P. F. (2022). Renewal and resurgence of severe problem behavior in an intensive outpatient setting: Prevalence, magnitude, and implications for practice. *Behavioral Interventions, 37*(3), 909–924. https://doi.org/10.1002/bin.1878

Falligant, J. M., Kranak, M. P., Piersma, D. E., Benson, R., Schmidt, J. D., & Frank-Crawford, M. A. (2024). Further evidence of renewal in automatically maintained behavior. *Journal of Applied Behavior Analysis, 57*(2), 490–501. https://doi.org/10.1002/jaba.1055

Fisher, W. W., Greer, B. D., Fuhrman, A. M., & Querim, A. C. (2015). Using multiple schedules during functional communication training to promote rapid transfer of treatment effects. *Journal of Applied Behavior Analysis, 48*(4), 713–733. https://doi.org/10.1002/jaba.254

Fisher, W. W., Greer, B. D., Fuhrman, A. M., Saini, V., & Simmons, C. A. (2018). Minimizing resurgence of destructive behavior using behavioral momentum theory. *Journal of Applied Behavior Analysis, 51*(4), 831–853. https://doi.org/10.1002/jaba.499

Greer, B. D., Fisher, W. W., Briggs, A. M., Lichtblau, K. R., Phillips, L. A., & Mitteer, D. R. (2019). Using schedule-correlated stimuli during functional communication training to promote the rapid transfer of treatment effects. *Behavioral Development, 24*(2), 100–119. https://doi.org/10.1037/bdb0000085

Hagopian, L. P. (2020). The consecutive controlled case series: Design, data-analytics, and reporting methods supporting the study of generality. *Journal of Applied Behavior Analysis, 53*(2), 596–619. https://doi.org/10.1002/jaba.691

Haney, S. D., Piazza, C. C., Peterson, K. M., & Greer, B. D. (2021). An evaluation of a renewalmitigation procedure for inappropriate mealtime behavior. *Journal of Applied Behavior Analysis, 54*(3), 903–927. https://doi.org/10.1002/jaba.815

Haney, S. D., Greer, B. D., Mitteer, D. R., & Randall, K. R. (2022). Relapse during the treatment of pediatric feeding disorders. *Journal of Applied Behavior Analysis, 55*(3), 704–726. https://doi.org/10.1002/jaba.913

Kimball, R. T., & Kranak, M. P. (2022). Six things practitioners should know about renewal. *Education & Treatment of Children, 45*(4), 395–410. https://doi.org/10.1007/s43494-022-00078-2

Kimball, R. T., Kelley, M. E., Podlesnik, C. A., Forton, A., & Hinkle, B. (2018). Resurgence with and without an alternative response. *Journal of Applied Behavior Analysis, 51*(4), 854–865. https://doi.org/10.1002/jaba.466

Kimball, R. T., Greer, B. D., Fuhrman, A. M., & Lambert, J. M. (2023). Relapse and its mitigation: Toward behavioral inoculation. *Journal of Applied Behavior Analysis, 56*(2), 282–301. https://doi.org/10.1002/jaba.971

Kimball, R. T., Kranak, M. P., Bernal-Gamboa, R., Gamez, A. M., Nieto, J., & Mason, T. (2025). Evaluating the combined effects of renewal and response-dependent reinstatement. *Journal of the Experimental Analysis of Behavior*. [manuscript in press].

Kincaid, S. L., Lattal, K. A., & Spence, J. (2015). Super-resurgence: ABA renewal increases resurgence. *Behavioural Processes, 115*, 70–73. https://doi.org/10.1016/j.beproc.2015.02.013

King, J. E., & Hayes, L. J. (2016). The role of discriminative stimuli on response patterns in resurgence. *The Psychological Record, 66*, 325–335. https://doi.org/10.1007/s40732-016-0175-2

King, H. C., Fischer, A. J., Houalihan, D. D., Davis, J. L., Radley, K. C., III, & Jenson, W. R. (2023). Caregiver telehealth training on antecedent strategies to increase children's instruction following in the home. *Journal of Behavioral Education*, 1–27. https://doi.org/10.1007/s10864-023-09528-2

King, H., Martone, L., Laureano, B., & Falligant, J. M. (2024). A systematic review of enhanced resurgence paradigms. *Journal of the Experimental Analysis of Behavior, 121*(2), 266–278. https://doi.org/10.1002/jeab.902

Kranak, M. P., & Falligant, J. M. (2021). Further investigation of resurgence following schedule thinning: Extension to an inpatient setting. *Behavioral Interventions, 36*(4), 1003–1012. https://doi.org/10.1002/bin.1831

Kranak, M. P., & Falligant, J. M. (2023). Treatment integrity, commission errors, and reinstatement: A primer. *Education and Treatment of Children, 46*(3), 249–262. https://doi.org/10.1007/s43494-023-00104-x

LaBrot, Z. C., Kupzyk, S., Strong-Bak, W., Bates-Brantley, K., & Caserta, A. (2022). Generalization and maintenance of caregivers' effective instruction delivery following group behavioral skills training. *Behavioral Interventions, 37*(3), 640–659. https://doi.org/10.1002/bin.1866

Lazareva, O. F. (2012). Relational learning in a context of transposition: A review. *Journal of the Experimental Analysis of Behavior, 97*(2), 231–248. https://doi.org/10.1901/jeab.2012.97-231

Mitteer, D. R., Greer, B. D., Fisher, W. W., Briggs, A. M., & Wacker, D. P. (2018). A laboratory model for evaluating relapse of undesirable caregiver behavior. *Journal of the Experimental Analysis of Behavior, 110*(2), 252–266. https://doi.org/10.1002/jeab.462

Mitteer, D. R., Greer, B. D., Randall, K. R., & Haney, S. D. (2022). On the scope and characteristics of relapse when treating severe destructive behavior. *Journal of Applied Behavior Analysis, 55*(3), 688–703. https://doi.org/10.1002/jaba.912

Neely, L., Garcia, E., Bankston, B., & Green, A. (2018). Generalization and maintenance of functional communication training for individuals with developmental disabilities: A systematic and quality review. *Research in Developmental Disabilities, 79*, 116–129. https://doi.org/10.1016/j.ridd.2018.02.002

Neely, L., Castro-Villarreal, F., Hong, E. R., Ponce, K., & Gerow, S. (2020). Clinic-based behavioral skills training to teach caregivers adaptive skill interventions for children with autism. *Advances in Neurodevelopmental Disorders, 4*(3), 295–307. https://doi.org/10.1007/s41252-020-00166-7

Nieto, J., Mason, T. A., Bernal-Gamboa, R., & Uengoer, M. (2020). The impacts of acquisition and extinction cues on ABC renewal of voluntary behaviors. *Learning & Memory, 27*(3), 114–118. https://doi.org/10.1101/lm.050831.119

Nieto, J., Mason, T. A., García-Salazar, J., Bernal-Gamboa, R., & Gámez, A. M. (2023). The impact of prolonging extinction on the ABC "super renewal" of instrumental responses in rats. *Behavioural Processes, 209*, 1–8. https://doi.org/10.1016/j.beproc.2023.104891

Nuta, R., Koudys, J., & O'Neill, P. (2021). Parent treatment integrity across multiple components of a behavioral intervention. *Behavioral Interventions, 36*(4), 796–816. https://doi.org/10.1002/bin.1817

Muething, C., Call, N., Pavlov, R. J., Gillespie, S., Clark, S., & Lomas Meyers, J. (2020). Prevalence of renewal of problem behavior during context changes. *Journal of Applied Behavior Analysis, 53*(3), 1485–1493. https://doi.org/10.1002/jaba.672

Muething, C., Call, N., Ritchey, C. M., Pavlov, A., Bernstein, A. M., & Podlesnik, C. A. (2022). Prevalence of relapse of automatically maintained behavior resulting from context changes. *Journal of Applied Behavior Analysis, 55*(1), 138–153. https://doi.org/10.1002/jaba.887

Patterson, M. L. (1982). A sequential functional model of nonverbal exchange. *Psychological Review, 89*(3), 231–249. https://doi.org/10.1037/0033-295X.89.3.231

Piazza, C. C., Fisher, W. W., Hagopian, L. P., Bowman, L. G., & Toole, L. (1996). Using a choice assessment to predict reinforcer effectiveness. *Journal of Applied Behavior Analysis, 29*(1), 1–9. https://doi.org/10.1901/jaba.1996.29-1

Podlesnik, C. A., & Fleet, J. D. (2014). Signaling added response-independent reinforcement to assess pavlovian processes in resistance to change and relapse. *Journal of the Experimental Analysis of Behavior, 102*(2), 179–197. https://doi.org/10.1002/jeab.96

Podlesnik, C. A., Kelly, M. E., Jimenez-Gomez, C., & Bouton, M. E. (2017). Renewed behavior for treatment and maintenance: A review. *Journal of Applied Behavior Analysis, 50*, 675–697. https://doi.org/10.1002/jaba.400

Preas, E. J., & Mathews, T. L. (2021). Evaluation of caregiver training procedures to teach activities of daily living skills. *Behavior Analysis in Practice, 14*(4), 958–973. https://doi.org/10.1007/s40617-020-00513-z

Randall, K. R., Arthur, S. A., Williams, J. L., & Kimball, R. T. (2024). A preliminary investigation of eye-tracking software to inform an ABA renewal mitigation procedure. *Learning and Motivation, 85*, 101946. https://doi.org/10.1016/j.lmot.2023.101946

Stocco, C. S., & Thompson, R. H. (2015). Contingency analysis of caregiver behavior: Implications for parent training and future directions. *Journal of Applied Behavior Analysis, 48*(2), 417–435. https://doi.org/10.1002/jaba.206

Stokes, T. F., & Baer, D. M. (1977). An implicit technology of generalization 1. *Journal of Applied Behavior Analysis, 10*(2), 349–367. https://doi.org/10.1901/jaba.1977.10-349

Swartzentruber, D. (1993). Transfer of contextual control across similarly trained conditioned stimuli. *Animal Learning & Behavior, 21*(1), 14–22. https://doi.org/10.3758/BF03197970

Wacker, D. P., Harding, J. W., Berg, W. K., Lee, J. F., Schieltz, K. M., Padilla, Y. C., Nevin, J. A., & Shahan, T. A. (2011). An evaluation of persistence of treatment effects during long-term treatment of destructive behavior. *Journal of the Experimental Analysis of Behavior, 96*(2), 261–282. https://doi.org/10.1901/jeab.2011.96-261

Wathen, S. N., & Podlesnik, C. A. (2018). Laboratory models of treatment relapse and mitigation techniques. *Behavior Analysis: Research and Practice, 18*(4), 362–387. https://doi.org/10.1037/bar0000119

Williams, C. L., & St. Peter, C. C. (2020). Resurgence of previously taught academic responses. *Journal of the Experimental Analysis of Behavior, 113*(1), 232–250. https://doi.org/10.1002/jeab.572

Chapter 5
Reinstatement and Reacquisition of Extinguished Behavior: Evidence from the Laboratory

Mark E. Bouton

Changing or modifying an established behavior can be difficult, and sustaining the change can be difficult, too (Bouton, 2014). One reason why behavior change is so hard to sustain is that the first behavior is rarely truly erased from the behavioral repertoire. Studies of *extinction*, a simple and representative example of behavior change, make this abundantly clear. The fact that extinction, the weakening of a behavior that occurs when its reinforcer is removed, does not necessarily create unlearning has been a theme of research on Pavlovian and operant extinction for decades (e.g., Bouton et al., 2021). Several well-known phenomena support the idea. In *spontaneous recovery*, extinguished responding can recover when time merely passes after extinction; in *renewal*, extinguished responding can recover when the background context (typically defined as the room or apparatus in which extinction has taken place) is changed; and in *resurgence*, an extinguished response can recover when reinforcement of an alternative behavior that has been reinforced to replace it is reduced or withdrawn (see Bouton et al., 2021, for one recent review). Each of these phenomena can also occur when the behavior is suppressed with other methods, including positive punishment (e.g., Bouton & Schepers, 2015; Broomer & Bouton, 2023a, 2024; Estes, 1944; Marchant et al., 2013; Sutton et al., 2021). Understanding the phenomena is thus potentially important in helping understand lapse and relapse after behavior change—and perhaps how to make behavior change more permanent.

My colleagues and I have long argued that one of the main principles underlying the various relapse effects is that extinction and behavior change are inherently

I thank Catalina Rey for her comments.

M. E. Bouton (✉)
Department of Psychological Science, University of Vermont, Burlington, VT, USA
e-mail: Mark.Bouton@uvm.edu

M. P. Kranak (ed.), *Behavioral Treatments for Individuals with Autism*, Autism and Child Psychopathology Series,
https://doi.org/10.1007/978-3-031-91965-7_5

context-specific—they are easily disrupted by changing the context. The principle is directly illustrated by the renewal effect (e.g., Bouton et al., 2011), where a behavior that has been learned in one context (Context A) and then extinguished in another (Context B) recovers (or "renews") when it is merely tested outside the extinction context (i.e., in either Context A or in a third context, Context C). Renewal also occurs if conditioning and extinction both occur in Context A and then testing is conducted in a second context. What organisms learn in extinction (as well as other methods that cause behavioral suppression, like punishment) is a form of inhibition that is inherently context-specific. Spontaneous recovery can be explained in these terms: It is the renewal effect that occurs when testing occurs in a new temporal context. And a wealth of evidence suggests that resurgence is at least partly the same: The extinguished response recovers when the participant is removed from the conditions in which it was extinguished and the alternative response is reinforced. In that case, the "context" is reinforcement of the alternative behavior. Although it is beyond the scope of this chapter, there is research to support these claims and a great deal of evidence suggesting that "context" can be broadly defined and may include (for example) drug state, deprivation state, stress state, social cues, and prior behaviors, among other things (e.g., see Bouton, 2019; Bouton et al., 2021 for review).

One feature of spontaneous recovery, renewal, and resurgence is that they are usually tested under conditions in which the response is not reinforced. That is, response recovery is typically observed in extinction. The method helps experimenters isolate the causal mechanisms by removing any effect of presenting the reinforcer itself. But in the natural world, the organism is also often exposed to the reinforcer again after extinction. Here there are two additional relapse paradigms that are highly relevant. In *reinstatement*, a response recovers when the reinforcer is simply presented again, not contingent on the behavior, after extinction (e.g., Reid, 1958). In *reacquisition*, the extinguished behavior can rapidly return if it is actually paired with the reinforcer again.[1] Either of these effects can result from *commission errors* in applied behavior analysis: That is, a problem behavior can return if a therapist accidentally presents the reinforcer during treatment (e.g., Kranak & Falligant, 2023). But the issue is also broader than that. A drinker, smoker, or drug user whose behavior has been reduced or eliminated by an effective behavioral treatment may similarly lapse or relapse when exposed to the reinforcer again. In the interest of understanding reinstatement and reacquisition, this chapter focuses on laboratory research with animals that has been directed at uncovering general learning principles that apply to these situations. (For a more applied focus, see Chap. 6, Stephens et al., this volume.) One of the main principles that basic research on reinstatement and reacquisition has uncovered is that the reinforcer (and perhaps even its pairings with a conditioned stimulus or an operant behavior) provides another kind of context that can renew extinguished behavior when it is encountered again.

[1] Reacquisition as defined here has occasionally been called "response-dependent" reinstatement (e.g., Kranak & Falligant, 2023; see also Podlesnik & Shahan, 2009). I will avoid this alternative, because it makes the term "reinstatement" less precise.

Reinstatement

Respondent Learning

Although the focus of the present book is primarily operant behavior, a great deal of relevant work on reinstatement has studied it in respondent (Pavlovian) conditioning. As will be seen, reinstatement in respondent and operant conditioning depends on similar principles, and it is useful to consider both. Pavlov (1927) was actually the first to report reinstatement in his original research on salivary conditioning with dogs. But it has since been studied especially intensively in Pavlovian fear conditioning in rats, where a conditional stimulus (CS), such as a tone, is paired with an aversive footshock unconditional stimulus (US). As a consequence of the pairings, the CS comes to arouse a response that is often called "fear." In a seminal set of experiments, Rescorla and Heth (1975) reported that after fear conditioning and then extinction (caused by repeatedly presenting the CS alone), one or two presentations of the US alone, without the CS, was sufficient to cause fear to return to the CS (see also Rescorla & Cunningham, 1977, 1978). They showed that reinstatement depended on prior conditioning of the CS, and was thus the recovery of the original learning. And they found that fear conditioned with a footshock US could be reinstated by exposure to another aversive event (a loud noise), and vice versa. It should be noted that, beginning with Rescorla and Heth (1975), studies of reinstatement in fear conditioning involve relatively few conditioning trials that are often widely distributed in time (e.g., separated by 20 min or more). And the extinction phase is typically conducted over several daily sessions. The reinstating USs are also typically presented in a unique session after extinction, and reinstated fear of the CS is tested in yet another session 24 hours later. The important point, though, is that the fear-reducing effects of extinction—which are thought to tap into mechanisms that underlie the effects of exposure therapy for human anxiety disorders (e.g., Craske et al., 2014)—are not permanent. Conditioned fear responding can return if the animal is merely re-exposed to the US.

Bouton and Bolles (1979) soon showed that the reinstatement effect after fear extinction depends critically on conditioning of the context that occurs during re-exposure to the US. To be specific, US exposures during reinstatement shocking are associated with the background context, making it fearful again, and such fear of the context is what causes fear of the CS to return. Two key findings supported this conclusion. First, exposures to the reinstating USs only reinstated fear of the CS if they were presented in the same context (Skinner box) in which the CS was to be tested—a finding that has been replicated in many experiments (e.g., animal fear conditioning: e.g., Bouton, 1984; Bouton & King, 1983, 1986; human fear conditioning: e.g., LaBar & Phelps, 2005; animal appetitive conditioning: Bouton & Peck, 1989). No reinstatement is observed if the US is presented in a different context. Second, multiple exposures to the context without shock after reinstatement shocking abolished the reinstatement effect (Bouton & Bolles, 1979). They arguably did so by reducing (extinguishing) fear of the context.

Later work developed a method that directly measured contextual conditioning and confirmed its crucial role. In "context preference tests," the rat was allowed to freely choose between lever pressing in the Skinner box and moving to a safe (unshocked) side box at the start of test sessions. Rats that were afraid of the context spent more time in the side box. Contextual conditioning measured this way correlated with (and thus predicted) the strength of the reinstatement effect in individual subjects (Bouton, 1984; Bouton & King, 1983, 1986). And other work discovered that a CS that had been through extinction was especially sensitive to the fear-augmenting effect of contextual conditioning—a CS that evoked fear, but had never been extinguished, was not affected by contextual conditioning created by post-conditioning presentation of shocks and confirmed by context preference testing (e.g., Bouton, 1984; Bouton & King, 1986). This was true even when the conditioned-only CS was arranged to evoke the same amount of fear as a partially extinguished CS; the partially extinguished CS, but not the conditioned-only CS, was augmented by contextual conditioning (Bouton, 1984). Contextual conditioning is thus crucial to reinstatement in Pavlovian fear conditioning. One interpretation is that contextual conditioning is itself a kind of cue that has been associated with conditioning; the rats were afraid of the context during fear conditioning. Returning contextual fear after extinction may thus cause an associative kind of renewal effect.

Operant Learning

Parallel research has documented a similar reinstatement effect after the extinction of operant conditioning. Reid (1958) was among the first to show that lever pressing reinforced with food pellets and then extinguished returned when the reinforcer was merely presented on its own (not contingent on lever pressing). Reinforcers presented contingent on a new second response are equally effective at reinstating the first response (Winterbauer & Bouton, 2011).[2] In an important follow-up to Reid's early work, Rescorla and Skucy (1969) showed that noncontingent presentations of the reinforcer after extinction indeed reinstated an extinguished response, and also retarded the loss of responding if they were presented during the course of extinction. This effect still happened when any response delayed the presentation of a scheduled reinforcer by 5 s. (This and other observations argued against a role for accidental pairings of the response and reinforcer.) Rescorla and Skucy also showed that reinstatement involves recovery of a previously learned response: Presenting noncontingent reinforcers caused a trained-then-extinguished response to recover, but had little effect on lever pressing that had never been reinforced. In a similar

---

[2] Presentations of a drug reinforcer can also reinstate extinguished drug self-administration behavior (e.g., rats lever pressing for intravenous delivery of drugs like cocaine or heroin, e.g., de Wit & Stewart, 1981, 1983). Like other types of operant behavior, extinguished "drug seeking" is also vulnerable to the other canonical relapse effects, but a discussion of drug self-administration is outside the scope of the present chapter. See Bouton et al. (2012) for one review.

vein, Franks and Lattal (1976) later established that reinstatement caused recovery of a high rate of responding when lever pressing had been reinforced on a variable ratio schedule, but a lower level of responding if it had been reinforced on differential reinforcement of low rate (DRL) schedule. Noncontingent reinforcers presented after extinction thus cause the recovery of a behavior (or behavior pattern) that had been learned before.

Is reinstatement after operant extinction due to contextual conditioning, the factor that plays such an important role in Pavlovian conditioning? The answer is at least partly "yes." Baker et al. (1991) studied reinstatement of extinguished lever pressing with a method more analogous to typical studies of Pavlovian conditioning, where the reinforcers were presented in a separate session with levers removed (and lever pressing thus prevented), rather than in a session where responding was available. When the extinguished response was tested the next day, the exposure to the reinforcers the day before increased (reinstated) responding compared to controls that did not receive them (see also Rescorla & Skucy, 1969). Moreover, that effect was diminished if the reinstating reinforcers were presented in a different context (a distinctively different Skinner box), or were followed by several sessions of extinction exposure to the context (without the lever available) before testing. Both effects were similar to those of Bouton and Bolles (1979) and consistent with a role for contextual conditioning. Baker et al. also found that reinstatement was diminished if the reinstating reinforcers were each signaled by a brief novel (3-s) visual stimulus—a third treatment that can decrease the resulting contextual conditioning (e.g., Rescorla & Wagner, 1972). (Many models of conditioning propose that signals compete with and "overshadow" contextual conditioning, which has been confirmed in several studies, e.g., Baker, 1990; Baker et al., 1981; Bouton, 1984; Odling-Smee, 1978; but see Balsam, 1985.) Contextual conditioning could invigorate operant responding through "Pavlovian-instrumental transfer" (e.g., Holmes et al., 2010; Rescorla & Solomon, 1967), or enter into associative control of the response (e.g., Trapold & Overmier, 1972) because of its unique presence during conditioning—in the manner suggested earlier for Pavlovian fear learning.

The effects of signaling the reinforcer confirmed the results of earlier operant studies (Baker, 1990) in which signaling noncontingent reinforcers that were being delivered while responding was being extinguished likewise reduced their response-augmenting effects. Interestingly, Baker (1990) also found that the same cue presented immediately *after* each reinforcer (i.e., in a "backward conditioning" arrangement) *enhanced* the free reinforcers' augmenting effect. This result was further consistent with the contextual conditioning account, because backward conditioning can make the stimulus a conditioned inhibitor, and Pavlovian inhibitors presented with a context can "protect" the context from undergoing extinction during the intervals between reinforcers (e.g., Fanselow, 1980; see also Rescorla, 2003), also consistent with models of associative learning (e.g., Rescorla & Wagner, 1972). There is thus a substantial amount of evidence supporting the view that reinstatement of extinguished operant responding is influenced by contextual conditioning created by the noncontingent reinforcers.

On the other hand, Baker et al. (1991) also found that there was more response recovery when the reinstating reinforcers were presented while the lever response was also available (see also Rescorla & Skucy, 1969). Although the results of Baker (1990) still indicate that contextual conditioning plays a role when the free reinforcers and response testing occur at the same time, another factor was clearly at work. One possibility is that the reinforcer itself can be a discriminative stimulus (S^D) that sets the occasion for the response. During operant conditioning, the animal is often reinforced for responding soon after delivery of another reinforcer. Extinction normally occurs without that stimulus, so when it is presented again, it can simply occasion the response. In his early paper, Reid (1958) had assumed exactly this mechanism (his paper was entitled "the reinforcer as a stimulus"). Thus, in addition to causing contextual conditioning, free reinforcers themselves may directly renew extinguished responding. In relevant Pavlovian research, noncontingent reinforcers in the test have been shown to occasion either responding or not responding to a CS—depending on whether they have been presented freely in the intertrial intervals of conditioning or extinction sessions (Bouton et al., 1993).

Several results support the S^D mechanism as a cause of reinstatement. Ostlund and Balleine (2007) trained rats to press two different levers in separate sessions. Pressing one lever was reinforced with a standard food pellet, and pressing the other was reinforced with a drop of a sucrose solution. In an extinction test, both responses were extinguished at the same time, and then one of the two reinforcers was presented noncontingently. The treatment caused a specific reinstatement of the response the reinforcer had been associated with. Another experiment pinpointed the reinforcer's S^D function. Two groups were trained with a new procedure in which a single reinforcer (either pellet or sucrose) was presented 4 s before the two levers were inserted into the operant chamber. The initial reinforcer signaled which lever response, R1 (response 1) or R2 (response 2), would be reinforced on that trial. For one group, the signaling outcome was the same as the reinforcing outcome (i.e., O1-R1-O1 and O2-R2-O2; where O1 refers to one outcome and O2 refers to a different outcome). For the other group, the signaling and reinforcing outcomes were different (i.e., O1-R1-O2 an O2-R2-O1). When the responses were both extinguished, presenting O1 or O2 noncontingently reinstated the response that had *followed* it in either group. Thus, the reinforcer's antecedent relation with the response, rather than its consequent relation, controlled the reinstatement effect. Reinstatement can be caused by the reinforcer serving as an S^D.[3]

[3]Outcome-specificity of reinstatement has also been reported in appetitive respondent conditioning: When one CS is associated with food pellets and another with sucrose, pellet or sucrose presentations after extinction can reinstate responding to the CS that specifically was associated with it (e.g., Delamater, 1997). That specificity was demonstrated in experiments that intermixed the two types of trials with sessions (unlike Ostlund and Balleine, who presented them in separate sessions), making the S^D explanation difficult there. Outcome-specificity of reinstatement in respondent appetitive conditioning further contrasts with respondent fear learning, where reinstatement is less outcome-specific. (Recall Rescorla and Heth's [1975] reinstatement across footshock and loud noise USs.)

Other important results also support the discriminative stimulus mechanism of operant reinstatement. Of particular note, if the animal receives a treatment in which the reinforcer is presented independently of the response during extinction, reinstatement does not occur when the reinforcer is presented again after responding has declined (e.g., Baker, 1990; Rescorla & Skucy, 1969; Winterbauer & Bouton, 2011). Theoretically, the animal has now learned to withhold its responding in the presence of the S^D; the S^D is now ineffective at occasioning the response. It is worth noting that, since the delivery of noncontingent reinforcers during extinction also slows down the loss of responding (Baker, 1990; Rescorla & Skucy, 1969), one might mistakenly conclude that adding noncontingent reinforcers to extinction provides an inferior extinction treatment. It is clearly not inferior in the sense that it protects the response from reinstatement.

Nevertheless, delivering noncontingent reinforcers during extinction does not create a blanket protection from relapse. For example, Nakajima et al. (2002) reported that ABA renewal of an operant response still occurs after extinction has included added noncontingent pellets. A similar point is made when responding has been eliminated by an omission contingency (differential reinforcement of other behavior, or DRO). Here responding is depressed when it postpones free reinforcers that are otherwise obtained. Uhl and Garcia (1969; see also Uhl, 1973, 1974; Uhl & Sherman, 1971) had established that a response suppressed by omission is not reinstated when noncontingent reinforcers are presented. But omission doesn't destroy the original learning. Rey et al. (2021) reinforced lever pressing in Context A and then eliminated it with extinction or omission training in Context B. Presenting noncontingent reinforcers then reinstated responding that had been eliminated by extinction, but had no effect on responding suppressed by omission. Yet, there was still a robust renewal of responding when the omission trained response was returned from Context B to Context A (see also Nakajima et al., 2002). Moreover, the level of that renewal was not different from that observed after simple extinction. Thus, neither omission nor noncontingent reinforcers in extinction can be said to erase the original learning or protect the response against all forms of relapse. But the *reinstating* effect of noncontingent reinforcers can be reduced with procedures that theoretically modify the reinforcer's function as an S^D.

Another elimination procedure that includes reinforcer exposures is differential reinforcement of alternative behavior, or DRA. DRA is commonly used in the clinical treatment of problem behavior (e.g., Wathen & Podlesnik, 2018). Here a new alternative response is reinforced at the same time the problem behavior is extinguished. The method not only teaches and strengthens a new (and often more appropriate) response, but may also weaken the S^D function of the reinforcer by now associating it with the inhibition of the problem behavior. The results of at least two studies suggest that DRA may indeed prevent reinstatement. Lieving and Lattal (2003) trained pigeons to peck a key for a food reinforcer (on VI 30) and then reinforced a new response, treadle pressing, on VI 30 while pecking was extinguished. Treadle pressing came to replace key pecking. When they now presented the reinforcer noncontingently (VT 30), the free reinforcers had no effect on behavior—and did *not* reinstate the extinguished key pecking. In contrast, when Lieving and Lattal removed all reinforcer presentations (and thus put both responses on extinction), keypecking resurged. The free reinforcers delivered during the test thus suppressed the resurgence effect. In a related experiment with rats, Bouton and Trask (2016) reinforced pressing one lever (R1) with one outcome (O1, either grain or sucrose pellets, each for half the rats, on a VI-30 schedule). In a second phase, while R1 was extinguished, pressing a second lever (R2) was reinforced with O2 (also on VI 30). R1 responding resurged when both responses were then extinguished. But noncontingent presentations of O2 (VT 30) continued to suppress R1 responding, thus not causing reinstatement, and again suppressing the resurgence effect (as in Lieving & Lattal, 2003). In contrast, noncontingent presentations of O1 did not suppress resurgence; unlike animals given O2, the animals receiving O1 performed R1 again in the test. Thus, the crucial thing suppressing resurgence is the reinforcer's presence during response elimination.[4] The results overall do suggest that presenting reinforcers in extinction—either noncontingently, on an omission schedule, or during a DRA treatment—can reduce the reinstatement effect that is normally produced by response-independent reinforcers. The treatments theoretically do so by reducing the reinforcer's discriminative, S^D, effect. Importantly, none of them, including DRA (e.g., Kimball et al., 2023), eliminate the renewal effect.

Summary

After extinction in both respondent and operant learning, presentation of reinforcers independently of the behavior (or perhaps contingent on another behavior) can cause a return or reinstatement of the extinguished response. Reinstatement in either respondent or operant learning is at least partly controlled by contextual conditioning created by the representation of the US or reinforcer. However, the reinforcer itself can also serve as an S^D or context that directly renews conditioned responding. Consistent with this mechanism, reinstatement is reduced or even eliminated with procedures that deliver the reinforcer in extinction.

[4]Companion studies by Trask and Bouton (2016) further suggested that presenting response-independent O2s during extinction likewise gives them the ability to suppress response recovery (e.g., presenting them during ABA renewal testing reduces the ABA renewal effect). In addition, presenting O2 noncontingently during extinction can reduce ***O1***'s ability to reinstate the extinguished response (as response-contingent O2s in DRA did for Bouton & Trask, 2016). This might be due to partial generalization between O1 and O2, which were different types of food pellets in all the experiments.

Reacquisition

A separate research literature has studied reacquisition, the (usually) rapid return of responding that occurs if response-reinforcer or CS-US pairings are resumed after extinction. There is a sense in which rapid reacquisition seems like an obvious consequence of the fact that at least some of the original learning (e.g., a response-reinforcer or CS-US association) is preserved through extinction—as reinstatement, renewal, spontaneous recovery, and resurgence all suggest. But why exactly should mere preservation of some of the previous learning make reacquisition occur so quickly? The evidence suggests that reacquisition is rapid if the reintroduced reinforcers, or response-reinforcer or CS-US pairings, can cause a renewal of conditioned responding.

Respondent Learning

Bouton (1986) noted that research prior to 1986 had not demonstrated a rapid reacquisition effect in Pavlovian learning that could be separated from other effects like simple spontaneous recovery occurring between extinction and the beginning of reacquisition. In two fear conditioning experiments, he studied reacquisition with a procedure that involved repeated daily extinction sessions that did not support much between-session spontaneous recovery by the end of extinction. He compared reacquisition of responding to a CS that had been conditioned and then extinguished with acquisition to a novel CS in a group that had received the same initial conditioning and extinction with a different CS. Surprisingly, he found that a moderate amount of extinction (16 or 24 extinction trials distributed over several daily sessions after 8 initial fear conditioning trials) yielded a CS whose reacquisition was neither faster nor slower than to a novel CS. And with more extended extinction training (72 extinction trials), reacquisition of the extinguished CS was significantly *slower*, not faster, than conditioning with the novel CS. In that experiment, reconditioning used a "partial reinforcement" procedure in which CS-US trials were alternated with CS-only trials. Among other things, this made the time between shock USs especially long (approximately 40 min). Reacquisition was slow even though Bouton used a conditioning and extinction procedure that had previously been shown to yield a CS with demonstrable excitation after extinction (e.g., Bouton & King, 1986). Although much of the original learning had thus presumably been preserved, it wasn't sufficient by itself to produce rapid reacquisition.

Bouton and Swartzentruber (1989) replicated and extended the slow reacquisition effect and confirmed that the slow-to-condition CS did still retain associative strength from the original acquisition phase. Thus, reacquisition was indeed slow even though the CS retained demonstrable conditioned properties. Furthermore, slow reacquisition occurred when reconditioning was conducted in the context (Skinner box) in which the CS had been extinguished; reacquisition was faster in other, non-extinction, contexts. And a return to the extinction context after reacquisition was complete in another context was also shown to recover extinction performance (i.e., the absence of fear). These and other results suggested that reacquisition was slow when the conditions cued (or "retrieved") extinction performance. And it was rapid when the conditions cued (or "retrieved") conditioning (fear) performance. The pattern fit a general pattern across many so-called interference paradigms in Pavlovian conditioning (e.g., extinction, latent inhibition, counterconditioning; Bouton, 1993). After fear extinction, the response to the CS can take either of two forms (fear or no fear) depending on what the current context retrieves.

Expanding on this point, Ricker and Bouton (1996) studied reacquisition in appetitive conditioning, where the CS is paired with a food-pellet US instead of footshock. Conditioned responding was indexed by anticipatory head entries in the cup where food was delivered. Ricker and Bouton hypothesized that rapid reacquisition, when it occurs, may be an ABA renewal effect that occurs when CS-US pairings (i.e., conditioning trials) have been associated with other upcoming conditioning trials during the original conditioning phase. As we saw in reinstatement, US presentations (and perhaps CS-US trials) can be considered a part of the conditioning context; after enough trials, the animal may learn that a conditioning trial signals other conditioning trials (cf. Capaldi, 1967, 1994). (Ricker and Bouton called this "trial-signaling.") Since CS-US pairings are absent in extinction, reintroducing them in reacquisition may simply cause renewal of the conditioned response. Ricker and Bouton reported at least two results that were consistent with this hypothesis. First, when reacquisition was conducted with alternating reinforced (CS-US) and nonreinforced (CS-no US) trials, high responding was observed during trials that followed reinforced trials, but not during trials that followed nonreinforced trials. The pattern was due to prior learning—it was not evident in naïve control groups that had not received initial conditioning and extinction. Second, either rapid or slow reacquisition could be produced in their method. Slow reacquisition occurred when there were only a few acquisition trials and many extinction trials (see also Bouton, 1986; Bouton & Swartzentruber, 1989). Rapid reacquisition occurred when there was a large number of conditioning trials (which provided more opportunity to learn that a reinforced trial signaled another reinforced trial). The picture that emerged was consistent with much of the Pavlovian literature, where rapid reacquisition has been reported in conditioning preparations involving many conditioning trials (appetitive conditioning, Ricker & Bouton, 1996; eyeblink conditioning, Napier et al., 1992; but see Leung et al., 2007, for an exception in fear conditioning) and slow reacquisition has occurred in conditioning preparations that typically involve very few conditioning trials (fear conditioning, Bouton, 1986, Bouton & Swartzentruber, 1989; Leung et al., 2007; taste aversion learning, e.g., Revusky & Coombes, 1979).

Bouton et al. (2004) put the trial signaling hypothesis to further test. If rapid reacquisition occurs because reintroducing CS-US trials causes renewal of the response, then inserting occasional CS-US trials in extinction might make them begin to signal extinction rather conditioning, and thus reduce the rapid reacquisition effect. Two appetitive conditioning experiments confirmed this counterintuitive prediction. In one, after conditioning with a procedure in which every CS presentation was reinforced, one group received simple extinction (CS-only trials) over a number of daily sessions while another group received a partial reinforcement procedure in which one out of every eight consecutive CS presentations was initially reinforced, then 1/12, and then finally 1/24. Not surprisingly, the loss of responding in the group that received occasional CS-US pairings was slower than that in the simple extinction group. But in a subsequent reacquisition phase, CS-US and CS-no US trials were alternated. Consistent with the trial-signaling hypothesis, reacquisition was significantly slower in the partial-reinforcement group than in the extinction-only group.[5] This result has been confirmed and extended in other methods (e.g., Gershman et al., 2013; Moris et al., 2017; Quintero et al., 2022; van den Akker et al., 2015; see Quintero et al., 2024 for a recent review). Of note is one model's idea that gradually thinning the number of reinforced trials might encourage the animal to update the original learning instead of encoding something separate and new (Gershman et al., 2010). This approach predicts that occasional reinforced trials in extinction should broadly prevent all the various relapse effects, a prediction that has met with mixed success (e.g., Quintero et al., 2024). According to a recent meta-analysis (Quintero et al., 2024), "the most consistent result [of providing occasional reinforced trials in extinction] seems to be the slowing down of the rate of reacquisition" (p. 15).

The Bouton et al. (2004) experiment also included another extinction group that received unpaired USs in the intertrial intervals at about the same time the partially reinforced group received their CS-US pairings. The unpaired-US treatment also slowed reacquisition (see also e.g., Frey & Butler, 1977; Rauhut et al., 2001), and its slowing effect was even deeper than that observed in the partially reinforced group. In fact, reacquisition occurred here at about the same rate as acquisition with a novel CS. Presumably, the difference lies in the fact that the CS-US pairings given the partially reinforced group transferred positively to reconditioning. Some investigators have also argued that an unpaired US procedure might be more effective than extinction at weakening the original association (e.g., see Thomas et al., 2005).

Overall, the results are consistent with the idea that rapid reacquisition after extinction is at least partly a renewal effect that is created by reintroduced exposures to the US or to CS-US pairings. Consistent with that view, it can be reduced with procedures that involve exposures to the US.

---

[5]As Ricker and Bouton had noted, the idea that reinforced and nonreinforced trials can signal upcoming trials has a history in learning theory. Capaldi (1967, 1994) put the idea to use in explaining the partial reinforcement extinction effect (PREE), where a partially reinforced response is slower to extinguish than a response that has always been reinforced. According to Capaldi (see also Harris, 2019), partial reinforcement associates nonreinforced (extinction) trials with upcoming reinforced trials, allowing better generalization of responding when the animal encounters nonreinforced trials in extinction. Slowing reacquisition after extinction by including reinforced trials in extinction (e.g., Bouton et al., 2004) is the complement of the PREE: It arguably associates reinforced trials with extinction and allows better generalization of extinction to reacquisition.

Operant Learning

There is a smaller but parallel literature on reacquisition in operant conditioning. Reacquisition after extinction here can also be rapid (e.g., Bullock & Smith, 1953; Willcocks & McNally, 2011). In an unpublished experiment conducted in my laboratory, Drina Vurbic (Vurbic, 2013) trained rats to either press a lever or pull a chain to receive food-pellet reinforcers (delivered on a VI 30 reinforcement schedule). The response was then extinguished over several daily sessions; between-session spontaneous recovery diminished to zero by the end of extinction. In a final phase, different groups received either reacquisition (on VI 30) with the conditioned-then-extinguished response or acquisition with the other untrained response (i.e., chain pulling if they had first learned lever pressing or lever pressing if they had first learned chain pulling). Reacquisition with the conditioned-then-extinguished response was faster than acquisition with the other response. The result demonstrated (perhaps for the first time) that rapid operant reacquisition entails actual recovery of a learned-then-extinguished response, rather than rapid learning that might occur with any response as a result of all the prior exposures to the reinforcer or all the time on the standard food-deprivation schedule. Nevertheless, acquisition with the untrained response was still faster than that seen in controls that had never had initial operant training. Its rapidity was in fact due to exposure to all the reinforcers that had been delivered during the initial training phase. In another experiment, different-response acquisition occurred at a rate that was equivalent to that of a group that received only noncontingent (yoked) reinforcers during the initial acquisition phase instead of actual operant training. Both of these groups demonstrated faster acquisition than a group that had not received reinforcer exposures in Phase 1. Vurbic's results suggest that rapid reacquisition can truly be due to the quick return of the previously learned response, although some rapidity can also result from mere exposure to reinforcers during the initial learning phase—which might invigorate responding, for example, by creating contextual conditioning (see above).

Vurbic (2013) also found that reintroducing response-reinforcer (VI 30) pairings in reacquisition caused more response recovery than the same reinforcers delivered noncontingently in a reinstatement treatment (a yoked group)—see Podlesnik & Shahan, 2009, for related pigeon results. The higher responding caused by response-contingent than response-independent reinforcers may not be especially surprising. Reinforcing the behavior could have a direct effect on response strength. And response-reinforcer pairings are themselves a possible cue that might signal other response-reinforcer pairings—analogous to trial-signaling in respondent learning (Ricker & Bouton, 1996).

In a further parallel with the Pavlovian work (Bouton & Swartzentruber, 1989), Todd, Winterbauer, and Bouton (2012) examined the effects of context switches on reacquisition of an extinguished operant. They studied the effects of sucrose and sweet-fatty reinforcers (perhaps analogous to rodent junk food) on lever pressing in non-hungry rats. As in the Pavlovian work, reacquisition was fastest if it occurred in the context in which extinction had *not* occurred: After conditioning in Context A and then extinction in Context B, reacquisition was faster in A than B; and after conditioning and extinction both in Context A, reacquisition was faster in a new context (B) than it was in Context A. As in fear conditioning (Bouton & Swartzentruber, 1989), the contexts also cued their corresponding conditioning and extinction performances. In contrast, Willcocks and McNally (2011) found no effect of context on the number of responses emitted during reacquisition, but they suggested that this could have been related to their use of a dense reinforcement schedule in hungry animals, which could have overwhelmed any effect of context. (They observed context effects analogous to Todd et al. when they analyzed the latency to the first response.) Despite the parallel between operant and classical conditioning, no one to my knowledge has tested or produced *slow* reacquisition in operant learning (cf. Bouton, 1986; Bouton & Swartzentruber, 1989; Ricker & Bouton, 1996). Based on what we know in respondent conditioning, slow operant reacquisition might be possible if the amount of operant training were minimal and the amount of extinction training were extensive, thus favoring the retrieval of extinction.

Research by Woods and Bouton (2007) further tested the parallel between Pavlovian and operant learning. They reasoned that a role for renewal by response-reinforcer pairings implies that providing some such pairings in extinction might associate them with extinction as well as conditioning, and thus reduce the source of the rapid reacquisition effect (cf. Bouton et al., 2004). Results of three experiments supported this view. In all of them, rats were trained to lever press on a VI 30 schedule and then received either extinction (over eight hour-long sessions) or a thinning partial reinforcement procedure that gradually increased the variable interval (starting with VI 4-min and then increasing every 30 min through VI 8, 12, 16, 20, 24, 28, and finally VI 32-min). This procedure slowed the loss of responding appreciably, and never completely eliminated responding. Most important, it also slowed reacquisition (compared with that after extinction) conducted with a lean VI 8-min reinforcement schedule. The effect was less evident when a richer VI 2-min schedule was used, perhaps because richer schedules begin to approximate the VI 30 schedule used in training. Slowed reacquisition was also easiest to observe in the minutes that followed each new response-reinforcer pairing. Thus, one effect of the thinning partial reinforcement procedure was to reduce the animal's immediate response to each reinforced response.

A final experiment compared the partial reinforcement schedule with one in which the pellet reinforcers were presented response-independently at similar time points within the response-elimination sessions. Noncontingent reinforcers and the sparse response-contingent reinforcers in the partial reinforcement procedure were both effective at slowing reacquisition, and there was no difference between the treatments. Thus, presenting a thinning number of reinforcers either response-contingently or noncontingently can slow the operant rapid reacquisition effect.

These findings are theoretically significant because they further support the idea that the reinforcer, or possibly the response-reinforcer pairing, is an event that can set the occasion for response recovery in the form of rapid reconditioning. But they are also important at a practical level, because they suggest that allowing a drinker, smoker, or drug user to occasionally experience the reinforcer—and connect it with continued extinction instead of bingeing—may be more effective than pure abstinence at discouraging relapse when a lapse leads to earning the reinforcer again. In the animal lab, either response-contingent or free reinforcers in extinction can help interfere with rapid reacquisition when an extinguished behavior is reinforced again.

The possibility that reinforcers delivered during a behavioral suppression treatment might help sustain behavior change is also consistent with recent research on positive punishment. Here, of course, an operant behavior is suppressed when an aversive stimulus like footshock is made a consequence of the response. Interestingly, despite the obvious differences between punishment and extinction, the two are similar in important ways. Punishment, like extinction, is sensitive to context change—Bouton and Schepers (2015) demonstrated that when lever pressing was reinforced in Context A and then punished (while also being reinforced) in Context B, tests of the response back in the original Context A or in a third Context C caused renewal of the punished response (ABA renewal, see also Marchant et al., 2013, and ABC renewal, respectively). Punished behavior is also vulnerable to spontaneous recovery (e.g., Estes, 1944). Broomer and Bouton (2023a) recently compared punishment (created by delivering response-contingent footshocks on a VI 90-s schedule) and simple extinction on ABA renewal and spontaneous recovery. With their method, renewal and spontaneous recovery were both evident, and apparently equivalent, after either punishment or extinction. However, the rate of reacquisition was a different story. When the original VI 30-s schedule was reinstituted after extinction, response recovery was almost immediate. But after punishment, which had taken place with the positive reinforcement contingency still in effect, response suppression persisted much longer. Broomer and Bouton argued that the punished animal had learned to suppress its behavior in the presence of recently earned reinforcers. Punishment was not merely "stronger" than extinction, because it had been equally vulnerable to renewal and spontaneous recovery. These results, like many others discussed in this chapter, suggest that reinforcers delivered during a behavioral suppression treatment can protect the animal from relapse when it is exposed to the reinforcer again.

Summary

After extinction in both respondent and operant learning, a reintroduction of CS-US (or response-reinforcer) pairings can cause a rapid return of the extinguished response. Organisms appear to retain both conditioning (or conditioning performance) and extinction (or extinction performance) after extinction. If conditions promote the retrieval of extinction, this can interfere with reacquisition; if conditions promote retrieval of conditioning, the response will return. The evidence suggests, again, that reintroducing the US or reinforcer itself, or CS-US or response-reinforcer pairings, may provide a cue that renews conditioning performance. As we saw in reinstatement, response elimination procedures that include presentations of the US or reinforcer can slow down or retard rapid reacquisition. This can even be true of extinction treatments that provide occasional CS-US or response-reinforcer pairings. Either kind of procedure is thought to associate the reinforcer with extinction rather than (or in addition to) conditioning.

Conclusions

Recent evidence suggests that operant extinction and punishment are response-specific as well as context-specific (Bouton & Schepers, 2015; Bouton et al., 2016; Broomer & Bouton, 2023b; Todd, 2013). For instance, when animals learn to make two different operant responses in the presence of one S^D, and then one of the responses is extinguished, the other behavior appears strong and largely unaffected (Bouton et al., 2016; Steinfeld & Bouton, 2022). Such results suggest that in operant extinction, the organism learns to inhibit a specific response. Together with work on the various relapse effects, this sort of finding suggests that after extinction, the behavior has a kind of bistable character—different circumstances can turn it on or turn it off.

The results described in this chapter all point to the fact that reinforcers presented after extinction, either response-contingently as in reacquisition or noncontingently as in reinstatement, can occasion or re-engage the learned response. This is especially true if the reinforcer is uniquely associated with conditioning. As we have seen, rapid reacquisition and reinstatement can both be reduced by including reinforcers in the behavioral suppression treatment. The two forms of relapse can be controlled, and behavior change sustained, by remembering the importance of the "reinforcer context."

References

Baker, A. G. (1990). Contextual conditioning during free-operant extinction: Unsignaled, signaled, and backward-signaled noncontingent food. *Animal Learning & Behavior, 18*, 199–218.

Baker, A. G., Mercier, P., Gabel, J., & Baker, P. A. (1981). Contextual conditioning and the US preexposure effect in conditioned fear. *Journal of Experimental Psychology: Animal Behavior Processes, 7*, 109–128.

Baker, A. G., Steinwald, H., & Bouton, M. E. (1991). Contextual conditioning and reinstatement of extinguished instrumental responding. *The Quarterly Journal of Experimental Psychology, 43B*, 199–218.

Balsam, P. D. (1985). The functions of context in learning and performance. In P. D. Balsam & A. Tomie (Eds.), *Context and learning* (pp. 1–1). Academic.

Bouton, M. E. (1984). Differential control by context in the inflation and reinstatement paradigms. *Journal of Experimental Psychology: Animal Behavior Processes, 10*, 56–74.

Bouton, M. E. (1986). Slow reacquisition following the extinction of conditioned suppression. *Learning and Motivation, 17*, 1–15.

Bouton, M. E. (1993). Context, time, and memory retrieval in the interference paradigms of Pavlovian learning. *Psychological Bulletin, 114*, 80–99.

Bouton, M. E. (2014). Why behavior change is difficult to sustain. *Preventive Medicine, 68*, 29–36.

Bouton, M. E. (2019). Extinction of instrumental (operant) learning: Interference, varieties of context, and mechanisms of contextual control. *Psychopharmacology, 236*, 7–19.

Bouton, M. E., & Bolles, R. C. (1979). Role of conditioned contextual stimuli in reinstatement of extinguished fear. *Journal of Experimental Psychology: Animal Behavior Processes, 5*, 368–378.

Bouton, M. E., & King, D. A. (1983). Contextual control of the extinction of conditioned fear: Tests for the associative value of the context. *Journal of Experimental Psychology: Animal Behavior Processes, 9*, 248–265.

Bouton, M. E., & King, D. A. (1986). Effect of context on performance to conditioned stimuli with mixed histories of reinforcement and nonreinforcement. *Journal of Experimental Psychology: Animal Behavior Processes, 12*, 4–15.

Bouton, M. E., & Peck, C. A. (1989). Context effects on conditioning, extinction, and reinstatement in an appetitive conditioning preparation. *Animal Learning & Behavior, 17*, 188–198.

Bouton, M. E., & Schepers, S. T. (2015). Renewal after the punishment of free operant behavior. *Journal of Experimental Psychology: Animal Learning and Cognition, 41*, 81–90.

Bouton, M. E., & Swartzentruber, D. (1989). Slow reacquisition following extinction: Context, encoding, and retrieval mechanisms. *Journal of Experimental Psychology: Animal Behavior Processes, 15*, 43–53.

Bouton, M. E., & Trask, S. (2016). Role of the discriminative properties of the reinforcer in resurgence. *Learning & Behavior, 44*, 137–150.

Bouton, M. E., Rosengard, C., Achenbach, G. G., Peck, C. A., & Brooks, D. C. (1993). Effects of contextual conditioning and unconditional stimulus presentation on performance in appetitive conditioning. *The Quarterly Journal of Experimental Psychology, 41B*, 63–95.

Bouton, M. E., Woods, A. M., & Pineño, O. (2004). Occasional reinforced trials during extinction can slow the rate of rapid reacquisition. *Learning and Motivation, 15*, 371–390.

Bouton, M. E., Todd, T. P., Vurbic, D., & Winterbauer, N. E. (2011). Renewal after the extinction of free operant behavior. *Learning & Behavior, 39*, 57–67.

Bouton, M. E., Winterbauer, N. E., & Vurbic, D. (2012). Context and extinction: Mechanisms of relapse in drug self-administration. In M. Haselgrove & L. Hogarth (Eds.), *Clinical applications of learning theory* (pp. 103–133). Psychology Press.

Bouton, M. E., Trask, S., & Carranza-Jasso, R. (2016). Learning to inhibit the response during instrumental (operant) extinction. *Journal of Experimental Psychology: Animal Learning and Cognition, 42*, 246–258.

Bouton, M. E., Maren, S., & McNally, G. P. (2021). Behavioral and neurobiological mechanisms of Pavlovian and instrumental extinction learning. *Physiological Reviews, 101*, 611–681.

Broomer, M. C., & Bouton, M. E. (2023a). A comparison of renewal, spontaneous recovery, and reacquisition after instrumental punishment and extinction. *Learning & Behavior, 51*, 262–273.

Broomer, M. C., & Bouton, M. E. (2023b). Response-specific effects of punishment of a discriminated operant response. *Learning and Motivation, 83*, 101907.

Broomer, M. C., & Bouton, M. E. (2024). Infralimbic cortex plays a similar role in the punishment and extinction of instrumental behavior. *Neurobiology of Learning and Memory, 211*, 107926.

Bullock, D. H., & Smith, W. C. (1953). The effect of repeated conditioning-extinction upon operant strength. *Journal of Experimental Psychology, 46*, 349–352.

Capaldi, E. J. (1967). A sequential hypothesis of instrumental learning. In K. W. Spence & J. T. Spence (Eds.), *Psychology of learning and motivation* (Vol. 1, pp. 67–156). Academic.

Capaldi, E. J. (1994). The sequential view: From rapidly fading stimulus traces to the organization of memory and the abstract concept of number. *Psychonomic Bulletin & Review, 1*, 156–181.

Craske, M. G., Treanor, M., Conway, C. C., Zbozinek, T., & Vervliet, B. (2014). Maximizing exposure therapy: An inhibitory learning approach. *Behaviour Research and Therapy, 58*, 10–23.

De Wit, H., & Stewart, J. (1981). Reinstatement of cocaine-reinforced responding in the rat. *Psychopharmacology, 75*, 134–143.
De Wit, H., & Stewart, J. (1983). Drug reinstatement of heroin-reinforced responding in the rat. *Psychopharmacology, 79*, 29–31.
Delamater, A. R. (1997). Selective reinstatement of stimulus–outcome associations. *Animal Learning & Behavior, 25*, 400–412.
Estes, W. K. (1944). An experimental study of punishment. *Psychological Monographs: General and Applied, 57*, i–40.
Fanselow, M. S. (1980). Signaled shock-free periods and preference for signaled shock. *Journal of Experimental Psychology: Animal Behavior Processes, 6*, 65–80.
Franks, G. J., & Lattal, K. A. (1976). Antecedent reinforcement schedule training and operant response reinstatement in rats. *Animal Learning & Behavior, 4*, 374–378.
Frey, P. W., & Butler, C. S. (1977). Extinction after aversive conditioning: An associative or nonassociative process? *Learning and Motivation, 8*, 1–17.
Gershman, S. J., Blei, D. M., & Niv, Y. (2010). Context, learning, and extinction. *Psychological Review, 117*, 197–209.
Gershman, S. J., Jones, C. E., Norman, K. A., Monfils, M.-H., & Niv, Y. (2013). Gradual extinction prevents the return of fear: Implications for the discovery of state. *Frontiers in Behavioral Neuroscience, 7*, 164.
Harris, J. A. (2019). The importance of trials. *Journal of Experimental Psychology: Animal Learning and Cognition, 45*, 390–404.
Holmes, N. M., Marchand, A. R., & Coutureau, E. (2010). Pavlovian to instrumental transfer: A neurobehavioural perspective. *Neuroscience and Biobehavioral Reviews, 34*, 1277–1295.
Kimball, R. T., Salvetti, E. L., Day, L. E., Karis, R., Silveira, J., & Kranak, M. P. (2023). Operant ABA renewal during dense and lean schedules of differential reinforcement. *Journal of the Experimental Analysis of Behavior, 119*, 529–538.
Kranak, M. P., & Falligant, J. M. (2023). Treatment integrity, commission errors, and reinstatement: A primer. *Education and Treatment of Children, 46*, 249–262.
LaBar, K. S., & Phelps, E. A. (2005). Reinstatement of conditioned fear in humans is context dependent and impaired in amnesia. *Behavioral Neuroscience, 119*, 677–686.
Leung, H. T., Bailey, G. K., Laurent, V., & Westbrook, R. F. (2007). Rapid reacquisition of fear to a completely extinguished context is replaced by transient impairment with additional extinction training. *Journal of Experimental Psychology: Animal Behavior Processes, 33*, 299–313.
Lieving, G. A., & Lattal, K. A. (2003). Recency, repeatability, and reinforcer retrenchment: An experimental analysis of resurgence. *Journal of the Experimental Analysis of Behavior, 80*, 217–233.
Marchant, N. J., Khuc, T. N., Pickens, C. L., Bonci, A., & Shaham, Y. (2013). Context-induced relapse to alcohol seeking after punishment in a rat model. *Biological Psychiatry, 73*, 256–262.
Moris, J., Barberia, I., Vadillo, M. A., Andrades, A., & López, F. J. (2017). Slower reacquisition after partial extinction in human contingency learning. *Journal of Experimental Psychology: Learning, Memory, and Cognition, 43*, 81–93.
Nakajima, S., Urushihara, K., & Masaki, T. (2002). Renewal of operant performance formerly eliminated by omission or noncontingency training upon return to the acquisition context. *Learning and Motivation, 33*, 510–525.
Napier, R. M., Macrae, M., & Kehoe, E. J. (1992). Rapid reacquisition in conditioning of the rabbit's nictitating membrane response. *Journal of Experimental Psychology: Animal Behavior Processes, 18*, 182–192.
Odling-Smee, F. J. (1978). The overshadowing of background stimuli by an informative CS in aversive Pavlovian conditioning with rats. *Animal Learning & Behavior, 6*, 43–51.
Ostlund, S. B., & Balleine, B. W. (2007). Selective reinstatement of instrumental performance depends on the discriminative stimulus properties of the mediating outcome. *Learning & Behavior, 35*, 43–52.
Pavlov, I. P. (1927). *Conditioned reflexes*. Oxford University Press.

Podlesnik, C. A., & Shahan, T. A. (2009). Behavioral momentum and relapse of extinguished operant responding. *Learning & Behavior, 37*, 357–364.

Quintero, M. J., Flores, A., Gutiérrez-Huerta, M. T., Molina-Guerrero, P., López, F. J., & Morís, J. (2022). Limitations of occasional reinforced extinction to alleviate spontaneous recovery and reinstatement effects: Evidence for a trial-signalling mechanism. *Quarterly Journal of Experimental Psychology, 75*, 765–783.

Quintero, M. J., López, F. J., Vadillo, M. A., & Morís, J. (2024). Occasional reinforced extinction as a method for relapse prevention: A critical systematic review and future directions. *Cognitive Therapy and Research, 48*, 1046.

Rauhut, A. S., Thomas, B. L., & Ayres, J. J. B. (2001). Treatments that weaken Pavlovian conditioned fear and thwart its renewal in rats: Implications for treating human phobias. *Journal of Experimental Psychology: Animal Behavior Processes, 27*, 99–114.

Reid, R. L. (1958). The role of the reinforcer as a stimulus. *British Journal of Psychology, 49*, 202–209.

Rescorla, R. A. (2003). Protection from extinction. *Learning & Behavior, 31*, 124–132.

Rescorla, R. A., & Cunningham, C. L. (1977). The erasure of reinstated fear. *Animal Learning & Behavior, 5*, 386–394.

Rescorla, R. A., & Cunningham, C. L. (1978). Recovery of the US representation over time during extinction. *Learning and Motivation, 9*, 373–391.

Rescorla, R. A., & Heth, C. D. (1975). Reinstatement of fear to an extinguished conditioned stimulus. *Journal of Experimental Psychology: Animal Behavior Processes, 1*, 88–96.

Rescorla, R. A., & Skucy, J. C. (1969). Effect of response-independent reinforcers during extinction. *Journal of Comparative and Physiological Psychology, 67*, 381–389.

Rescorla, R. A., & Solomon, R. L. (1967). Two-process learning theory: Relationships between Pavlovian conditioning and instrumental learning. *Psychological Review, 74*, 151–182.

Rescorla, R. A., & Wagner, A. R. (1972). A theory of Pavlovian conditioning: Variations in the effectiveness of reinforcement and nonreinforcement. In A. H. Black & W. K. Prokasy (Eds.), *Classical conditioning II: Current research and theory* (pp. 64–99). Appleton-Century-Crofts.

Revusky, S., & Coombes, S. (1979). Reacquisition of learned taste aversions. *Animal Learning & Behavior, 7*, 377–382.

Ricker, S. T., & Bouton, M. E. (1996). Reacquisition following extinction in appetitive conditioning. *Animal Learning & Behavior, 24*, 423–436.

Steinfeld, M. R., & Bouton, M. E. (2022). Inhibition in instrumental learning: Tests of response-specificity after feature-negative and extinction learning. *Journal of Experimental Psychology: Animal Learning and Cognition, 48*, 413–434.

Sutton, G. M., Nist, A. N., Nall, R. W., Browning, K. O., & Shahan, T. A. (2021). Resurgence of alcohol seeking following abstinence induced by punishment in male and female rats. *Behavioural Brain Research, 410*, 113345.

Thomas, B. L., Longo, C. L., & Ayres, J. J. B. (2005). Thwarting the renewal (relapse) of conditioned fear with the explicitly unpaired procedure: Possible interpretations and implications for treating human fears and phobias. *Learning and Motivation, 36*, 374–407.

Todd, T. P. (2013). Mechanisms of renewal after the extinction of instrumental behavior. *Journal of Experimental Psychology: Animal Behavior Processes, 39*, 193–207.

Todd, T. P., Winterbauer, N. E., & Bouton, M. E. (2012). Contextual control of appetite: Renewal of inhibited food-seeking behavior in sated rats after extinction. *Appetite, 58*, 484–489.

Trapold, M. A., & Overmier, J. B. (1972). The second learning process in instrumental learning. In A. H. Black & W. F. Prokasy (Eds.), *Classical conditioning Vol 2: Current research and theory* (pp. 427–452). Appleton-Century-Crofts.

Trask, S., & Bouton, M. E. (2016). Discriminative properties of the reinforcer can be used to attenuate the renewal of extinguished operant behavior. *Learning and Behavior, 44*, 151–161.

Uhl, C. N. (1973). Eliminating behavior with omission and extinction after varying amounts of training. *Animal Learning & Behavior, 1*, 237–240.

Uhl, C. N. (1974). Response elimination in rats with schedules of omission training, including yoked and response-independent reinforcement comparisons. *Learning and Motivation, 5*, 511–531.

Uhl, C. N., & Garcia, E. E. (1969). Comparison of omission with extinction in response elimination in rats. *Journal of Comparative and Physiological Psychology, 69*, 554–562.

Uhl, C. N., & Sherman, W. O. (1971). Comparison of combinations of omission punishment, and extinction methods in response elimination in rats. *Journal of Comparative and Physiological Psychology, 74*, 59–65.

van den Akker, K., Havermans, R. C., & Jansen, A. (2015). Effects of occasional reinforced trials during extinction on the reacquisition of conditioned responses to food cues. *Journal of Behavior Therapy and Experimental Psychiatry, 48*, 50–58.

Vurbic, D. (2013). *Rapid reacquisition of instrumental behavior after extinction*. Unpublished manuscript, University of Vermont.

Wathen, S. N., & Podlesnik, C. A. (2018). Laboratory models of treatment relapse and mitigation techniques. *Behavior Analysis: Research and Practice, 18*, 362–387.

Willcocks, A. L., & McNally, G. P. (2011). The role of context in re-acquisition of extinguished alcoholic beer-seeking. *Behavioral Neuroscience, 125*, 541–550.

Winterbauer, N. E., & Bouton, M. E. (2011). Mechanisms of resurgence II: Response-contingent reinforcers can reinstate a second extinguished behavior. *Learning and Motivation, 42*, 154–164.

Woods, A. M., & Bouton, M. E. (2007). Occasional reinforced responses during extinction can slow the rate of reacquisition of an operant response. *Learning and Motivation, 38*, 56–74.

Chapter 6
Reacquisition and Reinstatement of Problem Behavior: Knowns and Unknowns

Meredith J. Stephens, Megan A. Wessel, John Michael Falligant, and Michael P. Kranak

Although behavioral treatments can effectively reduce problem behavior under ideal conditions (e.g., dense schedules of reinforcement, perfect treatment integrity), desirable treatment gains must be generalized to real-world settings. As is the theme of this book, it is imperative that treatment gains be *durable* in the individual's everyday environment and when treatments are implemented by natural intervention agents (e.g., caregivers, teachers) or under less-than-perfect circumstances. One factor that will impact durability is the *procedural fidelity*[1] with which the treatment is being implemented. Procedural fidelity refers to the extent to which a treatment is being implemented as designed or prescribed (see Han et al., 2023; St. Peter et al., 2023). Researchers have shown that high or near-perfect levels of procedural fidelity lead to more durable outcomes (i.e., sustained reductions in problem behavior) compared to lower levels of procedural fidelity (e.g., Wacker et al., 2017).

Meredith Stephens and Megan Wessel share first-author status and are listed in alphabetical order by last name.

---

[1] Procedural fidelity has also been and is frequently referred to as treatment integrity, procedural integrity, and procedural adherence.

M. J. Stephens · M. A. Wessel
Oakland University, Rochester, MI, USA

J. M. Falligant
Auburn University, Auburn, AL, USA

M. P. Kranak (✉)
Oakland University and Oakland University Center for Autism, Rochester, MI, USA

Department of Human Development and Child Studies, Oakland University Center for Autism, Rochester, MI, USA
e-mail: kranak@oakland.edu

M. P. Kranak (ed.), *Behavioral Treatments for Individuals with Autism*, Autism and Child Psychopathology Series,
https://doi.org/10.1007/978-3-031-91965-7_6

In fact, even very minimal decreases in procedural fidelity have been shown to degrade treatment effects (e.g., Jones & St. Peter, 2022). Put simply, adequately high levels of procedural fidelity are essential to ensuring lasting treatment gains.

When procedural fidelity is poor, relapse of problem behavior will likely occur (Mace & Nevin, 2017). This is particularly concerning given that poor or inconsistent procedural fidelity is relatively common (e.g., Foreman et al., 2021). Generally speaking, there are two forms of procedural-fidelity errors: omission errors and commission errors. In brief, omission errors occur when an intervention agent fails to implement some aspect of the treatment as designed. For example, a caregiver might be attending to the needs of a sibling and is unable to honor the other child's mand, despite the mand being appropriate and the treatment indicating it should be reinforced. For additional discourse on omission errors and the type of relapse they might cause, see Chap. 1 (Mauzy et al., this volume) and Chap. 2 (Norris et al., this volume).

In contrast, commission errors occur when an intervention agent adds a step to the treatment that is not a part of the protocol. A very common commission error is when an intervention agent accidentally reinforces a problem behavior when the treatment plan outlines that a reinforcer should not be delivered. For example, a parent might reprimand or console their child when he is screaming, despite the treatment indicating that this behavior should be ignored (i.e., a commission error). Like omission errors, commission errors are also likely to lead to relapse. Relapse resulting from commission errors is called *reacquisition* or *response-dependent reinstatement*, equivalent terms that are used interchangeably in the literature (see Chap. 5, Bouton, this volume; see also Kranak & Falligant, 2023; Mitteer et al., 2021; Podlesnik & Shahan, 2009; Wathen & Podlesnik, 2018). Reacquisition occurs when a previously reinforced, but currently diminished, behavior recurs following the unexpected response-dependent delivery of reinforcers for the response. Continuing from the example in the preceding paragraph, suppose the caregiver had ceased delivering reprimands when their child screamed. However, one day they deliver a reprimand—either contingent on screaming or on some different behavior—and observe that the child's screaming, which was largely eliminated, instantly recurs at a high rate and intensity.

Mitigation Strategies for Reacquisition

In contrast to other forms of relapse, namely resurgence and renewal, there are no relapse-mitigation strategies designed explicitly for reacquisition that have been clinically validated (Kimball et al., 2023a, 2023b; see Kranak et al., 2022). Compared to the chapters on resurgence and renewal mitigation (Norris et al. and Grunewald et al., respectively), this chapter is understandably shorter. However, readers should take comfort in knowing that there are two primary recommendations, described in the following sections, that could serve as means of mitigating reacquisition. Moreover, procedures and data from basic and translational studies offer a promising approach for reacquisition mitigation.

Maintain High Procedural Fidelity

As mentioned, reacquisition occurs when a reinforcer is again provided contingently for a response (e.g., problem behavior) following its recurrence after a period of contacting extinction or has otherwise been reduced. Put simply, reacquisition cannot occur if commission errors do not occur. Thus, one way clinicians can mitigate reacquisition is by implementing treatments as they were prescribed, specifically by withholding reinforcement for the problem behavior when the treatment dictates it as such. As mentioned, treatments are more likely to have lasting and durable effects when they are implemented with higher procedural fidelity (Arkoosh et al., 2007; Fryling et al., 2012; Wacker et al., 2017). Importantly, the more commission errors that occur, the more (or greater) reacquisition will occur (Kranak & Falligant, 2023). Thus, when commission errors do occur, it is critical for intervention agents to implement the treatment with as high procedural fidelity as possible, as soon as possible (Mitteer et al., 2022).

Mitigate Resurgence and Renewal

Reacquisition cannot be the first type of relapse to occur, as its occurrence necessitates the recurrence of the problem behavior. In other words, commission errors cannot occur if the problem behavior has not already recurred via other forms of relapse. Two other common forms of relapse that occur in the context of problem behavior are resurgence (Lattal et al., 2017; Podlesnik et al., 2023) and renewal (Podlesnik & Kelley, 2015; Saini & Mitteer, 2020). Complete descriptions of resurgence and renewal are beyond the scope of this chapter. Readers are directed to Chap. 1, Mauzy et al. and Chap. 2, Norris et al. in this volume for basic information on and mitigation strategies for resurgence, respectively. Readers are directed to Chap. 3, Kimball et al. and Chap. 4, Grunewald et al. in this volume for basic information on and mitigation strategies for renewal, respectively.

Briefly, as they relate to the assessment and treatment of problem behavior, resurgence occurs due to a downshift in reinforcement for an alternative response (e.g., an omission reinforcement error for a functional communication response), whereas renewal occurs due to a change in stimulus conditions such as the location in which treatment is implemented or the person implementing treatment (i.e., a context change). When relapse of problem behavior occurs, caregivers and other natural intervention agents are likely to "give in" and reinforce the behavior. Thus, whenever an intervention agent engages in an omission error and resurgence of problem behavior occurs, that instance of resurgence presents an opportunity for a subsequent commission error to occur. Similarly, when a context change occurs and renewal happens, that instance of renewal presents an opportunity for a subsequent commission error to occur. Therefore, every instance of resurgence and renewal is an opportunity for reacquisition to occur.

In this sense, another recommendation for mitigating reacquisition is to mitigate other forms of relapse, namely resurgence and renewal. If there is no problem behavior occurring, then there are theoretically few, if any, opportunities for commission errors and subsequent reacquisition to occur. Fortunately, researchers and clinicians have developed a variety of methods for mitigating both resurgence and renewal (Kimball et al., 2023a, 2023b). To mitigate resurgence, for example, clinicians could incorporate competing stimuli or conduct schedule thinning (Fuhrman et al., 2018; Kranak & Brown, 2024). To mitigate renewal, for example, clinicians could incorporate supplemental discriminative stimuli, use extinction cues, or conduct multiple context training (Bernal-Gamboa et al., 2021; Greer et al., 2019; Kimball & Kranak, 2022). Readers interested in additional discourse on resurgence and renewal mitigation are again directed to Chap. 2, Norris et al. (this volume) and Chap. 4, Grunewald et al. (this volume), respectively.

As mentioned, no procedures for mitigating reacquisition specifically have been validated with clinically relevant behavior (i.e., problem behavior). However, basic and translational studies provide reasons to be optimistic about such a procedure. In a basic study with rats, Woods and Bouton (2007) found that exposing lever pressing to a progressively leaner schedule of reinforcement during response elimination—rather than placing lever pressing on extinction—resulted in less reacquisition during their reacquisition test compared to a group of rats whose lever pressing was placed on extinction during response elimination. Similarly, Kranak et al. (2022) conducted a proof-of-concept translational human-operant study with typically developing adults for a strategy to mitigate reacquisition: progressive ratio training. In brief, like the procedures in Woods and Bouton (2007), progressive ratio training entails exposing a target response to a progressively leaner schedule of reinforcement. Kranak et al. (2022) exposed a target response to a geometric progressive ratio schedule and paired that schedule with a discriminative stimulus. During their reacquisition test, reacquisition was less prevalent, and when it did occur, it occurred at lower rates when the stimulus paired with progressive ratio schedule was present compared to when it was absent. The results of Kranak et al. (2022) are promising but should be taken with caution, as that study was not conducted with relevant populations (e.g., individuals with intellectual and developmental disabilities) or topographies of behavior (e.g., aggression). Fortunately, our group is continuing work on progressive ratio training. At the time this chapter is being written, we are conducting a translational clinical trial (i.e., using proxy responses) to further validate progressive ratio training and move it closer to the applied end of the basic-translational-applied continuum by replicating and extending Kranak et al. (2022) with individuals with intellectual and developmental disabilities who engage in problem behavior, and the results are encouraging (Kranak, 2024–2026).

When planning for treatment to be implemented in an individual's natural environment by less-specialized intervention agents (e.g., caregivers), clinicians train those intervention agents on the treatment protocol, often with empirically validated training methods (e.g., behavioral skills training or BST; Schaefer & Andzik, 2021). Unfortunately, a difficult truth is that even after training caregivers to implement their loved one's treatment with high fidelity, it is very likely that commission errors are going to occur (Suess et al., 2014). For example, we analyzed a cohort of 304 caregivers trained using BST on their child's treatment plan, which largely consisted of functional communication training. Even after caregivers were trained to mastery, 88% (269 out of 304) of caregivers still made commission errors.

Because commission errors are very likely to occur in real-world settings, reacquisition is also very likely to occur in clinical practice. Although the true prevalence and other phenomenological aspects of reacquisition remain unknown (see Kranak & Falligant, 2023), researchers have documented substantial evidence surrounding the scope and characteristics of resurgence and renewal. To our knowledge, at this time, there have been at least 15 large-scale studies in which researchers have quantified and analyzed characteristics of resurgence and renewal (Briggs et al., 2018; Falligant et al., 2021, 2022, 2024; Haney et al., 2022; Kranak & Falligant, 2021; Laureano et al., 2024; Marshall et al., 2024; Mitteer et al., 2022; Muething et al., 2020, 2021, 2022; 2024; Podlesnik et al., 2024; Strohmeier et al., 2024). Collectively, the results of these studies indicate that relapse—specifically resurgence or renewal—occurs in majority of cases and applications of functional communication training, irrespective of function, setting, or topography. Considering the general commonality of documented prevalence estimates, it is therefore reasonable to posit that reacquisition also happens in majority of cases and applications of behavioral treatments like functional communication. This is especially reasonable given the likelihood of commission errors.

As discussed, currently, the two best ways for clinicians to prevent reacquisition of problem behavior are to (1) maintain high, near-perfect levels of procedural fidelity and (2) mitigate other forms of relapse. As work in this area continues, hopefully there will soon be a specific strategy for reacquisition mitigation that is validated and shown to be effective with problem behavior. Until then, we encourage readers to continue to implement treatment with as high procedural fidelity as possible and to be vigilant when other forms of relapse occur such that commission errors do not happen, leading to reacquisition and exacerbated relapse.

Conclusion

The reacquisition of problem behavior is a significant concern in behavioral interventions, particularly due to the prevalence of procedural fidelity errors. We know that this phenomenon is likely to occur under specific conditions, such as following operant renewal and resurgence. Additionally, translational research suggests that effective interventions will likely target the discriminative function of the reinforcement event by programming similarly unexpected reinforcer deliveries amidst prolonged periods of nonreinforcement. However, there are still several unknowns in this area. It remains unclear whether reacquisition is functionally different from response-dependent reinstatement, its overall prevalence, and what additional mitigation tactics might be effective.

Acknowledgments Chapter preparation was partially supported by grants 1R21HD113881-01, 1R21HD112724-01A1, and 1R21HD113794-01A1 from the National Institute of Child Health and Human Development (NICHD), as well as a NARSAD Young Investigator Grant from the Brain and Behavior Research Foundation (BBRF). The content is solely the responsibility of the authors and does not necessarily reflect the official views of the NICHD or BBRF.

References

Arkoosh, M. K., Derby, K. M., Wacker, D. P., Berg, W., McLaughlin, T. F., & Barretto, A. (2007). A descriptive evaluation of long-term treatment integrity. *Behavior Modification, 31*(6), 880–895. https://doi.org/10.1177/0145445507302254

Bernal-Gamboa, R., Almaguer-Azpeitia, M., Carreón, D., Nieto, J., & Uengoer, M. (2021). Positive affective states can play the role of context to renew extinguished instrumental behavior in rats. *Behavioural Processes, 187*, 104376.

Briggs, A. M., Fisher, W. W., Greer, B. D., & Kimball, R. T. (2018). Prevalence of resurgence of destructive behaviors when thinning reinforcement schedules during functional communication training. *Journal of Applied Behavior Analysis, 51*(3), 620–633. https://doi.org/10.1002/jaba.472

Falligant, J. M., Kranak, M. P., McNulty, M. K., Schmidt, J. D., Hausman, N. L., & Rooker, G. W. (2021). Prevalence of renewal of problem behavior: Replication and extension to an inpatient setting. *Journal of Applied Behavior Analysis, 54*(1), 367–373.

Falligant, J. M., Chin, M. D., & Kurtz, P. F. (2022). Renewal and resurgence of severe problem behavior in an intensive outpatient setting: Prevalence, magnitude, and implications for practice. *Behavioral Interventions, 37*(3), 909–924. https://doi.org/10.1002/bin.1878

Falligant, J. M., Kranak, M. P., Piersma, D. E., Benson, R., Schmidt, J. D., & Frank-Crawford, M. A. (2024). Further evidence of renewal in automatically maintained behavior. *Journal of Applied Behavior Analysis, 57*(2), 490–501. https://doi.org/10.1002/jaba.1055

Foreman, A. P., St. Peter, C. C., Mesches, G. A., Robinson, N., & Romano, L. M. (2021). Treatment integrity failures during timeout from play. *Behavior Modification, 45*(6), 988–1010. https://doi.org/10.1177/0145445520935392

Fryling, M. J., Wallace, M. D., & Yassine, J. N. (2012). Impact of treatment integrity on intervention effectiveness. *Journal of Applied Behavior Analysis, 45(*2), 449–453. https://doi.org/10.1901/jaba.2012.45-449

Fuhrman, A. M., Greer, B. D., Zangrillo, A. N., & Fisher, W. W. (2018). Evaluating competing activities to enhance functional communication training during reinforcement schedule thinning. *Journal of Applied Behavior Analysis, 51*(4), 931–942. https://doi.org/10.1002/jaba.486

Greer, B. D., Fisher, W. W., Briggs, A. M., Lichtblau, K. R., Phillips, L. A., & Mitteer, D. R. (2019). Using schedule-correlated stimuli during functional communication training to promote the rapid transfer of treatment effects. *Behavioral Development, 24*(2), 100–119. https://doi.org/10.1037/bdb0000085

Han, J. B., Bergmann, S., Brand, D., Wallace, M. D., St Peter, C. C., Feng, J., & Long, B. P. (2023). Trends in reporting procedural integrity: A comparison. *Behavior Analysis in Practice, 16*(2), 388–398. https://doi.org/10.1007/s40617-022-00741-5

Haney, S. D., Greer, B. D., Mitteer, D. R., & Randall, K. R. (2022). Relapse during the treatment of pediatric feeding disorders. *Journal of Applied Behavior Analysis, 55*(3), 704–726. https://doi.org/10.1002/jaba.913

Jones, S. H., & St. Peter, C. C. (2022). Nominally acceptable integrity failures negatively affect interventions involving intermittent reinforcement. *Journal of Applied Behavior Analysis, 55*(4), 1109–1123. https://doi.org/10.1002/jaba.944

Kimball, R. T., & Kranak, M. P. (2022). Six things practitioners should know about renewal. *Education & Treatment of Children, 45*(4), 395–410. https://doi.org/10.1007/s43494-022-00078-2

Kimball, R. T., Greer, B. D., Fuhrman, A. M., & Lambert, J. M. (2023a). Relapse and its mitigation: Toward behavioral inoculation. *Journal of Applied Behavior Analysis, 56*(2), 282–301. https://doi.org/10.1002/jaba.971

Kimball, R. T., Salvetti, E. L., Day, L. E., Karis, R., Silveira, J., & Kranak, M. P. (2023b). Operant ABA renewal during dense and lean schedules of differential reinforcement. *Journal of the Experimental Analysis of Behavior, 119*(3), 529–538. https://doi.org/10.1002/jeab.840

Kranak, M. P. (Principal Investigator). (2024–2026). *Using behavioral economics to mitigate relapse of problem behavior in an intellectual and developmental disabilities population* (Project No. 1R21HD113794-01A1) [Grant]. Eunice Kennedy Shriver National Institute of Child Health and Human Development. https://reporter.nih.gov/search/NtVOxAtaRUenSbIZ4Vk6bA/project-details/10986782

Kranak, M. P., & Falligant, J. M. (2021). Further investigation of resurgence following schedule thinning: Extension to an inpatient setting. *Behavioral Interventions, 36*(4), 1003–1012. https://doi.org/10.1002/bin.1831

Kranak, M., & Falligant, J. M. (2023). Treatment integrity, commission errors, and reinstatement: A primer. *Education and Treatment of Children, 46*(3), 249–262. https://doi.org/10.1007/s43494-023-00104-x

Kranak, M. P., & Brown, K. R. (2024). Updated recommendations for reinforcement schedule thinning following functional communication training. *Behavior Analysis in Practice, 17*(1), 87–106. https://doi.org/10.1007/s40617-023-00863-4

Kranak, M. P., Rooker, G. W., Arevalo, A. R., & Robinson, T. P. (2022). Mitigating reinstatement using progressive ratio schedules: A proof of concept. *Behavioral Development, 27*(1–2), 21–34. https://doi.org/10.1037/bdb0000108

Lattal, K. A., Cançado, C. R. X., Cook, J. E., Kincaid, S. L., Nighbor, T. D., & Oliver, A. C. (2017). On defining resurgence. *Behavioural Processes, 141(Pt 1)*, 85–91. https://doi.org/10.1016/j.beproc.2017.04.018

Laureano, B., Ringdahl, J., & Falligant, J. M. (2024). Examination of clinical variables affecting resurgence: A reanalysis of 46 applications. *Journal of Applied Behavior Analysis, 57*(3), 742–750. https://doi.org/10.1002/jaba.1091

Mace, F. C., & Nevin, J. A. (2017). Maintenance, generalization, and treatment relapse: A behavioral momentum analysis. *Education & Treatment of Children, 40*(1), 27–42. https://doi.org/10.1353/etc.2017.0001

Marshall, A. R., Mitteer, D. R., Greer, B. D., & Kishel, C. B. (2024). On the prevalence and magnitude of resurgence during delay-and-denial tolerance teaching. *Journal of Applied Behavior Analysis, 58*(1), 151–163. https://doi.org/10.1002/jaba.2930

Mitteer, D. R., Greer, B. D., Randall, K. R., Kimball, R. T., & Smith, S. W. (2021). Empirically deriving omission and commission errors for relapse tests: A demonstration of reverse translation. *Behavior Analysis: Research and Practice, 21*(4), 351–363. https://doi.org/10.1037/bar0000218

Mitteer, D. R., Greer, B. D., Randall, K. R., & Haney, S. D. (2022). On the scope and characteristics of relapse when treating severe destructive behavior. *Journal of Applied Behavior Analysis, 55*(3), 688–703. https://doi.org/10.1002/jaba.912

Muething, C., Call, N., Pavlov, A., Ringdahl, J., Gillespie, S., Clark, S., & Mevers, J. L. (2020). Prevalence of renewal of problem behavior during context changes. *Journal of Applied Behavior Analysis, 53*(3), 1485–1493. https://doi.org/10.1002/jaba.672

Muething, C., Pavlov, A., Call, N., Ringdahl, J., & Gillespie, S. (2021). Prevalence of resurgence during thinning of multiple schedules of reinforcement following functional communication training. *Journal of Applied Behavior Analysis, 54*(2), 813–823. https://doi.org/10.1002/jaba.791

Muething, C., Call, N., Ritchey, C. M., Pavlov, A., Bernstein, A. M., & Podlesnik, C. A. (2022). Prevalence of relapse of automatically maintained behavior resulting from context changes. *Journal of Applied Behavior Analysis, 55*(1), 138–153. https://doi.org/10.1002/jaba.887

Muething, C. S., Call, N., Ritchey, C. M., Pavlov, A., Bernstein, A. M., & Podlesnik, C. A. (2024). Prevalence of relapse of automatically maintained behavior resulting from context changes. *Journal of Applied Behavior Analysis, 55*(1), 138–153. https://doi.org/10.1002/jaba.887

Podlesnik, C. A., & Shahan, T. A. (2009). Behavioral momentum and relapse of extinguished operant responding. *Learning & Behavior, 37*(4), 357–364. https://doi.org/10.3758/LB.37.4.357

Podlesnik, C. A., & Kelley, M. E. (2015). Translational research on the relapse of operant behavior. *Revista Mexicana de Análisis de la Conducta, 41*(2), 226–251. https://doi.org/10.5514/rmac.v41.i2.63774

Podlesnik, C. A., Ritchey, C. M., Waits, J., & Gilroy, S. P. (2023). A comprehensive systematic review of procedures and analyses used in basic and preclinical studies of resurgence, 1970-2020. *Perspectives on Behavior Science, 46*(1), 137–184. https://doi.org/10.1007/s40614-022-00361-y

Podlesnik, C. A., Ritchey, C. M., Muething, C., & Falligant, J. M. (2024). Different criteria affect prevalence of relapse of behavior targeted for treatment. *Journal of Applied Behavior Analysis, 58*(1), 225–231. https://doi.org/10.1002/jaba.2927

Saini, V., & Mitteer, D. R. (2020). A review of investigations of operant renewal with human participants: Implications for theory and practice. *Journal of the Experimental Analysis of Behavior, 113*(1), 105–123. https://doi.org/10.1002/jeab.562

Schaefer, J. M., & Andzik, N. R. (2021). Evaluating behavioral skills training as an evidencebased practice when training parents to intervene with their children. *Behavior Modification, 45*(6), 887–910. https://doi.org/10.1177/0145445520923996

St. Peter, C. C., Brand, D., Jones, S. H., Wolgermuth, J. R., & Lipien, L. (2023). On a persisting curious double standard in behavior analysis: Behavioral scholars' perspectives on procedural integrity. *Journal of Applied Behavior Analysis, 56*(2), 336–351. https://doi.org/10.1002/jaba.974

Strohmeier, C. W., Cengher, M., Chin, M. D., & Falligant, J. M. (2024). Application of a terminal schedule probe method to inform schedule thinning with multiple schedules. *Journal of Applied Behavior Analysis, 57*(3), 676–694. https://doi.org/10.1002/jaba.1081

Suess, A. N., Romani, P. W., Wacker, D. P., Dyson, S. M., Kuhle, J. L., Lee, J. F., Lindgren, S. D., Kopelman, T. G., Pelzel, K. E., Waldron, D. B., & Waldron, D. B. (2014). Evaluating the treatment fidelity of parents who conduct in-home functional communication with coaching via telehealth. *Journal of Behavioral Education, 23*(1), 34–59. https://link.springer.com/article/10.1007/s10864-013-9183-3

Wacker, D. P., Schieltz, K. M., Berg, W. K., Harding, J. W., Dalmau, Y. C. P., & Lee, J. F. (2017). The long-term effects of functional communication training conducted in young children's home settings. *Education & Treatment of Children, 40*(1), 43–56. https://doi.org/10.1353/etc.2017.0003

Wathen, S. N., & Podlesnik, C. A. (2018). Laboratory models of treatment relapse and mitigation techniques. *Behavior Analysis: Research and Practice, 18*(4), 362–387. https://doi.org/10.1037/bar0000119

Woods, A. M., & Bouton, M. E. (2007). Occasional reinforced responses during extinction can slow the rate of reacquisition of an operant response. *Learning and Motivation, 38*(1), 56–74. https://doi.org/10.1016/j.lmot.2006.07.003

Chapter 7
Promoting Long-Term Behavior Change for Children with Autism and Feeding Difficulties

Emma M. Auten, Kathryn M. Peterson, and Jaime Crowley-Zalaket

Eating ensures individuals meet their needs through various physiological and biochemical processes (Gahagan, 2012). Everyone has different routines around mealtimes, such as eating with family or in certain locations, adhering to cultural or religious practices, or displaying preferences for certain combinations of foods. Eating evolves across the lifespan, beginning with breast- or bottle-feeding at birth and progressing to solid foods later in childhood (Carruth et al., 2004). Infants may experience feeding difficulties early in life, including poor latch, prolonged feeding times, impairments in sucking or swallowing, and insufficient milk intake (McGrattan et al., 2024). As children age, other feeding challenges may emerge. Commonly, children have "picky eating" phases. During these phases, children may be more selective with food choices and exhibit moderate challenging behavior or food refusal. These behaviors usually resolve with age and without direct intervention. However, other feeding difficulties can emerge for some children, including persistent inappropriate mealtime behaviors (e.g., tantrums), selective eating (i.e., only eating a few foods), failing to advance to higher or mixed textures (e.g., purees to table texture), frequent vomiting, inability to self-feed, oral-motor dysfunction, total food refusal, or a combination of these (Kerwin, 1999).

Kathryn Peterson is now at the Marcus Autism Center and Emory University.

E. M. Auten · K. M. Peterson (✉)
Children's Specialized Hospital, Somerset, NJ, USA

Division of Child Neurology and Neurodevelopmental Disabilities, Rutgers Robert Wood Johnson Medical School, New Brunswick, NJ, USA
e-mail: kathryn.peterson@choa.org

J. Crowley-Zalaket
Children's Specialized Hospital, Somerset, NJ, USA

M. P. Kranak (ed.), *Behavioral Treatments for Individuals with Autism*, Autism and Child Psychopathology Series,
https://doi.org/10.1007/978-3-031-91965-7_7

Studies have reported that children with autism spectrum disorder (ASD) do not consume as many vegetables as typically developing children and may primarily consume non-nutritious or "snack" foods (Evans et al., 2012). In particular, children with ASD mostly consume foods that are high in sodium, fat, or sugar (e.g., chips, fast food, candy) or rely on sweetened drinks for hydration (e.g., juice or soda; Hubbard et al., 2014; Volkert et al., 2016). Studies show that feeding difficulties are more prevalent among children with ASD than for children who are neurotypical (Schreck et al., 2004). Feeding difficulties among children with ASD have been linked to a core symptom of ASD—restricted, repetitive patterns of behavior. More specifically, children with ASD may engage in insistence on sameness, inflexible adherence to routines, or ritualized behavior patterns. In the context of eating, this might present as eating the same food every day, only consuming specific brands of food or foods from certain restaurants, or developing certain mealtime routines with an inability to adapt to change (Hubbard et al., 2014). Thus, children with ASD and feeding difficulties have been categorized as engaging in *change-resistant feeding behavior* (Crowley et al., 2020).

Change-resistant feeding behavior becomes problematic when it impedes growth (e.g., child does not meet energy, hydration, or nutritional needs) or results in inflexible or stressful mealtime practices (e.g., eating at home and never at school). For example, some children may refuse to eat a food unless it is prepared in a specific and familiar manner. Others may become dependent on supplemental nutrition, like expensive formulas (e.g., PediaSure®). Not only are formulas like PediaSure costly when purchased for frequent intake, but costs for the family could rise exponentially if the child is dependent on that formula to meet all of their nutrition and hydration needs (Ramstack & Listernick, 1991). For example, a 13-year-old child could require up to five bottles of formula per day to meet their calorie needs if they only consumed this one item during all meals. Although some insurance companies provide coverage for tube feedings (e.g., gastrostomy tube), there may not be insurance coverage for children who consume supplemental nutritional drinks by mouth (https://www.medicare.gov/). Further, changes in brand or availability of these nutritional sources may cause problems. During the COVID-19 pandemic, breakdowns in supply chains caused delays, shortages, and inconsistent availability of certain foods and beverages (Barman et al., 2021). In many cases, these circumstances left families unable to find or purchase necessary items. Notably, children with feeding difficulties often do not consume alternatives or "eat when they are hungry." Thus, inflexibility with mealtime routines can be detrimental to health in numerous ways.

Feeding challenges also may be underdiagnosed in this population if the child is growing properly or the family has other pressing goals (e.g., dangerous self-injurious behavior) on which to focus. Some children with feeding difficulties have complex medical histories or oral-motor deficits, while others appear to have primarily *behavioral* challenges. We use the term "feeding difficulties" more broadly to refer to the persistent and problematic feeding challenges that are displayed by individuals with ASD that may or may not be associated with underlying medical factors, skill deficits, or a formal feeding disorder diagnosis. Regardless of the topography or etiology, feeding difficulties present many concerns that warrant attention. Practitioners may consider severe food refusal as one form of self-injurious behavior, given that engaging in extreme food refusal can lead to physical injury, harm, or death in severe cases (Volkert & Piazza, 2012).

This chapter provides an outline for treatment of challenging mealtime behavior for children and adolescents with ASD. Another goal is to introduce practical recommendations for *long-term* behavior change. As such, we outline safety considerations for treating feeding difficulties, empirically supported behavior-change procedures, and discuss relapse during treatment for feeding disorders. Finally, we discuss practical ways to mitigate relapse of challenging mealtime behavior and review areas that warrant additional research.

Promoting Safety

Behavior analysts are likely to work with children with ASD that have some form of feeding difficulty, given the high prevalence among this population. Practitioners may be faced with determining their scope of competence for treating a child with feeding difficulties (Peterson et al., 2024). Therefore, when treating children with feeding difficulties, the first step to promoting long-term behavior change should be to ensure child safety and practitioner competency.

Although some children do not present with apparent health risks or medical conditions (Peterson et al., 2022), there may be masked health problems that arise or become apparent during treatment. For example, a child who has refused most foods may have unknown food allergies that do not appear until practitioners first expose the child to an offensive food (i.e., allergen). A child who is bottle-dependent may display swallow dysfunction when presented with the opportunity to drink thin liquids from an open cup. Thus, the first step to ensuring children are appropriate for feeding intervention is to seek approval/authorization from the child's medical team.

Medical providers should confirm that a child is medically stable for treatment and that there are no underlying medical conditions that may be contributing to the child's feeding difficulty. Physicians can determine whether additional medical tests or follow-up is necessary to minimize the likelihood of adverse reactions during treatment (e.g., unknown allergies, reflux). In addition, practitioners should always ensure that a child is a safe oral feeder by confirming with a professional who possesses pediatric swallow-safety expertise (e.g., speech-language pathologist). These experts may conduct bedside observations of a child eating or additional assessments, such as a modified barium swallow study. Behavior analysts should follow the recommendations of these experts regarding various meal components (e.g., changes to meal volume, bite or drink size, bite or drink pacing). Some children may engage in total refusal before treatment, resulting in inconclusive observations or swallow study results. Therefore, it is important in these situations that practitioners are trained to identify appropriate starting points and to detect signs that a child may be mismanaging solids or liquids and work closely with other providers.

Children who are medically cleared for treatment may still develop or display concerning behaviors in the course of treatment, such as inadequate chewing or swallowing. Others may engage in more challenging or maladaptive behavior (e.g., aggression, property destruction) as feeding demands increase. Consider the following example. A child (Edward) is an individual with ASD who eats a few foods/drinks across food groups (e.g., goldfish, crackers, pizza, milk, juice). Although Edward consumes a small range of different foods, his caregivers report that he will not try new foods, refuses to eat preferred foods if they are prepared differently, and has no fruits, vegetables, or healthy proteins in his diet. Edward's caregivers are interested in helping Edward eat a range of healthy foods to improve his nutrition and reduce mealtime rigidity. Edward's medical team identified no ongoing concerns and deemed him appropriate for feeding therapy. The behavior analyst and speech-language pathologist observed Edward engage in appropriate chewing with his preferred foods at the onset of treatment. Therefore, Edward was approved to start feeding treatment. Soon after treatment began, Edward started to engage in unsafe feeding behavior like mashing food on the roof of his mouth, overstuffing his mouth with food, and early swallowing (e.g., swallowing before chewing). All of these behaviors increased the risk of aspiration or choking and could indicate that Edward requires additional skill-building opportunities with target foods.

It is important to note that children who appear to manage food safely may engage in new or unexpected behaviors when challenged with different foods. Unsafe behaviors may occur with nonpreferred food to escape the bite or drink (e.g., not chewing broccoli to avoid the taste) or due to a history of limited practice with higher-textured foods (e.g., only consuming soft, meltable foods like crackers). Given the many safety considerations that are involved when working with children with ASD and feeding difficulties, behavior analysts should ensure they adhere to the Behavior Analyst Certification Board® (BACB®) Ethics code (BACB, 2020) and seek additional supervision to develop competence in this area from experienced providers. Further, providers should continue to collaborate and work with other disciplines to provide safe and comprehensive care.

Competency is also necessary to select and design appropriate interventions across different populations. As an additional example, a child (Sarah) chews her foods appropriately and has no recorded history of underlying medical problems. A behavior analyst consults the scientific literature and identifies simultaneous presentation as an antecedent-based treatment to introduce novel foods. However, even an antecedent-based strategy such as simultaneous presentation, which involves presenting pairings of a child's preferred food (e.g., pizza) with a target food (e.g., ham), may pose risks. If the child does not chew appropriately across all textures, the bite size of combined foods could be too large or too difficult to manage. Practitioners with little training on oral-motor skills and no supervision may not recognize when a child mismanages food. If repeated pairings of a preferred food with a nonpreferred food result in the child beginning to refuse their preferred foods, it could result in further limitations to the child's diet. Thus, for Sarah, the loss of her main source of protein and carbohydrates (i.e., pizza) could result in detrimental health effects. A practitioner with limited experience with food selectivity may lack the training and expertise to identify these risks as well as other effective interventions or solutions if the initial intervention is ineffective. The consequences of ineffective interventions are serious for this population. Weight loss and health effects can occur quickly, and the referral process to other providers is often lengthy (Sharp et al., 2024). Working with a multi- or interdisciplinary team helps ensure that a patient is receiving safe and complete care.

In addition to ensuring competency and medical/safety clearance, behavior analysts should consider several other steps before implementing an intervention to ensure they do not inadvertently worsen the feeding problems. First, practitioners should gather necessary resources, like a variety of safe seating options that can aid children in maintaining upright posture for an open airway. Practitioners should identify clean and hygienic spaces for which to conduct mealtime treatments and establish consistent food preparation protocols. It is important for practitioners to maintain consistency in food preparation to minimize the likelihood that errors could affect safety (e.g., heating a food in the microwave to unsafe temperatures, inadvertently presenting a texture that is too challenging for the child).

Practitioners also should ensure children have the appropriate prerequisite skills to begin feeding intervention. An initial goal could be for children to transition to the meal calmly and sit safely for the duration of the meal (e.g., 30–40 min). If a child is unable to sit during the mealtime, practitioners could target cooperation with sitting (e.g., feeding-chair fading) before feeding treatment. Practitioners should also be encouraged to regularly consult the scientific literature and seek professional development opportunities for updates to evidence-based assessment and treatment strategies. In cases in which the practitioner encounters unexpected challenges, they should refer the child to a provider with the appropriate expertise or seek consultative opportunities.

Day-Treatment Model

Intensive multidisciplinary programs delivered in a day-treatment or hospital setting are considered best practice for the assessment and treatment of pediatric feeding disorders (Sharp et al., 2017). Sharp et al. (2024) identified 16 day-treatment programs that operate within the United States and found that the primary interventions were behavioral treatments. Although the structure of day-treatment models may differ across sites, many have similar components. If a child is identified as potentially appropriate for the program, families are invited to an initial evaluation screening. During this time, the clinical team conducts structured and unstructured observations of the caregivers feeding their child to observe putative antecedents and consequences of the child's refusal behavior, such as caregiver-provided attention or escape. In addition, the team of providers assesses the child's oral-motor safety and reviews the child's complete feeding, medical, and oral-motor history to identify whether there are risks.

Based on the evaluation, the team of providers will make referrals for children to participate in feeding intervention if there are no concerns of safety or medical risk. Highly trained practitioners work with the other members of the multidisciplinary team (e.g., dieticians, gastroenterologists, speech therapists) to ensure child safety throughout the admission and to target specific feeding goals. After an effective intervention has been identified, the team begins to progress the child toward becoming a developmentally typical eater. That is, practitioners use an individualized and systematic approach to build upon the child's initial foundational skills. After a child meets their goals during day-treatment programs, children, ideally, would transition to follow-up services. Some programs refer to other community-based providers for follow-up services, while others maintain their own follow-up clients. During follow-up visits, the treatment team might focus on maintaining the child's initial progress while the child transitions to other settings (e.g., home, school) and eats with other people (e.g., caregivers, teachers, siblings). The team also focuses on skill building to increase mealtime flexibility (e.g., exposure to and practice with a variety of foods, brands, and textures). The terminal goal for children with feeding difficulties is to eat like same-age peers and meet their energy, nutrition, and hydration needs orally. Behavior-analytic treatments are the most effective interventions for accomplishing these goals (Kerwin, 1999; Volkert et al., 2016).

Empirically Supported Treatments

In general, behavior analysts develop goals to decrease *inappropriate mealtime behavior* (IMB), typically defined as behaviors that prevent the individual or feeder from depositing food or liquid into the mouth. These behaviors could include interfering behaviors such as batting the utensil away, covering the mouth, or turning one's head. Goals are also set to increase *acceptance* of target foods and liquids, defined as opening the mouth within a specific time criterion (e.g., 5 s) that allows the deposit of food or liquid (Piazza et al., 2003; Volkert & Piazza, 2012). Other challenging behaviors that often emerge throughout treatment include *expulsion,* defined as food or liquid exiting the mouth (not due to swallowing or vomiting). *Packing* occurs when individuals hold food or liquid in the oral cavity for extended periods (Patel, 2013). IMB, expel, and packing are all behaviors that may contact reinforcement, such as escape from the bite or drink, and be strengthened over time.

Behavior analysts conduct assessments before treatment to help identify the conditions during which problematic behavior may occur. Behavior analysts then arrange a functional analysis (Bachmeyer, 2009; Piazza et al., 2003) to deliver various consequences (e.g., tangible, attention, escape from the bite/drink) contingent on IMB and test which consequences may function as reinforcement. Kirkwood et al. (2021) showed that function-based treatments were more effective at reducing IMB than non-function-based treatments. Thus, interventions tailored to the individual and the maintaining consequences of their IMB are important for designing treatment plans.

Other assessments can also inform treatment. Even if a practitioner does not conduct a functional analysis, antecedent- or reinforcement-based assessment tools can be helpful to identify appropriate interventions and starting points. For example, Peterson et al. (2024) implemented a demand-fading and simultaneous-presentation treatment for two children with ASD and feeding difficulties. Before treatment, researchers conducted a demand hierarchy assessment to identify what steps the children would cooperate with in the absence of intervention (i.e., to identify a starting step for treatment). The researchers randomized steps of the response chain for eating, such as picking up the spoon, placing the bite in the mouth, chewing once, or chewing six times. Researchers selected the step in the chain that was most advanced (closest to the terminal response of eating) for which there was no challenging behavior and began a fading intervention at that step. The intervention involved reinforcing cooperation with eating steps until eventually, the children consumed bites of target foods. Additional research is warranted to continue to expand on assessment methodology, such as identifying effective interventions for expulsion or packing.

Outside of function-based treatment, there is a growing body of support for arbitrarily selected antecedent- and consequence-based interventions (Bachmeyer, 2009; Williams & Seiverling, 2023). Williams and Seiverling (2023) reviewed the behavior-analytic literature to identify advancements and the current state of the science for treatments for feeding difficulties. Some recent advancements in antecedent-based interventions included modeling (Hillman, 2019; O'Connor et al. 2020), stimulus fading (Patel et al., 2001), simultaneous presentation (Cho & Sonoyama, 2020; Peterson et al., 2024), utensil manipulations (Wilkins et al., 2014), and use of a high-probability instructional sequence (Patel et al., 2007). Consequence-based procedures included differential reinforcement (Berth et al., 2019; Patel et al., 2002), noncontingent access to preferred items/attention (Wilder et al., 2005), and nonremoval of the spoon (Peterson et al., 2018; Piazza et al., 2003).

Many studies have shown that one specific consequence-based procedure has been identified as the most effective for reducing IMB (Patel et al., 2002; Rivas et al., 2010). *Escape extinction* (EE) is a treatment used to reduce IMB after functional analysis results indicate that IMB is likely socially maintained through negative reinforcement (i.e., escape from the bite or drink). *Nonremoval of the spoon* is one type of extinction-based intervention during which the utensil is no longer removed contingent on IMB and remains at the lips. Patel et al. (2002) compared differential reinforcement of acceptance to differential reinforcement of mouth clean but found consumption only increased to high and stable levels once therapists added EE to the treatment package. The children in Patel et al. engaged in total food refusal, thus, they may have had few opportunities to contact the reinforcement contingencies in the absence of escape extinction. Similarly, Crowley et al. (2020) found that nonremoval of the spoon was necessary to increase consumption of novel foods for five of seven children with ASD and food selectivity. Intervention components were added sequentially, and the majority of children did not consume novel foods with differential reinforcement as an isolated intervention for consumption but did consume novel foods once exposed to nonremoval of the spoon. Ultimately, treatments for feeding difficulties should be individualized, assessment-informed, and guided by evidence as well as caregiver input.

Although many studies have shown that EE is effective at reducing IMB and increasing acceptance, researchers have cited temporary though undesirable side effects that include emotional responding (e.g., crying) or extinction bursts (Woods & Borrero, 2019). Another concern is the presumed difficulty associated with maintaining high levels of treatment fidelity that are likely necessary for the intervention to be optimally effective (Bachmeyer, 2009), especially for children who are older or larger in stature. Additional research is necessary to evaluate these concerns systematically with appropriate designs and study arrangements. To date, there has been no empirical evidence to suggest escape extinction procedures are less feasible with older individuals or are ineffective when implemented with reduced integrity. In addition, some research has shown that extinction bursts and emotional responding are less common than previously reported (Engler et al., 2023; Woods & Borrero, 2019). Thus, researchers should consider collecting more data on the feasibility of implementing extinction-based procedures, especially given that this treatment is highly effective and can be lifesaving for children with severe and pervasive feeding challenges.

Another reason that researchers should continue investigating extinction-based procedures is to better understand its long-term effects. Research has demonstrated robust and immediate outcomes following exposure to EE, but less is known about what happens for children with feeding difficulties after intensive treatment ends. Only a few studies have demonstrated that changes in feeding behavior maintained over time and resulted in long-lasting improvements to diet and health (e.g., Andersen et al., 2024; Sharp et al., 2017). However, there are many factors that could impede a child's ability to maintain skills or treatment gains over time. Eating is a behavior that must persist throughout the lifetime and must occur across many changing contexts (e.g., different people, settings, foods). Caregiver integrity with treatment protocols may drift and result in the child's challenging behavior returning. Additionally, it is not uncommon for challenging behavior to reemerge due to relapse (Haney et al., 2022; Ibañez et al., 2019). Relapse could include the recurrence of IMB, expulsion, packing, or other problematic behavior that was reduced during treatment.

Relapse of Inappropriate Mealtime Behavior

Treatment relapse is a well-studied phenomenon in behavior-analytic research (e.g., Kimball et al., 2023; Mitteer et al., 2022; Shahan, 2020). However, there have been fewer evaluations of the relapse of IMB (e.g., Haney et al., 2021, 2022; Ibañez et al., 2019; Kelley et al., 2018). Overall, IMB returning is problematic given that its occurrence often interferes with food or drink consumption and may persist if it contacts continued escape from the bite or drink.

Resurgence is one type of treatment relapse that occurs when a previously extinguished response (such as IMB) reoccurs following a degradation in reinforcement for the alternative response (e.g., quality, rate, magnitude). In basic and applied studies, resurgence is usually evaluated using a three-phase arrangement. During Phase 1, a target behavior (e.g., IMB) is reinforced. During Phase 2, the target behavior is placed on extinction and an alternative behavior is reinforced (e.g., bite or drink acceptance). During Phase 3, the alternative behavior is placed on extinction and resurgence is hypothesized to occur when the target behavior increases during this third phase (Sweeney & Shahan, 2013).

Resurgence of IMB may occur due to integrity errors. For example, a feeder that fails to provide reinforcement contingent on acceptance of the target bite may observe resurgence of IMB. Clinically, during follow-up services (after intensive treatment ends and the child and family are home conducting treatment independently), we often observe a number of treatment integrity errors and drift. For example, we might see that caregivers stop providing enthusiastic praise for each instance of bite acceptance or are simultaneously attending to other children or responsibilities. They may also inadvertently thin the reinforcement schedule or change the response effort by presenting multiple bite presentations without pausing to provide reinforcement or praise.

Feeding interventions, like other behavior-analytic treatments, often require a high level of response effort on the part of the caregivers. Integrity errors are likely affected by negative reinforcement (i.e., caregiver avoids child's vocal protests by using mostly preferred foods). Mitteer et al. (2018) studied caregiver errors and methods for increasing treatment adherence for severe challenging behavior, but more research is needed on caregiver behavior and integrity with implementing feeding interventions. In addition, researchers should continue to identify ways to make treatments feasible and ecologically valid so they can be implemented in the natural environment.

Resurgence may also be conceptualized as a worsening of conditions for the alternative response due to increased response effort rather than decreased reinforcement quality (Haney et al., 2022). In the basic literature, response effort has been defined as manipulating the effort associated with a response in terms of the physical force that is required to make the response, such as a key or lever press (Friman & Poling, 1995), or increasing the number of responses required to receive reinforcement (Williams et al., 2011). In the applied literature, response effort has been extended to other responses, including traveling a greater distance (Wilson et al., 2016), increasing the difficulty of academic tasks (Neef & Lutz, 2001), or engaging in tasks that necessitate greater precision or endurance (Walter & Dickson, 2023).

In the context of feeding treatment, researchers have conceptualized response-effort manipulations as changes (specifically, increases) to the bite/drink presentation rate (e.g., one bite every 30 s increased to one bite every 15 s), the number of bites/drinks consumed per session or meal, and the size of the bolus (Haney et al.,

2022). As an example, a practitioner may initially intervene by reinforcing acceptance of the bite or drink while extinguishing IMB. At first, the practitioner may present a level, small spoonful of pureed food during all bite presentations. After the child demonstrates success (i.e., reduction in IMB, increase in acceptance), the practitioner may attempt to increase the bolus to a heaping spoonful or a larger level spoonful. When the bolus is increased, IMB may reemerge.

Although plausible, the aforementioned examples of increased response effort cited by Haney et al. (2022) may not serve as increases in response effort for all individuals. Take the following example. To swallow one leveled spoonful of yogurt, a smooth, uniform-textured food, an individual must open to accept the bite, close their lips around the bowl of the spoon, pull the yogurt off the spoon by coordinating a sweeping and suction of the lips, and then propel the bolus back toward the pharynx to swallow. Say that after the individual successfully takes and swallows the bite of yogurt, the practitioner adds volume to the spoon for the next bite presentation (i.e., increasing from a small, level spoonful of yogurt to a heaping spoonful of yogurt). From an observer's perspective, it might be difficult to determine whether the increase in the amount of food on the spoon is tantamount to an increase in response effort. If challenging behavior re-emerges in these cases, the practitioner may be left to wonder whether more of the "aversive" stimulus is less preferred to the individual (i.e., worsening of conditions) or if more of the stimulus is "more effortful" to manage/swallow (i.e., increase in response effort).

The same could be true when evaluating different textures of foods. It may be more plausible to assume there is an increase in response effort associated with increasing the texture from a smooth, uniform consistency (e.g., applesauce) to higher or mixed textures (e.g., raw apple slice). The child will now need to lateralize the bite to the molars, engage in rotary and circular chews to break the food apart while keeping the food on the teeth, and then re-form the masticated pieces into a bolus to prepare for swallowing. Clinically, we observe that children consuming pureed foods will engage in higher levels of IMB and refuse those same foods when they are later presented in a table-textured format, even when the child does not have oral-motor skill deficits.

Although there are likely differences in response effort associated with textural variations, it is difficult to confirm a quantitative value of effort across foods or food types (e.g., meat-based proteins versus raw vegetables versus crackers versus bread). As a few examples, an individual may need to engage in additional tongue movements to successfully manage smaller pieces of dense, table-textured foods, given that pieces could be more likely to stick to the molars (e.g., chewy/leathery foods) or to the roof of the mouth (e.g., soft breads). Alternatively, it may be less effortful for an individual to manage a larger piece of meltable, table-textured food (e.g., cracker, Cheeto puff) with minimal bite pressure. The amount of effort associated with safe and appropriate management of different textures likely depends on the child's oral-motor status, history with chewing, physiology and anatomy (e.g., number of teeth), and preferences. In addition, it is difficult to predict what changes to effort (e.g., texture, size) will lead to resurgence. To the authors' knowledge, there are no standardized tools to assess the impact of these variables on resurgence of IMB among children with feeding difficulties. In many of the above examples, IMB could reemerge due to context changes (i.e., changes to size, texture) rather than an increase in response effort. That is, a recurrence of IMB could instead be conceptualized as renewal.

Renewal is another type of treatment relapse that occurs when a previously extinguished response (e.g., IMB) reoccurs following a context change (Podlesnik et al., 2017). When considering the mealtime, context changes are exceedingly common. Mealtime context changes could include changes in food (e.g., type or texture), volume (e.g., amount of food or drink presented), utensils (e.g., spoon or fork), settings (e.g., home or clinic), or feeders (e.g., caregivers, teachers), to name a few. Even small changes to the environment (e.g., background music, presence of siblings or other individuals, color of bowls/cups) can serve as context changes. These stimuli or contexts could signal to the child that reinforcement (e.g., escape) is once again available for IMB.

After successful treatment has been identified during a day-treatment program, practitioners aim to teach caregivers to implement the intervention and feed their child as a critical next step. Changing the feeder from a trained therapist to a caregiver could function as a context change for the child. Ibañez et al. (2019) tested for renewal by treating the food selectivity of three children. During the first context, caregivers served as the feeders and reinforced IMB in a simulated home setting. During the second context, treatment was implemented (i.e., extinction) in a clinical setting with a trained therapist as the feeder. During the return to the first context, extinction was implemented by the caregiver in the simulated home setting. Renewal was observed during these transitions for three children despite high levels of treatment integrity by the caregivers.

Haney et al. (2021) further demonstrated that renewal of IMB can occur when caregivers become feeders, even when those caregivers implement extinction with high levels of treatment integrity in the same clinic setting. Inappropriate mealtime behavior reemerged for two out of four participants in this study when the caregivers took over as feeders. Haney et al. also found that changes to the setting alone (i.e., clinic session room to simulated home environment) can be a context change that leads to the renewal of IMB and demonstrated this for one participant with a feeding disorder. Researchers hypothesized that the addition of new foods would evoke the renewal of IMB and evaluated this in a renewal test for one participant, however, renewal did not occur. Additional research is needed to continue to evaluate mitigation strategies for both resurgence and renewal, especially given the likelihood of changes occurring throughout a child's feeding routines and the impact these phenomena can have on feeding success.

Clinically, we observe the reemergence of IMB when we attempt to add novel foods or drinks, following the child's success with initial targeted foods or drinks. Our team has begun to systematically evaluate this phenomenon by separating the target foods into pairs according to food groups (i.e., fruits, vegetables, proteins, starches) and adding the pairs into treatment separately. Unlike Haney et al. (2021), we have observed the renewal of IMB for some children in our clinical evaluations. It is unclear if the reemergence of IMB was due to the context changes (i.e., transitioning from fruits after treating vegetables) or due to other factors (e.g., idiosyncratic food preferences across children). Overall, it appears that context changes are generally idiosyncratic. Practitioners should be cautious and prepare caregivers for the possibility of renewal while they attempt to further advance children toward developmentally appropriate feeding routines. Future researchers should also develop assessment tools to determine which context changes may be most critical to address for individuals before beginning feeding intervention.

Spontaneous recovery is a third type of relapse that occurs when an extinguished behavior re-emerges after the passage of time or a period of time away from extinction and usually occurs during the next session of extinction (Rescorla, 2004). During treatment for feeding difficulties, this could occur from one mealtime to the next mealtime (e.g., breakfast to lunch) or following a break in treatment. For example, children who are tube-dependent may receive tube feedings over the weekend and only experience intervention for their feeding difficulties at the clinic during the week. At the start of each week, practitioners may see a reemergence of IMB even if there were low levels during the previous week. To date, there are no studies that have specifically evaluated the occurrence of spontaneous recovery of IMB or identified the conditions in which it is most likely to occur.

Mitigating Relapse

Unfortunately, relapse can be detrimental to advancing a child toward developmentally appropriate feeding routines if problematic behavior reoccurs, contacts reinforcement, and is maintained over time (Haney et al., 2022). Eating is crucial for survival, learning, development, and maintaining optimal health. Eating and drinking occur across many contexts. In fact, it may be nearly impossible to hold food or liquid and the entire mealtime environment as a constant, unchanging stimulus. Therefore, an important goal of day-treatment programs should be to identify and implement methods for mitigating relapse. Below, we outline several strategies for consideration. First, we review strategies for practitioners to consider embedding in their treatment process to mitigate relapse. Next, we discuss the importance of prevention and planning.

Designing Treatment

An important aspect of designing treatment is ensuring that the mealtime context is structured and consistent and that mealtime changes are made systematically. Consistency with mealtime structure ensures that behavior change is measurable. It also ensures that behavior changes are most likely due to the intervention and not due to the influence of uncontrolled variables (e.g., the number of bites presented).

Recall that any changes in mealtime structure could function as a context change or serve as increases in response effort, which could result in relapse.

As one mitigation strategy, the authors recommend practitioners begin intervention with a consistent meal schedule in a well-controlled environment. Unless using differential negative reinforcement, it is best to keep meal termination time-based. Meal lengths should be age and developmentally appropriate. Practitioners should also structure the mealtime using consistent trial presentations that are evenly paced (e.g., 5-bite sessions with fixed-time 30-s presentation schedules). Additionally, the bite or drink size (i.e., bolus) should be held constant across trials. The easiest way to ensure consistency is to teach feeders how to measure the bolus sizes. For example, using a ruler to cut bites of table-textured foods, using a specific utensil for all presentations (e.g., small maroon spoon), and leveling the bolus (when using pureed food) or using a syringe to pull specific amounts of liquid for each drink presentation. Foods or drinks should be prepared the same way from session to session.

Training

Teaching caregivers, family members, or other providers to implement treatment protocols is vital, as these individuals will serve as feeders or meal facilitators in the natural environment (e.g., at home or school). Caregivers who are taught to implement treatment when IMB occurs at high rates may obtain relevant experience and practice, preparing them for relapse that could later occur. Alternatively, caregivers who are taught to implement treatment after IMB has contacted extinction and occurs at low rates may be less prepared to manage challenging mealtime behavior when it occurs. Pairing caregivers with extinction could mitigate the likelihood of relapse in the future. It is also an opportunity to address caregiver errors with integrity in an environment that is safe and when errors may be corrected quickly with practitioner support. Therefore, we recommend beginning training for caregivers as soon as it is safe for them to begin implementing the intervention.

Training research in feeding indicates that lengthy training procedures are not necessary for caregivers to implement extinction-based interventions with high levels of treatment integrity. Bachmeyer et al. (2020) demonstrated that caregivers can reach high levels of integrity implementing escape extinction in feeding with in vivo feedback alone. Alternatively, other researchers suggest that gradually fading caregivers into feeding sessions may mitigate renewal (Haney et al., 2021). With fading, context changes may be less discriminable to the child because changes are made incrementally. As an example, fading steps could include: (a) therapist feeds child while caregiver delivers consequence for appropriate behavior (e.g., praise bite acceptance); (b) therapist feeds child while caregiver delivers verbal instructions (e.g., "take a bite") and consequence for appropriate behavior; (c) caregiver feeds child with therapist sitting next to caregiver; and (d) therapist gradually fades distance away from caregiver and child (e.g., across table, by clinic room door, out of room). All of these steps would be implemented following predetermined fading criteria (e.g., specific level of IMB and consumption). Additional research is necessary to explore mitigation strategies during treatment of feeding difficulties and caregiver training.

Similar to explaining the risks and benefits of intervention options to caregivers, the authors recommend discussing the possibility of relapse before beginning intervention. Unpredictable context changes may occur (e.g., feeding the child in ER waiting room) or spontaneous recovery may be a factor for that child. It is important to explain the potential for relapse to caregivers and to emphasize the importance of remaining consistent with the treatment protocol. Clinically, we see that when relapse occurs, many caregivers then begin making integrity errors, either because they are not fully prepared to respond to IMB or because they believe that relapse indicates that the intervention is not working. Education on relapse and in vivo training while IMB is still occurring should be evaluated as strategies to prevent future integrity errors. We encourage practitioners to identify additional methods for making the treatment protocols as feasible as possible to minimize the likelihood that caregivers will have difficulties persisting with the treatment.

Programming for Generalization

Another consideration for treatment includes planning for generalization by training across different contexts. Research has shown that responding that contacts extinction across multiple contexts may mitigate renewal (Kimball et al., 2023). As an example, when considering food variety (i.e., different foods) as a context change (Bouton, 2019), practitioners might consider introducing greater food variety early in treatment rather than sequentially as a potential mitigation strategy when implementing extinction.

Research is needed to further understand the effects of programming common stimuli across contexts as one method of generalization (e.g., Haney et al., 2021). For example, during mitigation, Haney et al. (2021) incorporated items from the child's home mealtime environment (e.g., plant, lamp, centerpiece) into the clinic treatment room during extinction to create context similarity. Haney et al. also projected an image of the child's home mealtime environment on the wall in the clinic treatment room during extinction sessions. Our team has used similar strategies during clinical evaluations to create context similarity. For one child with a severe feeding disorder and ASD, we successfully increased his consumption of 16 target foods in the clinic setting using extinction-based treatment. For half of those foods (eight foods), whenever we conducted treatment, we also projected an image of his home (where meals occur) on the wall of the treatment room, with the goal of pairing effective treatment with home-related stimuli. Next, we asked his mother to present all 16 foods to him at home, but without treatment in place. Interestingly, the child only consumed the eight foods at home that we had previously paired with the home-projected image and did not consume the other eight foods. The findings of that clinical evaluation suggest that practitioners could use similar context stimuli to assist with generalization before transitioning the treatment into the home setting.

Another way to prepare for a transition to different settings is to conduct generalization probes (mealtime sessions in different settings) throughout treatment. For example, say that the practitioner first implements an effective treatment in the child's treatment room. After the practitioner observes low levels of IMB in the treatment room, they might conduct sessions in a different location of the clinic (e.g., another treatment session, lunch room, conference room). If renewal occurs, clinicians could return to the previous context (i.e., the treatment room) and make additional manipulations (e.g., change features of the treatment room to resemble other rooms in the clinic). If renewal does not occur, practitioners could conduct generalization probes in additional alternative settings (e.g., school, home) while evaluating the child's behavior.

Systematic Changes to Intervention Components

As previously mentioned, mealtime structure should remain consistent across therapeutic meals initially. As a child makes progress with their feeding goals, changes to the foods, bolus sizes, presentation rates, or other structural elements can be made. These changes are important to build toward more naturalistic feeding routines. However, it is important to make these changes one at a time, to understand what effect each change has on the child's behavior. If relapse is a concern, the authors recommend that mealtime structure changes should be small (at first) to minimize the likelihood of relapse. For example, changing the rate of bite presentations from every 30 s to 15 s could be one way for modestly increasing meal efficiency. At other times, treatment effects may be durable enough to withstand larger changes and relapse may not occur. That is, practitioners could consider conducting terminal probes to assess if smaller changes are necessary or if larger changes can be made to save time. For example, when advancing to a full-portioned meal, a practitioner may choose to conduct a probe of a full portion before sequentially increasing the number of bites on the plate. There are no assessments that exist to evaluate the likelihood of relapse based on the type of change to the mealtime structure; however, researchers could consider evaluating this further to inform treatment progressions.

There are many variables to consider when making changes to mealtime structure. For example, the rate of presentation, the bolus size, the types of targeted foods or drinks, the preparation method of foods (e.g., transition to the methods that caregivers use in the home to cook or prepare the foods), the feeder, the meal setting, the texture, and many others. The order in which these types of structural changes are made is not standardized. Rather, these changes often depend on the child, their skills, and the caregivers' goals. For example, one family may be more concerned with nutrition and food variety; thus, they will wish to prioritize changes to food type to include more healthy options first. For another family, calories, volume, and weight gain may be most crucial; therefore, increasing the bite size, presentation rate, or overall meal volume may be most important. In our clinical experience, we encounter many caregivers who seem eager to introduce table-textured foods or for their child to begin self-feeding. However, it is important that practitioners assess when a child is ready for those changes, especially considering there may be critical increases in response effort, which could lead to resurgence.

Another consideration is reinforcement schedule thinning. Schedule thinning may inadvertently result in two changes being made at the same time. Take, for example, a scenario in which the practitioner plans to advance a child from individual bite presentations to a meal-based format, in which multiple different foods are presented on a single plate. If attempting to thin the schedule to reach this more advanced goal, the practitioner may inevitably increase the response effort and reduce the immediacy or quantity of reinforcement. Practitioners may need to exercise caution and creativity to ensure ratio strain or resurgence does not occur. The authors recommend gradually thinning the schedule of reinforcement based on previously set criteria or using probes to determine the next schedule, as is recommended for chained schedules for other responses (Hagopian et al., 2011). However, there is no research specifically on schedule thinning in feeding, and even for well-studied responses (i.e., functional communication training), the method of schedule thinning is not standardized across researchers or practitioners (Hagopian et al.). Jumping to the terminal schedule and risking even a temporary increase in IMB and decrease in consumption is not recommended due to the potential impact on the child's health and well-being if they are not eating. Overall, practitioners should be prepared that any change during feeding intervention could lead to relapse and have a treatment in place to address IMB and other challenging behaviors to minimize the impact on the child and their progress.

Intervention Feasibility

Another factor for practitioners to consider when designing a feeding intervention is the feasibility of the intervention in other settings and with other feeders. Cumbersome treatments that are difficult to implement with high integrity may be prone to errors. However, eating involves a complex set of responses, and, as challenges emerge, precise treatment components may be necessary to address the challenges (e.g., Nuk deposit to address swallowing; Ibañez et al., 2021). For example, a caregiver may have a difficult time using a Nuk brush to deposit a bite of food into the mouth; thus, practitioners could consider transitioning to a spoon as long as the treatment effects persist. These procedures may have been necessary initially to reduce problematic behaviors (e.g., packing); therefore, practitioners need to balance progress with feasibility and generalization to the natural setting. This may mean working on simplifying an intervention as opposed to increasing response effort, while making changes systematically.

Conclusion

Many children with ASD have feeding difficulties that necessitate treatment. Even after treatment leads to improvements in eating (e.g., reduction in IMB; consumption of a range of healthy foods and liquids), relapse of challenging behavior could occur. It is critical that practitioners are aware of relapse, the conditions in which it is likely to occur, and how to plan for its mitigation. In this chapter, we outlined several steps that practitioners could take to prevent or mitigate relapse and provided recommendations for practitioners to consider when treating individuals with feeding difficulties.

Of the highest priority for creating durable behavior change is to prioritize safety. To promote safety, it is critical that practitioners obtain the necessary experience, education, and training to become competent professionals in this specialized area. Meaningful behavior change cannot happen without first identifying that an individual is ready and appropriate for treatment to prevent injury or harm. A practitioner who is unprepared to treat a child with feeding difficulties may cause further problems, including an increase in inappropriate behaviors over time and perhaps resistance to effective treatments. Practitioners should refer children to specialized providers if they do not possess the necessary training and experience to safely address feeding concerns.

Second, it is important that practitioners design durable treatments for individuals with ASD and feeding difficulties. Durability may require that practitioners teach caregivers how to implement the intervention in natural settings and to program methods for generalization. Teaching caregivers how to use treatments and how to implement them with high degrees of fidelity can minimize the likelihood that relapse will occur due to integrity errors. Practitioners should also include caregivers in the treatment-planning and goal-setting process. Caregivers may wish to prioritize certain goals over others based on their concerns for child health. Alternatively, caregivers may wish to pursue some goals over others based on their cultural preferences, religious beliefs, or general routines. These are important considerations to increase caregiver participation, which, in turn, may contribute to long-term maintenance.

In addition, practitioners should actively plan for generalization by programming common stimuli, conducting treatment in alternative settings, and systematically introducing changes to the treatment. Practitioners should use feasible interventions or at least take steps to reduce the complexity of interventions before teaching caregivers. It could be that caregivers are more likely to continue with treatment in the natural setting if it requires lower levels of response effort. It could also be that caregivers are less likely to make errors in the treatment protocol if it is simpler and involves fewer steps. However, of greatest importance is long-term maintenance of improved child behavior; thus, feasibility of intervention steps should come second to this more crucial goal.

Although researchers have recently begun to evaluate relapse in the context of treating feeding difficulties, there is much research to be done in this area to learn more about when relapse is likely to occur and how to mitigate its occurrence. Relapse of IMB could result in detrimental effects such as weight loss, dehydration, impairments in cognitive or emotional functioning, hospitalization, weakened immune system, recurrent infections, or death in extreme cases (Peterson et al., 2018). Researchers should continue to identify strategies for the identification and mitigation of relapse. These steps will help to promote long-term behavior change that leads to improved health and quality of life for children with ASD and feeding difficulties, as well as for their families.

References

Andersen, A. S., Crowley-Zalaket, J. G., Engler, C. W., Zeleny, J. R., Peterson, K. M., Miles, A. G., & Piazza, C. C. (2024). Long-term outcomes after behavior-analytic intervention for pediatric feeding disorders. *Journal of Developmental and Physical Disabilities*, 1–16. https://doi.org/10.1007/s10882-024-09960-w

Bachmeyer, M. H. (2009). Treatment of selective and inadequate food intake in children: A review and practical guide. *Behavior Analysis in Practice, 2*, 43–50. https://doi.org/10.1007/BF03391736

Bachmeyer-Lee, M. H., Kirkwood, C. A., Sheehan, C. M., Gibson, A. L., Shuler, N. J., & Keane, J. A. (2020). Utilizing in-vivo feedback for caregiver training of pediatric feeding protocols. *Journal of Applied Behavior Analysis, 53*(3), 1622–1637. https://doi.org/10.1002/jaba.693

Barman, A., Das, R., & De, P. K. (2021). Impact of COVID-19 in food supply chain: Disruptions and recovery strategy. *Current Research in Behavioral Sciences, 2*, 100017. https://doi.org/10.1016/j.crbeha.2021.100017

Behavior Analyst Certification Board. (2020). *Ethics code for behavior analysts*. https://bacb.com/wp-content/ethics-code-for-behavior-analysts/

Berth, D. P., Bachmeyer, M. H., Kirkwood, C. A., Mauzy, C. R., IV, Retzlaff, B. J., & Gibson, A. L. (2019). Noncontingent and differential reinforcement in the treatment of pediatric feeding problems. *Journal of Applied Behavior Analysis, 52*(3), 622–641. https://doi.org/10.1002/jaba.562

Bouton, M. E. (2019). Extinction of instrumental (operant) learning: Interference, varieties of context, and mechanisms of contextual control. *Psychopharmacology, 236*(1), 7–19. https://doi.org/10.1007/s00213-018-5076-4

Carruth, B. R., Ziegler, P. J., Gordon, A., & Hendricks, K. (2004). Developmental milestones and self-feeding behaviors in infants and toddlers. *Journal of the American Dietetic Association, 104*, 51–56. https://doi.org/10.1016/j.jada.2003.10.019

Cho, S., & Sonoyama, S. (2020). Combining stimulus fading with simultaneous stimulus presentation in a school setting for food selectivity in a child with autism spectrum disorder. *Education and Treatment of Children, 43*(4), 335–345. https://doi.org/10.1007/s43494-020-00011-5

Crowley, J. G., Peterson, K. M., Fisher, W. W., & Piazza, C. C. (2020). Treating food selectivity as resistance to change in children with autism spectrum disorder. *Journal of Applied Behavior Analysis, 53*(4), 2002–2023. https://doi.org/10.1002/jaba.711

Engler, C. W., Ibañez, V. F., Peterson, K. M., & Andersen, A. S. (2023). Further examination of behavior during extinction-based treatment of pediatric food refusal. *Behavioral Interventions, 38*(4), 1–28. https://doi.org/10.1002/bin.1974

Evans, E. W., Must, A., Anderson, S. E., Curtin, C., Scampini, R., Maslin, M., & Bandini, L. (2012). Dietary patterns and body mass index in children with autism and typically developing children. *Research in Autism Spectrum Disorders, 6*(1), 399–405. https://doi.org/10.1016/j.rasd.2011.06.014

Friman, P. C., & Poling, A. (1995). Making life easier with effort: Basic findings and applied research on response effort. *Journal of Applied Behavior Analysis, 28*(4), 583–590. https://doi.org/10.1901/jaba.1995.28-583

Gahagan, S. (2012). Development of eating behavior: Biology and context. *Journal of Developmental & Behavioral Pediatrics, 33*(3), 261–271. https://doi.org/10.1097/DBP.0b013e31824a7baa

Hagopian, L. P., Boelter, E. W., & Jarmolowicz, D. P. (2011). Reinforcement schedule thinning following functional communication training: Review and recommendations. *Behavior Analysis in Practice, 4*, 4–16. https://doi.org/10.1007/BF03391770

Haney, S. D., Piazza, C. C., Peterson, K. M., & Greer, B. D. (2021). An evaluation of a renewal-mitigation procedure for inappropriate mealtime behavior. *Journal of Applied Behavior Analysis, 54*(3), 903–927. https://doi.org/10.1002/jaba.815

Haney, S. D., Greer, B. D., Mitteer, D. R., & Randall, K. R. (2022). Relapse during the treatment of pediatric feeding disorders. *Journal of Applied Behavior Analysis, 55*(3), 704–726. https://doi.org/10.1002/jaba.913

Hillman, H. (2019). Home-based video modeling on food selectivity of children with an autism spectrum disorder. *Physical & Occupational Therapy in Pediatrics, 39*(6), 629–641. https://doi.org/10.1080/01942638.2019.1610139

Hubbard, K. L., Anderson, S. E., Curtin, C., Must, A., & Bandini, L. G. (2014). A comparison of food refusal related to characteristics of food in children with autism spectrum disorder and typically developing children. *Journal of the Academy of Nutrition and Dietetics, 114*(12), 1981–1987. https://doi.org/10.1016/j.jand.2014.04.017

Ibañez, V. F., Piazza, C. C., & Peterson, K. M. (2019). A translational evaluation of renewal of inappropriate mealtime behavior. *Journal of Applied Behavior Analysis, 52*(4), 1005–1020. https://doi.org/10.1002/jaba.647

Ibañez, V. F., Peters, K. P., St Paul, J. A., & Vollmer, T. R. (2021). Further evaluation of modified-bolus-placement methods during initial treatment of pediatric feeding disorders. *Journal of Applied Behavior Analysis, 54*(1), 287–308. https://doi.org/10.1002/jaba.748

Kelley, M. E., Jimenez-Gomez, C., Podlesnik, C. A., & Morgan, A. (2018). Evaluation of renewal mitigation of negatively reinforced socially significant operant behavior. *Learning and Motivation, 63*, 133–141. https://doi.org/10.1016/j.lmot.2018.05.003

Kerwin, M. E. (1999). Empirically supported treatments in pediatric psychology: Severe feeding problems. *Journal of Pediatric Psychology, 24*(3), 193–214. https://doi.org/10.1093/jpepsy/24.3.193

Kimball, R. T., Greer, B. D., Fuhrman, A. M., & Lambert, J. M. (2023). Relapse and its mitigation: Toward behavioral inoculation. *Journal of Applied Behavior Analysis, 56*(2), 282–301. https://doi.org/10.1002/jaba.971

Kirkwood, C. A., Piazza, C. C., & Peterson, K. M. (2021). A comparison of function-and nonfunction-based extinction treatments for inappropriate mealtime behavior. *Journal of Applied Behavior Analysis, 54*(3), 928–945. https://doi.org/10.1002/jaba.825

McGrattan, K. E., Hammell, A. E., Turski, M. E., Klein, K. K., Delaware, E., McCormick, J., Weikle, E., Broderick, E., Ramel, S. E., & Mohr, A. H. (2024). Feeding characteristics of healthy infants without reported feeding impairments throughout the first month of life. *Journal of Perinatology, 44*, 71–77. https://doi.org/10.1038/s41372-023-01760-y

Mitteer, D. R., Greer, B. D., Fisher, W. W., Briggs, A. M., & Wacker, D. P. (2018). A laboratory model for evaluating relapse of undesirable caregiver behavior. *Journal of the Experimental Analysis of Behavior, 110*(2), 252–266. https://doi.org/10.1002/jeab.462

Mitteer, D. R., Greer, B. D., Randall, K. R., & Haney, S. D. (2022). On the scope and characteristics of relapse when treating severe destructive behavior. *Journal of Applied Behavior Analysis, 55*(3), 688–703. https://doi.org/10.1002/jaba.912

Neef, N. A., & Lutz, M. N. (2001). A brief computer-based assessment of reinforcer dimensions affecting choice. *Journal of Applied Behavior Analysis, 34*(1), 57–60. https://doi.org/10.1901/jaba.2001.34-57

O'Connor, E., Cividini-Motta, C., & MacNaul, H. (2020). Treatment of food selectivity: An evaluation of video modeling of contingencies. *Behavioral Interventions, 35*(1), 57–75. https://doi.org/10.1002/bin.1693

Patel, M. R. (2013). Assessment of pediatric feeding disorders. In *Handbook of crisis intervention and developmental disabilities* (pp. 169–182). Springer New York. https://doi.org/10.1007/978-1-4614-6531-7_10

Patel, M. R., Piazza, C. C., Kelly, M. L., Ochsner, C. A., & Santana, C. M. (2001). Using a fading procedure to increase fluid consumption in a child with feeding problems. *Journal of Applied Behavior Analysis, 34*(3), 357–360. https://doi.org/10.1901/jaba.2001.34-357

Patel, M., Piazza, C. C., Martinez, C. J., Volkert, V. M., & Santana, C. M. (2002). An evaluation of two differential reinforcement procedures with escape extinction to treat food refusal. *Journal of Applied Behavior Analysis, 35*(4), 363–374. https://doi.org/10.1901/jaba.2002.35-363

Patel, M., Reed, G. K., Piazza, C. C., Mueller, M., Bachmeyer, M. H., & Layer, S. A. (2007). Use of a high-probability instructional sequence to increase compliance to feeding demands in the absence of escape extinction. *Behavioral Interventions: Theory & Practice in Residential & Community-Based Clinical Programs, 22*(4), 305–310. https://doi.org/10.1002/bin.251

Peterson, K. M., Ibañez, V. F., Kirkwood, C. A., Crowley, J. G., & Piazza, C. C. (2018). Assessment of pediatric feeding disorders. In *Handbook of childhood psychopathology and developmental disabilities assessment* (pp. 415–431). Springer Nature. https://doi.org/10.1007/978-3-319-93542-3_22

Peterson, K. M., Phipps, L., & Ibañez, V. F. (2022). Food-related disorders and applied behavior analysis. In *Handbook of autism and pervasive developmental disorder: Assessment, diagnosis, and treatment* (pp. 1017–1036). Springer International Publishing.

Peterson, K. M., Crowley-Zalaket, J. G., & Ibañez, V. F. (2024). Simultaneous presentation and differential reinforcement to increase consumption. *Behavioral Interventions*, e2044. https://doi.org/10.1002/bin.2044

Piazza, C. C., Fisher, W. W., Brown, K. A., Shore, B. A., Patel, M. R., Katz, R. M., Sevin, B. M., Gulotta, C. S., & Blakely-Smith, A. (2003). Functional analysis of inappropriate mealtime behaviors. *Journal of Applied Behavior Analysis, 36*(2), 187–204. https://doi.org/10.1901/jaba.2003.36-187

Podlesnik, C. A., Kelley, M. E., Jimenez-Gomez, C., & Bouton, M. E. (2017). Renewed behavior produced by context change and its implications for treatment maintenance: A review. *Journal of Applied Behavior Analysis, 50*(3), 675–697. https://doi.org/10.1002/jaba.400

Ramstack, M., & Listernick, R. (1991). Safety and efficacy of a new pediatric enteral product in the young child. *Journal of Parenteral and Enteral Nutrition, 15*(1), 89–92. https://doi.org/10.1177/014860719101500189

Rescorla, R. A. (2004). Spontaneous recovery. *Learning & Memory, 11*(5), 501–509. https://doi.org/10.1101/lm.77504

Rivas, K. D., Piazza, C. C., Patel, M. R., & Bachmeyer, M. H. (2010). Spoon distance fading with and without escape extinction as treatment for food refusal. *Journal of Applied Behavior Analysis, 43*(4), 673–683. https://doi.org/10.1901/jaba.2010.43-673

Schreck, K. A., Williams, K., & Smith, A. F. (2004). A comparison of eating behaviors between children with and without autism. *Journal of Autism and Developmental Disorders, 34*, 433–438. https://doi.org/10.1023/B:JADD.0000037419.78531.86

Shahan, T. A. (2020). Relapse: An introduction. *Journal of the Experimental Analysis of Behavior, 113*(1), 8–14. https://doi.org/10.1002/jeab.578

Sharp, W. G., Volkert, V. M., Scahill, L., McCracken, C. E., & McElhanon, B. (2017). A systematic review and meta-analysis of intensive multidisciplinary intervention for pediatric feeding disorders: How standard is the standard of care? *The Journal of Pediatrics, 181*, 116–124. https://doi.org/10.1016/j.jpeds.2016.10.002

Sharp, W. G., Malugen, E., Pederson, J., Martin-Halpine, L., Dempster, R., Baranwal, N., … & Volkert, V. M. (2024). Intensive multidisciplinary feeding day programs in the United States:

A report regarding the treatment landscape. *The Journal of Pediatrics*, 114–126. https://doi.org/10.1016/j.jpeds.2024.114126.

Sweeney, M. M., & Shahan, T. A. (2013). Effects of high, low, and thinning rates of alternative reinforcement on response elimination and resurgence. *Journal of the Experimental Analysis of Behavior, 100*(1), 102–116. https://doi.org/10.1002/jeab.26

Volkert, V. M., & Piazza, C. C. (2012). Pediatric feeding disorders. In P. Sturmey & M. Hersen (Eds.), *Handbook of evidence-based practice in clinical psychology, Vol. 1. Child and adolescent disorders* (pp. 323–337). Wiley. https://doi.org/10.1002/9781118156391.ebcp001013

Volkert, V. M., Patel, M. R., & Peterson, K. M. (2016). Food refusal and selective eating. In *Behavioral health promotion and intervention in intellectual and developmental disabilities* (pp. 137–161). Springer International Publishing. https://doi.org/10.1007/978-3-319-27297-9_7

Walter, K. M., & Dickson, C. A. (2023). Response effort and resurgence. *Journal of the Experimental Analysis of Behavior, 119*(2), 373–391. https://doi.org/10.1002/jeab.835

Wilder, D. A., Normand, M., & Atwell, J. (2005). Noncontingent reinforcement as treatment for food refusal and associated self-injury. *Journal of Applied Behavior Analysis, 38*(4), 549–553. https://doi.org/10.1901/jaba.2005.132-04

Wilkins, J. W., Piazza, C. C., Groff, R. A., Volkert, V. M., Kozisek, J. M., & Milnes, S. M. (2014). Utensil manipulation during initial treatment of pediatric feeding problems. *Journal of Applied Behavior Analysis, 47*(4), 694–709. https://doi.org/10.1002/jaba.169

Williams, K., & Seiverling, L. (2023). Behavior analytic feeding interventions: Current state of the literature. *Behavior Modification, 47*(4), 983–1011. https://doi.org/10.1177/01454455221098118

Williams, D. C., Saunders, K. J., & Perone, M. (2011). Extended pausing by humans on multiple fixed-ratio schedules with varied reinforcer magnitude and response requirements. *Journal of the Experimental Analysis of Behavior, 95*(2), 203–220. https://doi.org/10.1901/jeab.2011.95-203

Wilson, A. N., Glassford, T. S., & Koerkenmeier, S. M. (2016). Effects of response effort on resurgence. *Behavior Analysis in Practice, 9*, 174–178. https://doi.org/10.1007/s40617-016-0122-3

Woods, J. N., & Borrero, C. S. (2019). Examining extinction bursts in the treatment of pediatric food refusal. *Behavioral Interventions, 34*(3), 307–322. https://doi.org/10.1002/bin.1672

Chapter 8
Persistence of Desirable Behavior

Kelly M. Schieltz, Joel E. Ringdahl, and Matthew J. O'Brien

Persistence of Desirable Behavior

Behaviors of social significance such as aggression, self-injury, and destruction (henceforth referred to as *challenging behavior* for the purposes of this chapter) provide the impetus for service delivery in many applied settings. Treatments that produce a reduction in challenging behavior often are most effective when alternative behavior (e.g., communication, task engagement, social engagement; henceforth referred to as *desirable behavior*) is established and strengthened. To establish desirable behavior, practitioners often use differential reinforcement procedures, whereby the desirable behavior is reinforced, and the challenging behavior is placed on extinction or produces some less potent form of reinforcement. Historically, clinical services end or shift to other goals when the desirable behavior is established and the challenging behavior is reduced or eliminated. However, this practice of shifting clinical services or goals once desirable behavior is established and challenging behavior is reduced may be limiting when considering persistence of the

This chapter was supported by Grant R01HD069377 from the Eunice Kennedy Shriver National Institute of Child Health and Human Development (NICHD). The content is solely the responsibility of the authors and does not necessarily represent the official views of the NICHD.
The authors have no relevant financial or non-financial interests to disclose.

K. M. Schieltz (✉) · M. J. O'Brien
Stead Family Department of Pediatrics, The University of Iowa, Carver College of Medicine, Iowa City, IA, USA
e-mail: Kelly-schieltz@uiowa.edu

J. E. Ringdahl
Department of Communication Sciences and Special Education, University of Georgia, College of Education, Athens, GA, USA

M. P. Kranak (ed.), *Behavioral Treatments for Individuals with Autism*, Autism and Child Psychopathology Series,
https://doi.org/10.1007/978-3-031-91965-7_8

desirable behavior over time. Nevin and Wacker (2013) defined persistence of the desired behavior as one of two necessary components of long-term maintenance of treatment effects, with the second component consisting of a lack of recurrence of the challenging behavior. Combined, these two components demonstrate durability of treatment effects under treatment disruption (e.g., communication device is broken, substitute teacher does not know to implement the treatment plan, a favorite TV show comes on when instructed to leave the house), which is inevitable in daily life. In this chapter, we focus on one component of long-term maintenance: the persistence of desirable behavior.

A colloquial way to view the impacts of reinforcement and extinction is that the former "strengthens" behavior while the latter "weakens" behavior. Both of these processes (strengthening and weakening) are tied to response rate (Nevin, 1974). That is, response rate increases with reinforcement and decreases with extinction. When a response occurs at a higher rate, with more intensity, or more persistently, it is concluded that the response has greater *response strength* than a different response that does not show the same rate, intensity, or persistence (Kling, 1971). This notion of "strength" dates back to Skinner (1938) who wrote of the strength of a behavior as a reflection of response rate and the number of responses emitted in extinction. Others have conceptualized "strength" in terms of the matching law (Hernstein, 1970) or behavioral momentum theory (Nevin & Grace, 2000), whereby the strength of a response changes as a function of variations in reinforcement rate or by its reinforcement history, respectively. Further, a response that is more resistant to change (i.e., persists) during disruption when compared to its baseline levels is considered to have greater strength or be more durable. Thus, one might consider persistence of a response under treatment disruption as a measure of "strength" (see Shahan, 2017, for a discussion of moving beyond the primary notion of reinforcement and response-strengthening).

Response strength has been shown to be affected by varying dimensions of reinforcement. For example, in a series of experiments with pigeons, Nevin (1974) showed that reinforcement rate, magnitude, and delays influenced the rate of responding. Specifically, denser rates of reinforcement (e.g., variable interval [VI] 1 min), larger reinforcement magnitudes (e.g., 7.5-s access), and shorter delays to reinforcement (e.g., 2.5-s wait) resulted in greater response rates under disruption when compared to leaner rates of reinforcement (e.g., VI 3 min), smaller reinforcement magnitudes (e.g., 2.5-s access), and longer delays to reinforcement (e.g., 7.5-s wait), respectively. Similar applied and translational findings have been demonstrated relative to rate (e.g., Romani et al., 2016) and magnitude (e.g., McComas et al., 2008) of reinforcement. Taken together, these studies suggest that varying the dimensions of reinforcement along the lines of rate, magnitude, and immediacy influence the strength of a response and its persistence (or resistance to change).

Although much of the focus on response strength has emphasized the influence of reinforcement parameters and history (or the response-reinforcer relation), others have evaluated the influence of stimulus-reinforcer relations. For example, Nevin et al. (1990) showed that persistence occurred at higher levels in contexts associated with higher overall amounts of reinforcement. Specifically, when contexts resulted in the same amount of reinforcement regardless of reinforcement delivery occurring contingently or with an added noncontingent presentation, pigeon key pecks persisted to a greater extent in contexts associated with higher overall amounts of reinforcement when compared to contexts with lower overall amounts of contingent reinforcement, suggesting that stimulus-reinforcer relations influence response persistence.

Between response-reinforcer and stimulus-reinforcer relations, the research literature on persistence that shifts toward the applied end of the research continuum (i.e., translational research using human operant paradigms, applied-translational research) has largely focused on persistence of the target behavior (i.e., challenging behavior). These studies are often interested in *treatment relapse*, which is defined as the re-emergence of a reduced or eliminated behavior following treatment (Lattal & Wacker, 2015; Pritchard et al., 2014; Shahan, 2020; Wathen & Podlesnkik, 2018). Treatment relapse occurs under varying conditions, with the most commonly studied types consisting of *resurgence* (see Chaps. 1 and 2), *renewal* (see Chaps. 3 and 4), and *reinstatement/rapid reacquisition* (see Chaps. 5 and 6). When studying variables impacting treatment longevity, studies on treatment relapse have been important for better understanding what, when, and how it occurs, which has led to systematic lines of research on how to mitigate its occurrence (Fisher et al., 2020; Kimball et al., 2023; Kranak et al., 2022; Suess et al., 2020; Wathen & Podlesnkik, 2018). From an applied perspective, these lines of research are important for practice because service delivery goals are meant to reduce or eliminate challenging behavior, not to have it return following treatment or discharge from services. However, persistence of desired behavior represents an equally important yet understudied aspect of treatment even though teaching and reinforcing desired behaviors are often included in such treatment programs. To fully understand and guide practitioners toward incorporating long-term maintenance goals that achieve both a lack of relapse of challenging behavior and persistence of desired behavior during everyday disruptions to the prescribed treatment program, a more complete understanding of how to achieve persistence of desired behavior is needed, which is the focus of this chapter. Given both the stimulus-reinforcer and response-reinforcer relations associated with behavioral persistence, we focus on how the variables associated with the three-term contingency influence persistence of desired behavior. That is, we discuss considerations related to *antecedents*, *behaviors*, and *consequences*.

Antecedent Considerations

Antecedent Strategies to Promote Persistence

Antecedents are stimuli that precede the behavior of interest. When assessing challenging behavior or teaching communication, an event that establishes, or otherwise increases, the value of consequences as reinforcers (i.e., establishing operations) serves as the antecedent. For example, when teaching an individual to request a break, academic instruction might serve as an antecedent to the behavior of activating a voice output communication device that plays the message, "break please." However, establishing operations represents only one type of antecedent. Antecedents also include stimuli, such as prompts (to communicate), contingency-specifying statements (e.g., "Touch the card if you want a break."), and signals indicating the availability or unavailability of a reinforcer (i.e., discriminative stimuli).

Prompts

Cooper et al. (2020) define *prompts* as any additional assistance provided to promote a desired response. When teaching communication, or other desired responses, a prompt might include a vocal statement by the therapist (e.g., "If you want a break, let me know") or a model of the response (e.g., the therapist activates a microswitch that plays the message "break please" while adding the vocal prompt, "If you want a break, press the button like this"). The use of prompts to bring about responding seems intuitive to most behavior analysts. Nonetheless, some studies have directly demonstrated the benefit of prompts during communication training (i.e., functional communication training [FCT] or mand training), resulting then in explorations of prompting as a variable that impacts persistence of the desired behavior.

Falcomata et al. (2010) evaluated the impact of prompt rates on appropriate communicative responses exhibited by individuals with intellectual and developmental disabilities (IDD). Their study demonstrated that the rate of various communication modalities (i.e., vocal, microswitch activation, and card touch) exhibited by the participants varied with therapist prompt rate. That is, when a single communication modality produced reinforcement, its rate of use was higher when therapist prompts were delivered at a rate of 2.0 per min when compared to 0.5 prompts per min. This finding was replicated across all three modalities. In addition, this study demonstrated the same relation between prompt rate and communication when all three communication modalities produced reinforcement (i.e., a concurrent reinforcement schedule was in place). These results were replicated by Romani et al. (2013) across two individuals with IDD (Experiment 1).

Romani et al. (2013) then extended the results of Falcomata et al. (2010) by evaluating for the persistence of communication responses exhibited by one individual with IDD while also evaluating for the likelihood of prompt dependency (Experiment 2). This evaluation was conducted in two phases. In Phase 1, mand training occurred under alternating dense (2.0 per min) and lean (0.5 per min) prompting schedules signaled by different colored boards. In Phase 2, manding was placed on extinction while prompting schedules remained in place. Results showed that during mand training, communicative responding was not emitted in a one-to-one relation with prompts, suggesting that manding was not prompt dependent. Additionally, under treatment disruption (i.e., extinction) mands persisted at higher rates during the dense prompting schedule, suggesting that prompting schedules could have a differential effect on response persistence of a desired behavior (i.e., manding). However, the obtained reinforcement rate across prompt rate conditions was not controlled for. Thus, these findings could be explained as a function of already known impacts of reinforcement rate on persistence (c.f., Nevin, 1974; Nevin et al., 1990).

Ringdahl et al. (2023) further explored the relation between prompt rate and response persistence. In their study, these researchers replicated and extended the findings of Romani et al. (2013) by holding the reinforcement rate similar across the two prompt rate conditions. In addition, Ringdahl et al. evaluated the response persistence effects of prompt rate across two clinical presentations: (a) individuals referred for communication training in the absence of co-occurring challenging behavior (i.e., mand training), and (b) individuals referred for communication training in the context of treatment for challenging behavior (i.e., FCT). Results of Ringdahl et al. varied by clinical profile. For the individuals referred for mand training, a relation between prompt rate and response persistence emerged. These findings replicated Romani et al. and did so while controlling for known consequence-related confounds, specifically reinforcement rate. For the individuals referred for FCT, the results were less evident. Three of the five participants in this portion of the study exhibited more response persistence during the dense prompt rate condition. However, those differences were minimal for two of the three participants. For the remaining two individuals, one exhibited a minimal increase in responding during the lean prompt density condition, while the other exhibited much greater responding during that condition. Overall, the results suggested (a) prompt density had an impact on response persistence for one clinical population (those without co-occurring challenging behavior), and (b) prompt density lead to less evident differences in response persistence for a different clinical population (those with co-occurring challenging behavior). This second finding suggested that variables such as history of reinforcement and response class size and membership might interact with antecedents to influence response persistence. Further, and in consideration of uncontrolled variables such as reinforcement history within applied populations, small differences in responding should not be discounted, as those differences may be more common among applied populations (Romani et al., 2016; Schieltz et al., 2017).

Discriminative Stimuli

Discriminative stimuli include any stimulus with a discriminative function (Catania, 2013), which often serve as signals of the availability or absence of reinforcement for a particular behavior. In behavior treatments, discriminative stimuli play an important role in teaching individuals when a desired behavior is likely to contact reinforcement (S^D) or extinction (S^Δ). For example, in FCT, a signal (e.g., a green card, an instruction) may be used to indicate that a mand will be reinforced and another signal (e.g., a red card, a different instruction) may be used to indicate that the mand will be placed on extinction.

Discriminative stimuli are often incorporated within a multiple schedule during FCT schedule thinning. In this approach, reinforcement and extinction components may alternate, with distinctive discriminative stimuli at the outset of the reinforcement (S^D) and extinction (S^Δ) components (Mitteer et al., 2020). By signaling each component, an individual discriminates the conditions under which a mand will be reinforced or not and in so doing the discriminative stimuli exert control over an individual's behavior. This discrimination, in turn, allows the reinforcement schedule to be thinned through a gradual increase in the duration of the extinction component.

The use of discriminative stimuli during schedule thinning may offer several benefits, including a more palatable reinforcement schedule for implementers and the mitigation of the recurrence of challenging behavior during disruptions to treatment (Mitteer et al., 2020); however, such signals may produce a more nuanced result in terms of persistence of communication. Fisher et al. (2020) demonstrated this nuance in a study with four children who exhibited challenging behavior. Each participant received FCT in two distinct contexts (i.e., different colored rooms with implementers wearing different colors of clothing), one associated with multiple-schedule FCT with discriminative stimuli (S^Ds and S^Δs were different colored index cards or posterboards) and one with traditional FCT without discriminative stimuli. During multiple-schedule FCT, the S^D signaled the availability of reinforcement contingent on manding and the S^Δ signaled that reinforcement was unavailable even if manding occurred (i.e., extinction). Both types of FCT were conducted within a multielement design. Following FCT, an extinction disruption was implemented in which challenging behavior and manding were placed on extinction in the presence or absence of the S^Δ. For each of the four participants, less recurrence of the challenging behavior was observed in the context where the S^Δ was present, which suggests that challenging behavior had come under the control of the discriminative stimuli; however, manding also persisted to a lesser degree in the presence of discriminative stimuli, suggesting that it too had come under the control of the discriminative stimuli. Thus, if one goal of an FCT treatment is to reduce the probability of the recurrence of challenging behavior when extinction occurs, then the use of discriminative stimuli may produce that effect; however, if another goal of FCT is to ensure that manding has greater persistence during extinction, then the use of discriminative stimuli may have countertherapeutic effects. Thus, discriminative stimuli may reduce the probability that challenging behavior will recur when a signal is used to indicate reinforcement is unavailable (S^Δ), but so too will the probability that manding will recur. The trade-off to implementing FCT without signals is that both challenging behavior and manding are likely to recur and persist to a greater extent.

One alternative that may increase the likelihood of persistence of desired behavior during treatment disruption is to maintain the presence of S^Ds for desired behavior during periods of disruption, which was not evaluated in the study conducted by Fisher et al. (2020). For example, Suess et al. (2020) used common stimuli (i.e., work picture card, specific location illustrated by a picture card for leisure activities to be placed during the work period ["safe spot"]) to train multiple desired behaviors (i.e., task completion, manding) within an FCT treatment program for four young children with autism spectrum disorder who engaged in escape maintained challenging behavior. Prior to implementing common stimuli within the escape context of FCT, the stimuli were initially trained within a play context that did not have a known history of reinforcement for challenging behavior. Following successful training, all desired and challenging behaviors were placed on extinction. Specifically, during the extinction disruptor phase, common stimuli continued to be presented (i.e., work card, placing leisure activities on the "safe spot"); however, demands continued to be presented regardless of the occurrence of challenging or desired behavior. Relative to desired behavior, results showed that task completion persisted at high levels for all four participants, and although manding decreased when compared to levels during the FCT phase, manding persisted at higher levels for three of the four participants when compared to the initial extinction phase (prior to training). Taken together, results suggest that the presence of common stimuli for desired behavior during treatment disruptions may be beneficial for promoting the persistence of desired behavior. These findings should be considered in light of more nuanced findings from basic research laboratories (e.g., Browning & Shahan, 2021).

Rules

Verbal antecedents, or rules, which establish contingencies may exert control over one's behaviors, resulting in what is considered *rule-governed behavior* (Catania, 2013). For example, a parent may tell a child, "If you ask nicely, I'll buy you candy," and the child may respond accordingly. Rules and the subsequent effects of rule-governed behavior may affect the persistence of behaviors. In their study on the effects of discriminative stimuli during FCT, Fisher et al. (2020) suggested that the discriminative stimuli may not have been the only antecedent to impact behavioral persistence. They noted that during multiple-schedule FCT with discriminative stimuli, sessions began with the therapist delivering rules describing the contingencies for each discriminative stimulus. As a result, they suggested that the rules may have contributed to the decrease in persistence of challenging behavior and manding.

A limited number of translational studies have evaluated the effects of rules on behavioral persistence (e.g., Baumann et al., 2009; LeFrancois et al., 1988; Rosenfarb et al., 1992). In one such study, Podlesnik and Chase (2006) examined the persistence of responding to simple math problems by six college students following training that involved either minimal instructions (MI) or complete instructions (CI) for the task. Using a computer program, three participants assigned to the MI group were only provided with information on the exchange rate for points associated with correct responses (one point = 5 cents). By contrast, three participants assigned to the CI group were given instructions on how to enter their answers to the math problems, the exchange rate for points, and details on the reinforcement schedule. More specifically, participants in the CI group were informed how often, on average, they should respond to obtain points (based on a VI schedule that was yoked to the responding of a matched participant in the MI group). During training, the two groups had similar rates of reinforcement. To evaluate the persistence of responding to math problems, a disruptor assessment was conducted at least twice for each participant. In the disruptor assessment, a sitcom television show chosen by the respective participant played on a nearby television while the participant continued with either the MI or CI procedures. For 14 out of 15 disruptor assessments, participants in the CI group exhibited greater persistence of responding and thus demonstrated the behavior-strengthening effect of instructions.

In an unpublished dissertation study, Trump (2019) evaluated the effects of instructions on the persistence of correct responding during various academic tasks for four young children receiving special education services. In the baseline phase of this study, each participant was presented with academic tasks under two training conditions within a multielement design. In one condition, an experimenter provided instructions that explained the reinforcement contingency for completing the academic work, and, in the other condition, the same academic work was presented without instructions. A VI 12-s reinforcement schedule was used in both conditions, and data were collected on participants' correct and incorrect responding for academic tasks for which they had previously demonstrated proficiency. To evaluate the persistence of total (correct and incorrect) responding, "instruction" and "no instruction" sessions were repeated five times but with a disruptor test embedded each time. The disruptor test entailed playing a cartoon video while the participant was expected to complete the academic task. The results were inconsistent across participants. For one participant, total responding persisted to a greater extent in the "instructions" condition during four of the five disruptor sessions, whereas for another participant, total responding persisted more in the "no instructions" condition for three of the five disruptor sessions. For the remaining two participants, persistence of total responding was equivocal for both conditions across the five disruptor sessions. Despite inconsistent findings, for one of the participants, the use of instructions led to greater persistence of total responding, which suggests that the use of rules may influence persistence for some individuals.

In sum, a few translational and applied studies provide preliminary evidence that rules regarding reinforcement contingencies may affect the persistence of some behaviors. Although studies by Fisher et al. (2020) and Trump (2019) provide either limited or mixed support for the notion that rules may enhance the behavioral persistence of some behaviors, translational studies, such as the one conducted by Podlesnik and Chase (2006), offer stronger evidence of this relationship. More research, including applied studies, is needed to confirm this hypothesis.

Clinical Implications of Antecedent Influences on Persistence

More research is needed to better understand how antecedent strategies may enhance the persistence of desired behaviors; however, some clinical considerations may be gleaned from what research has been conducted. With regard to prompt density, studies by Romani et al. (2013) and Ringdahl et al. (2023) provide preliminary support for the use of a dense prompting schedule to enhance the persistence of communication. Studies by Fisher et al. (2020) and Suess et al. (2020) showed that discriminative stimuli have the potential to influence behavioral persistence, with the latter study demonstrating greater persistence of two desired behavioral topographies (task completion and manding). Finally, despite mixed results in at least one study on the influence of rules on behavioral persistence (i.e., Trump, 2019), unequivocal findings by Podlesnik and Chase (2006) suggest that rules may enhance behavioral persistence of desired behaviors.

Behavior Considerations

Historically, evaluations of variables impacting response persistence have largely focused on consequence-related variables (covered in the following section of this chapter; antecedent variables previously covered provide some exceptions to this focus). Often, evaluations of response persistence include non-human basic investigations that utilize a single response allocated to different apparatuses (e.g., key pecks on a green or red key). However, in applied behavior analytic contexts, clinicians and implementers often focus on more than one response modality. For example, interest may be paid to multiple members of a response class, including challenging and desired behavior, such as when attempting to reduce challenging behavior through the use of a differential reinforcement of alternative behavior program. Similarly, implementers might be interested in teaching multiple response modalities, such as when teaching communication using a multimodal approach (e.g., Diehl & Wallace, 2018) or when teaching communication variability using lag schedules (e.g., Adami et al., 2017).

Given different response modalities within applied behavior analytic evaluations, it may be important to focus on how behavior-related variables impact both initial clinical outcomes as well as longer term maintenance of those clinical outcomes. One behavior-related variable that has been shown in the literature to impact clinical outcomes is response proficiency. *Proficiency*, in this context, refers to the level of prompting required to bring about a (communicative) response. As an example, if an individual exhibits one communication modality (e.g., microswitch activation) without any therapist prompts, and that same individual requires a model prompt to exhibit a second communication modality (e.g., manual sign), the first modality would be considered "high proficiency" and the second communication modality "low proficiency." Ringdahl et al. (2009) demonstrated that FCT implemented with a high-proficiency communication modality produced better initial FCT outcomes than FCT implemented with a low-proficiency communication modality. This finding was later replicated by Falcomata et al. (2017) across different response classes.

Response effort or efficiency represents a second behavior-related variable that may impact clinical outcomes. For example, Horner and Day (1991) conducted FCT under two conditions. In one condition, the individual was taught to manually sign the sentence "I want a break please." During implementation, treatment gains were initially observed. However, these gains were short-lived and deteriorated across sessions. In the second FCT condition, the participant obtained reinforcement by exhibiting a one-word manual sign, "please." During this condition, immediate and sustained reductions in challenging behavior occurred. Buckley and Newchok (2005) replicated the findings reported by Horner and Day. These authors also implemented FCT with an individual utilizing two different approaches: low-effort FCT (handing a small picture of a preferred stimulus to the therapist) and high-effort FCT (get out of seat, walk to a felt board located across the room, remove the small picture of the preferred stimulus, return to seat, and hand the picture to the therapist). Following FCT with challenging behavior placed on extinction, both low-effort and high-effort approaches were alternated in an ABAB fashion. During these implementations, the communicative response and aggression produced access to the programmed reinforcer. That is, FCT was conducted without extinction of challenging behavior in both approaches during this portion of the study. This investigation noted that FCT with the low-effort communication response resulted in sustained communication and low levels of aggression. This outcome was achieved even though the FCT arrangement programmed reinforcement for aggression. However, when FCT was conducted with the high-effort communication response, the participant exhibited low levels of communication and increased aggression.

Richman et al. (2001) also investigated response effort as a variable impacting treatment. Specifically, their study investigated three different concurrent schedule arrangements on response allocation. In two of the arrangements, a single communication response (either saying "please" or touching a card) produced reinforcement, as did exhibiting aggression. In the third arrangement, the therapist provided reinforcement for saying "please," touching the card, or exhibiting aggression. Results demonstrated that responding allocated to either saying "please" or touching the card when either was the sole available communication modality, while aggression remained low. Further, when both communication modalities produced reinforcement, the participant allocated responding to saying "please," while card touching and aggression remained low. Although Richman et al. interpreted these findings as a demonstration of response efficiency, they may instead be a demonstration that the individual preferred communicating vocally relative to the card.

Although each of these response-related variables—proficiency, efficiency, and preference—have been investigated with respect to their impact on initial clinical impact, their influence on long-term treatment implementation and maintenance of treatment effects has not been as thoroughly studied. *Preference* represents one exception. While response proficiency and response efficiency seem to differentially impact initial clinical outcomes, response preference does not. Winborn-Kemmerer et al. (2009) demonstrated that FCT conducted individually with two separate communication responses produced similar, efficacious outcomes for each of the two participants. However, when the researchers implemented FCT with both communication modalities available and programmed to produce reinforcement, the participants allocated responding to one of the communication modalities, while challenging behavior remained low.

Ringdahl et al. (2018) expanded on these findings. In their study, communicative responding was similar across two similarly proficient and efficient communication modalities. For a subset of participants, reductions in challenging behavior were also observed across FCT conditions with single communication modalities. A concurrent schedule arrangement, similar to the one explored by Richman et al. (2001) and Winborn-Kemmerer et al., (2009) identified a preferred communication modality for each participant. Following similar histories of reinforcement for each communicative response, reinforcement was subsequently withheld (i.e., communication was placed on extinction). Results demonstrated that the higher preferred communication modality persisted during this treatment disruption to a greater extent than the lower preferred communication modality. The findings were not uniform; however, the positive correlation between relative preference and relative persistence was noted for seven of the eight participants included in the study's two experiments.

Clinical Implications of Behavior Influences on Persistence

Clinically, these studies suggest enough of a relation between communication modality and efficacy, in both the near and long term, to warrant clinicians taking an intentional approach to determining what communication modality to include in the treatments they design. Communication modalities that are efficient (i.e., low effort) and shown to be highly proficient (i.e., requiring limited external prompts) should be selected to maximize initial treatment outcomes, particularly in the context of FCT. The relation between these variables and response persistence has not been thoroughly investigated. However, questions about those relations might be moot, as establishing treatment effects with modalities that are inefficient (i.e., high effort) or shown to be minimally proficient (i.e., requiring invasive prompts) is difficult to achieve. In the absence of building a successful history of reinforcement, questions about persistence of the response are premature. While similarly efficient and proficient response modalities might bring about initial treatment effects, extant data suggests that modalities preferred by the individual are more persistent when reinforcement delivery is disrupted (Ringdahl et al., 2018). Thus, gaining a priori information regarding communication modalities that are efficient, proficient, and preferred allows clinicians to build communication-based programs that will be optimally successful in the short term and produce resilient responding. This second outcome has relevance for schedule thinning, which is likely to produce unreinforced responding, and transfer of treatment to novel implementers and novel environments where mistakes in procedural fidelity are also likely to produce unreinforced responding.

Consequence Considerations

Consequence Strategies to Promote Persistence

Consequences are stimulus changes (i.e., presentation or removal) following a behavior that may increase (reinforcement) or decrease (punishment) the probability of that behavior recurring. Of particular importance to the discussion of behavioral persistence are consequences that serve to reinforce a preceding behavior and the various dimensions of those reinforcing consequences (i.e., rate, quality, magnitude, delay). While early studies on the influence of dimensions of reinforcement on behavioral persistence were largely confined to basic laboratories (see Mace, 2018, for a discussion on the work of Tony Nevin), recent research from translational and applied studies has replicated and extended some of the basic research findings.

Rate of Reinforcement

Largely influenced by Tony Nevin's work on behavioral momentum theory, several studies have evaluated the influence that rate of reinforcement (i.e., the number of reinforcers over time) has on behavioral persistence. For example, Nevin et al. (1990) compared the persistence of key pecking in pigeons following a two-component multiple schedule (signaled with red and green lights) where one component used a VI 1 min schedule of reinforcement for key pecking and the other component used a VI 1 min schedule of reinforcement plus delivery of reinforcers independent of responding on a variable time (VT) 30 s schedule. Results showed that pigeons displayed higher response rates in the VI only component. However, when key pecking was placed on extinction in each signaled component, key pecking persisted to a greater extent in the VI + VT component than in the VI only component, suggesting that the greater rate of reinforcement was associated with greater persistence. Although no inherent appropriate/inappropriate dichotomy exists in some basic studies like Nevin et al., the results have implications for how reinforcement histories could be arranged to bring about persistent responding of the desired behavior in applied studies and contexts.

For example, Mace et al. (1990) replicated the results of Nevin et al. (1990) in a translational study with two adults with disabilities. Using a silverware sorting task, participants were reinforced according to a VI 1 min schedule of reinforcement in one component of a multiple schedule and a VI 1 min plus a VT 30 s schedule in the other component. Unlike the Nevin et al. study, persistence of sorting was measured using a video distraction condition where a music/dance video played in each component. For both participants, persistence was greater in the component that incorporated the dense (i.e., VI + VT) schedule.

Similarly, but in the context of negative reinforcement, Romani et al. (2016) examined the persistence of task completion for three young children who displayed escape motivated challenging behavior. Following a functional analysis, compliance training was conducted with each participant. During compliance training, task completion was on a fixed ratio 1 reinforcement (i.e., work break) schedule and challenging behavior was placed on extinction. When stability was established for challenging behavior and task completion, a schedule manipulation phase was conducted whereby each participant completed demands on lean (VI only) and dense (VI + FT) negative reinforcement (i.e., work breaks) schedules signaled by different colored tasks. In a subsequent extinction phase where both challenging behavior and task completion were placed on extinction, task completion was more persistent following dense reinforcement schedules; however, the authors noted that the effect was modest (in comparison to the larger effects observed in non-human animal studies), which may be a more common result with applied populations due to uncontrolled prior reinforcement histories.

Findings regarding the influence of the rate of reinforcement on behavioral persistence have been relatively consistent in showing that higher rates of reinforcement lead to greater response persistence; however, there are exceptions. For example, Lionello-Denolf and Dube (2011) evaluated and compared behavioral persistence using multiple-schedule and single-schedule training. Twelve children with intellectual disabilities tapped on icons on a touch screen and received tokens or food items on a VI schedule (lean schedule) or on a schedule that included both contingent and noncontingent delivery of reinforcers (VI + VT; dense schedule). For six children, a two-component multiple-schedule arrangement was used during training, with one component associated with the dense schedule of reinforcement (VI + VT) and one component associated with the lean schedule of reinforcement (VI only). For the other six children, training occurred on two single schedules with one lean and one dense schedule. Following training for each paradigm, disruptor tests were conducted and showed that for those who participated in the multiple-schedule training, behavioral persistence was greater in the presence of the stimulus associated with the dense reinforcement component; however, for participants in the single-schedule training, there was no consistent difference in persistence between the dense and lean conditions. Thus, the use of single schedules in training may result in different outcomes related to persistence than when a multiple-schedule arrangement is used.

Another example was seen by Helvey et al. (2023) who evaluated the recurrence of challenging behavior for four children following FCT. In this study, each child received FCT across lean and dense reinforcement schedule conditions conducted within a multielement design with discriminative stimuli associated with each condition. Following FCT, an extinction disruption test was conducted where challenging behavior and manding were both placed on extinction in the presence of the different discriminative stimuli associated with the lean and dense reinforcement schedules. Not only was there no discernible difference in recurrence of challenging behavior between the lean and dense schedules of reinforcement, for two participants, manding persisted to a greater extent during the extinction disruption in the condition associated with the dense schedule of reinforcement, and for the other two participants, greater persistence of manding was observed in the condition associated with the lean schedule of reinforcement.

Reinforcer Quality

The influence that reinforcer quality (i.e., the degree of preference of the reinforcer type) has on behavioral persistence has been studied in basic and applied research. For example, across two experiments, one applied and one basic, Mace et al. (1997) demonstrated the effects of reinforcer quality on behavioral persistence. In the first experiment, two adolescent males receiving treatment for noncompliance were treated using a high-probability (high-*p*) sequence. In this treatment, a low-probability (low-*p*; i.e., those previously shown to result in noncompliance) demand was preceded by a series of high-*p* demands (i.e., those previously shown to result in high compliance), with each of the high-*p* demands resulting in one of three types of reinforcers: (a) praise, (b) food, or (c) praise and food. For both participants, it was determined that food was preferred over praise. In this arrangement, the low-*p* demand functioned as the disruptor following various histories of reinforcement that differed along the dimension of reinforcer quality. The results showed that compliance to many of the low-*p* demands increased with the high-*p* treatment that was paired with only praise (i.e., relatively low-quality reinforcer); however, when the high-*p* treatment was ineffective for bringing about an increase in compliance to low-*p* demands, the effectiveness of the high-*p* treatment was further increased by pairing it with food and praise or food alone (i.e., relatively high-quality reinforcers). This finding suggests that a higher-quality reinforcer may produce more behavioral persistence (i.e., continued compliance in the context of a low-*p* demand [disruptor]) than a lower-quality reinforcer. These results were replicated in Mace et al.'s second experiment with rats.

Reinforcer Magnitude

Another dimension of reinforcement that may impact behavioral persistence is magnitude. The magnitude of reinforcement refers to the size or amount of reinforcement (e.g., the duration of play time or the size of the bowl of ice cream). Studies interested in the effect of reinforcer magnitude on behavioral persistence have largely been conducted in basic research labs with non-human animals. For example, in one of the earliest studies on the effects of reinforcer magnitude on behavioral persistence, Nevin (1974) compared the persistence of key pecking by two pigeons following training with different reinforcer magnitudes. Both pigeons were trained using a two-component multiple schedule in which each component was associated with a different magnitude (i.e., durations of access) of food. To evaluate persistence, a response-independent feeding schedule was implemented for each component. Key pecking persisted to a greater degree in the component associated with the longer (i.e., greater magnitude) reinforcement.

Grimes and Shull (2001) conducted a study on behavioral persistence that combined aspects of reinforcer magnitude and reinforcer quality. In this study, food pellets were used to reinforce rats' lever presses on a VI 100 s schedule across two components of a multiple schedule; however, in one of the components, response-independent delivery (VT schedule) of sweetened condensed milk was added to the VI schedule of food pellets. The results suggested that the persistence of lever pressing when placed on extinction was greater in a component associated with the VI + VT reinforcement that used different types of reinforcers than the component associated with only the VI reinforcement schedule involving food pellets.

Given the paucity of applied research on the effects of reinforcer magnitude on behavioral persistence McComas et al. (2008) offer a translational study using three college students. In this study, persistence of responding (right or left side mouse clicks) to visual stimuli on a computer task was evaluated. Points, which were later exchanged for money, were used as reinforcers. In an initial phase, a multiple concurrent VI 30 s reinforcement schedule was used in two components. In one component, the reinforcement magnitude for clicking on the right side of the screen was held constant (1 pt) while the magnitude for clicking on the left side of the screen was twice as much. In the other component, the reinforcement magnitude for clicking on the right side of the screen was held constant (1 pt) but clicking on the left side resulted in reinforcement that was eight times as much. When mouse clicks were placed on extinction, responding was more persistent for two of three participants in the component associated with the greater magnitude reinforcer.

Delay of Reinforcement

Like other dimensions of reinforcement, reinforcement delays (i.e., the latency from a behavior offset to the point of reinforcer presentation) have the potential to positively or negatively affect the rate of responding (see Lattal, 2010, for discussion on delayed reinforcement of operant behavior) and has been shown to impact behavioral persistence (Grace et al., 1998). Following an initial experimental phase that showed pigeons preferred shorter delays to feeding following key pecking, Grace et al. implemented training using a two-component multiple schedule where four pigeons received immediate feeding in one component and a 3-s delay to feeding in the other component. As expected, the rates of responding were higher during the "no delay" component. When key pecking was placed on extinction in each component, responding persisted to a greater extent for three of four pigeons in the "no delay" component, suggesting that training under shorter delays to reinforcement increases the persistence of the trained behavior. Similar findings have been obtained in other basic studies (e.g., Bell, 1999; Podlesnik et al., 2006) but have yet to be explored in applied-translational studies.

Reinforcement History Enhancements

Beyond understanding the influence of specific dimensions of reinforcement on the persistence of desired behavior, Wacker et al. (2011) evaluated the effects of building reinforcement histories for desired behavior over time. In this study, FCT using a two-step chained procedure (task completion first, manding second) was implemented across eight young children with developmental disabilities who engaged in escape maintained challenging behavior. Extinction disruptor tests were intermittently probed throughout FCT and FCT schedule thinning to evaluate for the recurrence of challenging behavior and persistence of desired behavior. Across participants, challenging behavior failed to recur only after many months of FCT (up to 18 months). Relative to persistence of desired behavior, task completion generally did not persist until the final extinction disruptor phase (which coincided with the lack of challenging behavior recurrence), whereas manding either did not persist or persisted at very low levels during the final extinction disruptor phase. Relative to this latter outcome, most participants in this study did not have vocal repertoires, and the trained communication modality was not present during these disruptor phases. Thus, interpretations of the persistence of manding should be cautiously considered. When long-term maintenance was achieved (no recurrence of challenging behavior, persistence of desired behavior), Wacker et al. further evaluated long-term maintenance under additional treatment disruptions (i.e., extended sessions of extinction, novel task, competing reinforcement, absence of the communication modality). During these disruptor tests, task completion persisted at high levels across all disruptions, and manding was variable. Taken together, results suggest that continuing treatment for longer periods of time may be effective at promoting the persistence of desired behavior.

Another potential solution for promoting the persistence of desired behavior includes enhancing the reinforcement history for the desired response. In our recent work (Ringdahl, 2018), we have evaluated the impact of two types of reinforcement history enhancements on the persistence of communicative behavior. These enhancements include such manipulations as differences in rate and magnitude of reinforcement. Results of our investigations have been equivocal to date. While rate and magnitude enhancements appear to increase the persistence of single communicative responses, this finding has not been uniform across participants. Thus, it may be that sensitivity to various contingency parameters, such as rate and magnitude, varies from individual to individual and that programming enhancements to increase persistence will first require identification of the relevant parameter to which behavior is sensitive. When applying rate and magnitude enhancements in an attempt to increase the persistence of the identified low-preferred communication modality for any given individual, we have also obtained equivocal results. However, in these investigations, the preponderance of individuals demonstrated that rate and magnitude enhancements do not increase the persistence of the low-preferred response. That is, the high-preferred response remains the most persistent, even after an enhanced reinforcement history is developed for the low-preferred response. Thus, it may be that preference (as discussed previously) outweighs reinforcement history when determining relative preference across responses in a response class.

Clinical Implications of Consequence Considerations on Persistence

Consequence-based strategies involving manipulations of dimensions of reinforcement may offer the greatest opportunity to enhance behavioral persistence. Informed by a combination of basic, translational, and applied studies, clinicians may consider "boosting" reinforcement in several ways to increase the persistence of desired behaviors. While this defies the convention of using the minimum sufficient reinforcement, treatments that include higher quality and greater magnitude reinforcers that are provided more immediately may find that desired behaviors persist to a greater extent under various treatment disruptions. For treatments employing a multiple-schedule paradigm, it appears that increasing the rate of reinforcement in the presence of the desired behavior, whether contingently or noncontingently, may produce greater persistence; however, this same benefit may not hold true in single-schedule approaches.

Conclusion

Developing and teaching desired behaviors is often a clinical goal in treatment plans that seek to reduce the occurrence of challenging behavior. A less common clinical goal is demonstrating long-term maintenance of challenging and desired behaviors when treatment plans are disrupted. That is, demonstrating a lack of recurrence of challenging behavior and persistence of desired behavior in the face of treatment disruptions. Although much of the extant literature on long-term maintenance focuses on mitigating the recurrence of challenging behavior, this chapter focused on variables related to the persistence of desired behavior across the three-term contingency. Like the literature on challenging behavior, results are often mixed in relation to behavioral mechanisms that promote the persistence of desired behavior. However, behavioral mechanisms such as prompts, discriminative stimuli, rules, response preference, and reinforcer dimensions show preliminary promise toward promoting the persistence of desired behavior. Moving forward, practitioners are encouraged to incorporate a broader goal within their treatment programs that includes strengthening desirable behavior until it persists in the face of naturally occurring disruptions, and in so doing may consider some of the antecedent, behavior, and consequence strategies discussed in this chapter. Additionally, because persistence of desired behavior is often not the primary target in long-term maintenance studies, researchers are encouraged to consider studying both mitigation strategies for reducing relapse of challenging behavior *and* promotion strategies for encouraging the persistence of desired behavior during treatment disruptions.

References

Adami, S., Falcomata, T. S., Muething, C. S., & Hoffman, K. (2017). An evaluation of lag schedules of reinforcement during functional communication training: Effects on varied mand responding and challenging behavior. *Behavior Analysis in Practice, 10*(3), 209–213. https://doi.org/10.1007/s40617-017-0179-7

Baumann, A. A., Abreu-Rodrigues, J., & da Souza, A. S. (2009). Rules and self-rules: Effects of variation upon behavioral sensitivity to change. *The Psychological Record, 59*(4), 641–670. https://doi.org/10.1007/BF03395685

Bell, M. C. (1999). Pavlovian contingencies and resistance to change in a multiple schedule. *Journal of the Experimental Analysis of Behavior, 72*(1), 81–96. https://doi.org/10.1901/jeab.1999.72-81

Browning, K. O., & Shahan, T. A. (2021). Examination of alternative-response discrimination training and resurgence in rats. *Learning & Behavior, 49*(4), 379–396. https://doi.org/10.3758/s13420-021-00470-9

Buckley, S. D., & Newchok, D. K. (2005). Differential impact of response effort within a response chain on use of mands in a student with autism. *Research in Developmental Disabilities, 26*(1), 77–85. https://doi.org/10.1016/j.ridd.2004.07.004

Catania, A. C. (2013). *Learning* (5th ed.). Sloan.

Cooper, J. O., Heron, T. E., & Heward, W. L. (2020). *Applied behavior analysis* (3rd ed.). Pearson Education.

Diehl, S. K., & Wallace, S. E. (2018). A modified multimodal communication treatment for individuals with traumatic brain injury. *Augmentative and Alternative Communication, 34*(4), 323–334. https://doi.org/10.1080/07434618.1523224

Falcomata, T. S., Ringdahl, J. E., Christensen, T. J., & Boelter, E. W. (2010). An evaluation of prompt schedules and mand reference during functional communication training. *Behavior Analyst Today, 11*(1), 77–84. https://doi.org/10.1037/h0100690

Falcomata, T. S., Shpall, C. S., Ringdahl, J. E., Ferguson, R. H., Wingate, H. V., & Swinnea, S. B. (2017). A comparison of high and low-proficiency mands during functional communication training across multiple functions of problem behavior. *Journal of Developmental and Physical Disabilities, 29*(6), 983–1002. https://doi.org/10.1007/s10882-017-9571-z

Fisher, W. W., Fuhrman, A. M., Greer, B. D., Mitteer, D. R., & Piazza, C. C. (2020). Mitigating resurgence of destructive behavior using the discriminative stimuli of a multiple schedule. *Journal of the Experimental Analysis of Behavior, 113*(1), 263–277. https://doi.org/10.1002/jeab.552

Grace, R. C., Schwendiman, J. W., & Nevin, J. A. (1998). Effects of unsignaled delay of reinforcement on preference and resistance to change. *Journal of the Experimental Analysis of Behavior, 69*(3), 247–261. https://doi.org/10.1901/jeab.1998.69-247

Grimes, J. A., & Shull, R. L. (2001). Response-independent milk delivery enhances persistence of pellet-reinforced lever pressing by rats. *Journal of the Experimental Analysis of Behavior, 76*(2), 179–194. https://doi.org/10.1901/jeab.2001.76-179

Helvey, C. I., Fisher, W. W., Greer, B. D., Fuhrman, A. M., & Mitteer, D. R. (2023). Resurgence of destructive behavior following differential rates of alternative reinforcement. *Journal of Applied Behavior Analysis, 56*(4), 804–815. https://doi.org/10.1002/jaba.1010

Hernstein, R. J. (1970). On the law of effect. *Journal of the Experimental Analysis of Behavior, 13*(2), 243–266. https://doi.org/10.1901/jeab.1970.13-243

Horner, R. H., & Day, H. M. (1991). The effects of response efficiency on functionally equivalent competing behaviors. *Journal of Applied Behavior Analysis, 24*(4), 719–732. https://doi.org/10.1901/jaba.1991.24-719

Kimball, R. T., Greer, B. D., Fuhrman, A. M., & Lambert, J. M. (2023). Relapse and its mitigation: Toward behavioral inoculation. *Journal of Applied Behavior Analysis, 56*(2), 282–301. https://doi.org/10.1002/jaba.971

Kling, J. W. (1971). Learning: Introductory survey. In J. W. Kling & L. A. Riggs (Eds.), *Experimental psychology* (pp. 551–613). Holt.

Kranak, M. P., Rooker, G. W., Arevalo, A. R., & Robison, T. P. (2022). Mitigating reinstatement using progressive ratio schedules: A proof of concept. *Behavioral Development, 27*(1–2), 21–34. https://doi.org/10.1037/bdb0000108

Lattal, K. A. (2010). Delayed reinforcement of operant behavior. *Journal of the Experimental Analysis of Behavior, 93*(1), 129–139. https://doi.org/10.1901/jeab.2010.93-129

Lattal, K. A., & Wacker, D. (2015). Some dimensions of recurrent operant behavior. *Mexican Journal of Behavior Analysis, 41*(2), 1–13. https://doi.org/10.5514/rmac.v41.i2.63716

LeFrancois, J. R., Chase, P. N., & Joyce, J. H. (1988). The effects of a variety of instructions on human fixed-interval performance. *Journal of the Experimental Analysis of Behavior, 49*(3), 383–393. https://doi.org/10.1901/jeab.1988.49-383

Lionello-Denolf, K. M., & Dube, W. V. (2011). Contextual influences on resistance to disruption in children with intellectual disabilities. *Journal of the Experimental Analysis of Behavior, 96*(3), 317–327. https://doi.org/10.1901/jeab.2011.96-317

Mace, F. C. (2018). Tony Nevin: The embrace of translational work by a basic scientist. *Journal of the Experimental Analysis of Behavior, 109*(1), 56–65. https://doi.org/10.1002/jeab.297

Mace, F. C., Lalli, J. S., Shea, M. C., Lalli, E. P., West, B. J., Roberts, M., & Nevin, J. A. (1990). The momentum of human behavior in a natural setting. *Journal of the Experimental Analysis of Behavior, 54*(3), 163–172. https://doi.org/10.1901/jeab.1990.54-163

Mace, F. C., Mauro, B. C., Boyajian, A. E., & Eckert, T. L. (1997). Effects of reinforcer quality on behavioral momentum: Coordinated applied and basic research. *Journal of Applied Behavior Analysis, 30*(1), 1–20. https://doi.org/10.1901/jaba.1997.30-1

McComas, J. J., Hartman, E. C., & Jimenez, A. (2008). Some effects of magnitude of reinforcement on persistence of responding. *Psychological Record, 58*(4), 517–527. https://doi.org/10.1007/BF03395635

Mitteer, D. R., Randall, K. R., Van Winkle, L. J., & Greer, B. D. (2020). Incorporating discriminative stimuli into functional communication training with augmentative and alternative communication devices: A tutorial. *Augmentative and Alternative Communication, 36*(1), 63–70. https://doi.org/10.1080/07434618.2020.1731761

Nevin, J. A. (1974). Response strength in multiple schedules. *Journal of the Experimental Analysis of Behavior, 21*(3), 389–408. https://doi.org/10.1901/jeab.1974.21-389

Nevin, J. A., & Grace, R. C. (2000). Behavioral momentum and the law of effect. *Behavioral and Brain Sciences, 23*(1), 73–130. https://doi.org/10.1017/s0140525x00002405

Nevin, J. A., & Wacker, D. P. (2013). Response strength and persistence. In G. J. Madden (Editor-in-Chief), *APA handbook of behavior analysis: Vol. 2. Translating principles into practice* (pp. 109–128). American Psychological Association.

Nevin, J. A., Tota, M. E., Torquato, R. D., & Shull, R. L. (1990). Alternative reinforcement increases resistance to change: Pavlovian or operant contingencies? *Journal of the Experimental Analysis of Behavior, 53*(3), 359–379. https://doi.org/10.1901/jeab.1990.53-359

Podlesnik, C. A., & Chase, P. N. (2006). Sensitivity and strength: Effects of instructions on resistance to change. *The Psychological Record, 56*(2), 303–320. https://doi.org/10.1007/BF03395552

Podlesnik, C. A., Jimenez-Gomez, C., Ward, R. D., & Shahan, T. A. (2006). Resistance to change of responding maintained by unsignaled delays to reinforcement: A response-bout analysis. *Journal of the Experimental Analysis of Behavior, 85*(3), 329–347. https://doi.org/10.1901/jeab.2006.47-05

Pritchard, D., Hoerger, M., & Mace, F. C. (2014). Treatment relapse and behavioral momentum theory. *Journal of Applied Behavior Analysis, 47*(4), 814–833. https://doi.org/10.1002/jaba.163

Richman, D. M., Wacker, D. P., & Winborn, L. (2001). Response efficiency during functional communication training: Effects of effort on response allocation. *Journal of Applied Behavior Analysis, 34*(1), 73–76. https://doi.org/10.1901/jaba.2001.34-73

Ringdahl, J. (2018). *Effects of reinforcer and extinction factors on response strength of behavior*. US Department of Health and Human Services, National Institutes of Health, National Institute of Child Health and Human Development.

Ringdahl, J. E., Falcomata, T. S., Christensen, T. J., Bass-Ringdahl, S. M., Lentz, A., Dutt, A., & Schuh-Claus, J. (2009). Evaluation of a pre-treatment assessment to select mand topographies for functional communication training. *Research in Developmental Disabilities, 30*(2), 330–341. https://doi.org/10.1016/j.ridd.2008.06.002

Ringdahl, J. E., Berg, W. K., Wacker, D. P., Crook, K., Molony, M. A., Vargo, K. K., Neurnberger, J. E., Zabala, K., & Taylor, C. J. (2018). Effects of response preference on resistance to change. *Journal of the Experimental Analysis of Behavior, 109*(1), 265–280. https://doi.org/10.1002/jeab.308

Ringdahl, J. E., Crook, K., Berg, W. K., Wacker, D. P., Molony, M., Romani, P., Ryan, S., Ryan, A., & Zabala, K. (2023). Further evaluation of prompt density, rate of reinforcement, and the persistence of manding. *Behavioral Interventions, 38*(3), 538–553. https://doi.org/10.1002/bin.1944

Romani, P. W., Suess, A. N., Whittington, H., Kopelman, C., Ringdahl, J. E., Vinquist, K. M., & Dutt, A. (2013). Prompt density, rate of reinforcement, and the persistence of manding. *The Psychological Record, 63*(4), 821–834. https://doi.org/10.11133/j.tpr.2013.63.4.008

Romani, P. W., Ringdahl, J. E., Wacker, D. P., Lustig, N. H., Vinquist, K. M., Northup, J., Kane, A. M., & Carrion, D. P. (2016). Relations between rate of negative reinforcement and the persistence of task completion. *Journal of Applied Behavior Analysis, 49*(1), 122–137. https://doi.org/10.1002/jaba.252

Rosenfarb, I. S., Newland, M. C., Brannon, S. E., & Howey, D. S. (1992). Effects of self-generated rules on the development of schedule-controlled behavior. *Journal of the Experimental Analysis of Behavior, 58*(1), 107–121. https://doi.org/10.1901/jeab.1992.58-107

Schieltz, K. M., Wacker, D. P., Ringdahl, J. E., & Berg, W. K. (2017). Basing assessment and treatment of problem behavior on behavioral momentum theory: Analyses of behavioral persistence. *Behavioural Processes, 141*(Pt 1), 75–84. https://doi.org/10.1016/j.bbeproc.2017.02.013

Shahan, T. A. (2017). Moving beyond reinforcement and response strength. *Behavior Analyst, 40*, 107–121. https://doi.org/10.1007/s40614-017-0092-y

Shahan, T. A. (2020). Relapse: An introduction. *Journal of the Experimental Analysis of Behavior, 113*(1), 8–14. https://doi.org/10.1002/jeab.578

Skinner, B. F. (1938). *The behavior of organisms*. Appleton-Century-Crofts.

Suess, A. N., Schieltz, K. S., Wacker, D. P., Detrick, J., & Podlesnik, C. A. (2020). An evaluation of resurgence following functional communication training conducted in alternative antecedent contexts via telehealth. *Journal of the Experimental Analysis of Behavior, 113*(1), 278–301. https://doi.org/10.1002/jeab.551

Trump, C. E. (2019). *Evaluating the effect of instructions on response persistence through the framework of behavioral momentum theory* [Doctoral dissertation, University of Georgia]. ProQuest Dissertations & Theses Global.

Wacker, D. P., Harding, J. W., Berg, W. K., Lee, J. F., Schieltz, K. M., Padilla, Y. C., Nevin, J. A., & Shahan, T. (2011). An evaluation of persistence of treatment effects during long-term treatment of destructive behavior. *Journal of the Experimental Analysis of Behavior, 96*(2), 261–282. https://doi.org/10.1901/jeab.2011.96-261

Wathen, S. N., & Podlesnkik, C. A. (2018). Laboratory models of treatment relapse and mitigation techniques. *Behavior Analysis: Research and Practice, 18*(4), 362–387. https://doi.org/10.1037/bar0000119

Winborn-Kemmerer, L., Ringdahl, J. E., Wacker, D. P., & Kitsukawa, K. (2009). A demonstration of individual preference for novel mands during functional communication training. *Journal of Applied Behavior Analysis, 42*(1), 185–189. https://doi.org/10.1901/jaba.2009.42-185

Chapter 9
Strategies for Promoting and Ensuring Client and Staff Safety During the Treatment of Severe Behavior

Ashley M. Fuhrman, Landon S. Cowan, Lauren A. Phillips, and Chelsea C. Elwood

Common reasons that caregivers may seek behavioral treatment for a loved one with autism spectrum disorder (ASD) include concerns about aggressive behaviors such as hitting, kicking, or biting (Kanne & Mazurek, 2011); self-injurious behaviors (SIB) such as head banging, biting oneself, or hitting oneself (Haddock & Hagopian, 2020); and destructive behaviors such as throwing, kicking, or destroying items or property. In an evaluation of psychiatric-related emergency room (ER) visits conducted by Kalb et al. (2012), researchers found that children with ASD were nine times more likely to visit an ER for psychiatric concerns than children without ASD. Severe behaviors such as hurting oneself or others or running away are often the main reason for these ER visits (Kalb et al., 2012). Although the frequency and severity of these behaviors may vary across individuals, SIB can pose significant risk of injury to clients, aggression can pose significant risk of injury to staff, and destructive behavior can result in significant damage to property and risk of injury to those in the environment. SIB and aggression can result in lacerations, bruising, head injuries, and many other types of severe injuries that require medical intervention. Destructive behavior can result in broken items (e.g., glass) that can pose additional risks of injury to those in the immediate environment. In addition, pica (e.g., consumption of toxic cleaners) and elopement (e.g., running into a busy street with oncoming traffic) can present serious risk of injury or death to clients.

The number of inpatient and intensive outpatient programs that exist to uniquely serve individuals impacted by ASD and severe behavior is limited. Caregivers may often face barriers in identifying providers who can safely and effectively provide

A. M. Fuhrman (✉) · L. S. Cowan · L. A. Phillips · C. C. Elwood
Trumpet Behavioral Health, Dublin, CA, USA

BlueSprig Pediatrics, Houston, TX, USA
e-mail: ashley.fuhrman@bluesprigpediatrics.com

M. P. Kranak (ed.), *Behavioral Treatments for Individuals with Autism*, Autism and Child Psychopathology Series,
https://doi.org/10.1007/978-3-031-91965-7_9

treatment for their loved ones' severe behavior or may be faced with an option to place their loved one in a residential facility or increase pharmaceutical treatment of the behavior, which may often come with undesired side effects (Hess et al., 2010). These variables may often lead caregivers to seek out less intensive outpatient providers, such as behavior analysts, to assist with the treatment of their loved ones' severe behavior. As such, it is not uncommon for behavior-analytic organizations to receive requests for services from caregivers whose referral concerns for their loved ones include one or many of the abovementioned topographies of severe behavior that can pose immediate risk of harm to clients and staff.

When delivering treatment for severe behavior, organizations must ensure that they are equipped to provide safe and effective care to the clients they serve. It is essential for organizations to build a culture focused on the prevention of client and staff injuries and to establish policies, procedures, and resources to equip their providers to prioritize safety. In this chapter, we provide recommendations for several possible safeguard recommendations for practitioners to consider when conducting the assessment and treatment of severe behavior, such as antecedent strategies (e.g., screening procedures, environmental considerations, safety resources and procedures), training considerations, and safe responses to severe behavior when it does occur. The extent to which the following recommendations may apply can depend on the number of learners a facility may serve and whether there is a focus for all learners on the treatment of severe behavior. For example, a center primarily providing early intensive behavioral intervention for young children with ASD, some of whom may have mild to moderate behavior concerns, may only need to consider a few of the following recommendations (e.g., staff training, safety resources and procedures). Whereas a center that is focusing on the assessment and treatment of severe behavior with a wider age range of learners may likely need to consider all the following recommendations to ensure safe and effective care.

Antecedent Considerations

When it comes to behaviors that can pose serious risk of harm to self, others, and the environment, we recommend that practitioners always program preventative strategies as a first step to ensure client and staff safety. In the following sections, we provide recommendations specific to antecedent strategies that practitioners may consider in terms of awareness, environmental considerations, safety resources and procedures (e.g., protective equipment, dress code), and training considerations. If practitioners emphasize these proactive antecedent strategies, events with the potential for client and staff injuries will be less likely to occur, and the need for building systems to respond to behavioral escalations and client or staff injuries will be lessened.

Preparedness

First, it is important to have procedures in place to ensure awareness of several important variables that will contribute to being prepared to safely serve clients impacted by severe behavior. Before each client's first appointment, staff should be aware of any referral concerns surrounding severe behaviors. A screening form or phone call are two possible ways to gather information about severe behavior referral concerns prior to a first appointment. If practitioners do not ask caregivers specific questions or ask using language that may be inconsistent with the caregiver's understanding of the behaviors, they may not gather all the necessary information to ensure preparedness. For example, if a practitioner asks about concerns of aggression, one caregiver may include instances of cursing as a form of aggression while another caregiver may not. Another caregiver may consider the throwing of objects at individuals as property destruction instead of aggression. In addition, caregivers may underreport severe behavior if they have contacted the contingency of other providers turning them away due to safety concerns surrounding the behaviors. Thus, screening procedures should include specific questions and definitions for caregivers to discriminate between different types of severe behavior and an assurance that the information gathered will be used to ensure safe and effective assessment.

Gathering information on the frequency (e.g., daily, hourly) and the severity of the outcomes (e.g., produces red marks, results in bruising) of the severe behavior can provide additional information to help prepare safeguards for care. For example, the Destructive Behavior Severity Scale (Fisher et al., 2013, 2022) includes a section that quantifies frequency and severity according to the physical impacts of various topographies of destructive behavior (e.g., injury, elopement impacts, physical property damage) on a four-point scale. Using a scale such as this will help practitioners be aware of all the possible topographies of severe behavior, the frequency of each topography, and the potential risk of each topography that will require safeguards to ensure safe and effective care.

Environmental Considerations

Service Setting Location

When conducting treatment of severe behavior, it is important to consider the space in which the service delivery will take place. Establishing a safe setting is critical to ensure the safety and well-being of clients and staff. Severe behaviors require a controlled environment to minimize risks and provide effective interventions. As such, practitioners should consider what service settings (e.g., center, home, school) allow for that control and safety and make the appropriate recommendations for treatment. Given that most topographies of severe behavior can present imminent risk of harm to clients themselves or others, we recommend an environment that is (a) arranged to allow clients to have individual therapy and single-occupancy bathroom spaces as well as large shared free spaces (e.g., gym, playground), (b) free of unnecessary furniture and materials that may be thrown, broken, or used during SIB, (c) nearby other trained team members who can support with the safe management of severe behavior, and (d) not adjacent to a busy street (i.e., to prevent increased danger following successful elopement). As such, center- or hospital-based services are often the best environment to ensure safe and effective care in the treatment of severe behavior. It is important to note that providing clients with their own dedicated therapy space often decreases the maximum number of clients able to be served in a center relative to centers that serve early learners in shared classrooms and group settings.

Organizations providing both early intensive behavioral interventions and severe behavior services in the same building should also consider the arrangement of treatment spaces to minimize or avoid instances where clients can access the other treatment area (i.e., avoiding instances where clients with severe behavior might elope to an area with young early learners). Examples of ways organizations might separate these clinical areas include badge-access doors between the clinical spaces and separate entrances and lobby spaces.

Therapy Space

In addition to the service setting location, practitioners must make several considerations surrounding the arrangement and design of the therapy space as another proactive safety strategy (Fisher et al., 2022). In fact, some of the billing codes that organizations may use to bill for the assessment and treatment of severe behavior with higher staffing ratios require a customized environment that is configured to allow for the safe implementation of procedures.

By providing an individual with their own therapeutic space designed in a way to allow their severe behavior to occur as safely as possible, practitioners can decrease the possibility of injury and property damage while conducting individualized assessment and treatment procedures that involve the need for observation of the dangerous behaviors. These measures can also decrease the need for more restrictive interventions (e.g., restraint) to maintain safety in escalated behavior scenarios.

Protective Padding

Installation of protective padding on the walls (e.g., wood-backed wall padding like that used in basketball gymnasiums) and rubberized or padded flooring in therapy rooms is one crucial consideration for the spaces where practitioners plan to conduct treatment of SIB, aggression, and property destruction. The protective padding and softer flooring can help prevent (a) client injuries from head banging, body slamming, and flopping, (b) staff injuries from pushing or shoving, and (c) property damage from kicking or throwing objects at walls. This safeguard against injuries and property damage reduces the potential need for more restrictive or intrusive procedures to maintain safety. Although protective padding in therapy spaces has strong practical benefits in terms of safety, it is reasonable that some caregivers and clients may associate padded walls with an institutional feel or stigmatization of their behaviors. Thus, we recommend that practitioners consider modifications to create a more welcoming and personalized environment (e.g., padding with screen-printed images, wall decals featuring favorite themes of the clients, decorative lighting that clients can control and choose colors of, light covers or skylights with plexiglass).

Observation and Communication Systems

It is critical to have an environment that facilitates effective communication and continuous monitoring such that practitioners can always observe and participate in therapy sessions and support during escalated behavior events. One-way observation windows in therapy rooms allow staff to monitor clients safely and unobtrusively. This feature ensures that staff can observe and collect data on behaviors without having extra data collection materials and extra staff in close physical proximity to the client, which can be essential for the precise data collection necessary for the safe and effective treatment of severe behavior. Moreover, it helps to maintain the clients' privacy and allows them the opportunity to request space from staff while still being safely monitored.

Additional ways to facilitate effective communication and continuous monitoring include two-way intercom systems and camera systems. Intercom systems enable immediate communication between the client, staff, and the supervising clinicians, which is often vital during crises or when immediate intervention is needed. Camera systems allow for real-time monitoring and support (e.g., from a practitioner on-site or remotely), the ability to review incidents to better understand behavioral events, the context in which they occur, and how to increase safety for all involved. These technological supports help facilitate both proactive and reactive strategies in safe behavior management.

Elopement Safeguards

To mitigate the risk of elopement, which is a common and life-threatening concern for individuals with ASD (Anderson et al., 2012; Mouridsen et al., 2008), a secure environment is essential. Securing the environment to mitigate elopement can include alarmed doors, delayed egress, secure fencing, and protocols for quickly locating and retrieving clients who engage in elopement attempts. Ensuring these safeguards are in place can increase the safety of clients and staff who could be seriously injured in successful elopement (e.g., vehicle accidents, trips, and falls).

Staffing Ratios and Workspace

It is an essential safety consideration to maintain a higher staffing ratio, such as at least a 2:1 ratio of behavior technicians with each client receiving treatment for severe behavior. A higher staffing ratio ensures that each client receives the intensive support and supervision necessary to manage and reduce severe behaviors safely and effectively. For example, with 2:1 support, one behavior technician can conduct treatment procedures in the room with the client while the second behavior technician is positioned behind the one-way observation window collecting continuous and precise data, communicating protocol procedures, gathering additional materials, safety equipment, or clinical oversight needed, and jumping into the session to support the safe management of escalated behavior episodes. Higher staffing ratios also allow for more prompt intervention and support during behavioral crises, improving overall safety and effectiveness of service delivery.

Additionally, smaller caseloads and the close physical proximity of supervising behavior analysts are crucial, as they allow for more thorough assessment, detailed behavior intervention planning, and continuous supervision and support for the behavior technicians and clients. The behavior analysts should be on-site and immediately available during all client service hours, as is required by some of the billing codes that organizations use for the assessment and treatment of severe behavior with an increased staffing ratio. Positioning behavior analyst's office space in the same space as therapy rooms allows for them to quickly respond and provide oversight during client appointments. This increased staff-to-client ratio and associated level of oversight can facilitate improved treatment outcomes and ensure that interventions are implemented consistently and accurately. In addition, higher staffing ratios and smaller caseloads may also reduce staff burnout and increase retention for these critical positions (Plantiveau et al., 2018).

Safety Resources and Standard Operating Procedures

After ensuring that the service setting and facility are equipped for the safe and effective delivery of treatment for severe behavior, organizations should work to establish and maintain safety resources and standard operating procedures (SOPs) for staff. Examples of these resources and SOPs include the use of personal protective padding and equipment, two-way radio communication systems, and team member dress code.

Personal Protective Padding and Equipment

Personal protective padding (PPP) is staff-worn safety gear commonly used to minimize injury across various situations that could lead to injury. Fisher et al. (2013) provides everyday examples of protective measures, including roller-coaster harnesses, football helmets, and boxing gloves; these safety measures exist to protect an individual from injury. Similarly, staff who work with individuals who engage in severe behavior should wear PPP to protect themselves from injury that could be sustained from aggression. Personal protective padding and equipment are critical antecedent manipulation to increase staff safety when working with clients with aggression, just as wearing a seatbelt in a moving vehicle is a critical requirement that avoids significant injury in the event of an accident.

We recommend that organizations working with clients with severe behavior have several types and sizes of PPP available to staff and purchase new types and sizes of PPP when needed to mitigate injury risk. There are a variety of forms of PPP that staff can wear to protect most areas of their body that could be at risk of injury from aggression. One of the most useful pieces of PPP for staff members is padded arm guards that individuals typically use for martial arts. Padded arm guards reach from the top of the knuckles to the elbow to protect the lower arm and hand. The arm guards remain intact well, can be easily washed and sanitized, and protect the arm and hand from aggression such as biting, hitting, pinching, and scratching. With clients who engage in biting, we recommend an additional layer of protection by placing youth soccer shin guards on the top and bottom of the forearms prior to placing the padded arm guards on. Staff should never wear any hard-shell protective equipment (e.g., shin guards, helmet) without some form of padding over the top of it such that the protection for staff does not present risk of injury to the clients (e.g., mouth/teeth injury from biting a shin guard, hand injury from hitting a hard helmet). To protect the biceps and triceps from similar topographies of aggression, staff can wear large, padded shin guards on the upper arm.

Padded helmets, typically used for sparring in martial arts, may be used to avoid hair pulls or injury from head-directed aggression (e.g., hitting, throwing items). Padded sparring helmets allow for the addition of a plastic face shield to further protect the face from aggression or bodily fluids (e.g., spit, eye-directed aggression). With clients for whom hair pulling is a concern but there is not a need for a full helmet, scrub caps, skull caps, or swim caps are less restrictive alternatives; staff can also place these items underneath a helmet as an extra layer of protection from hair pulls that could occur if a client grabs the top of a helmet. To protect the chest, shoulders, and ribs of staff members from aggression or throwing of items, an individual may wear a padded chest plate typically used in various sports such as lacrosse or hockey. Additionally, padded shin guards and volleyball kneepads can protect the shins and knees from kicks. Cut-resistant gloves can protect the staff from scratches and bites to the hand and fingers and can protect the client from a staff's fingernails. Staff can wear a compression shirt over all the upper body PPP to keep the gear intact and more concealed.

In some cases when the frequency and severity of SIB regularly presents imminent risk of harm, client-worn protection may be necessary to maintain client safety. Client-worn protection can include a helmet, cut-resistant gloves, or mechanical restraint due to the continuous nature and high risk of harm due to the severity of SIB (APBA, 2010). APBA (2010) identified two devices used for mechanical restraint, including arm splints and hand mitts. They further indicate the use of such restraints only be implemented following a set of guidelines, such as collaborating with a medical professional, completion of a functional behavior assessment, and demonstration of less restrictive interventions that were proven ineffective (APBA, 2010). If a client's SIB warrants client-worn protection or mechanical restraint, their behavior intervention plan (BIP) should always include information on its proper use and a fading plan.

Various types of blocking pads can serve as additional PPP to reduce injury and the need for more restrictive interventions. First, a large martial arts kick pad with straps on the back side can block attempts at various types of aggression toward staff. These blocking pads can protect nearly any part of a staff's body by moving it to protect any body part targeted. Smaller blocking pads, such as those used as hand targets in martial arts, are easier to hold and can block client SIB (e.g., head banging, self-hitting, self-hair pulling) and staff-directed aggression. To further protect a client from possible injuries that can be sustained from head banging, staff can use items such as nap mats, corner guards, and pool noodles to cover hard surfaces such as tables, windows, floors, or walls.

Personal protective equipment (PPE), items often used in a medical setting, can protect individuals from transmission of bodily fluids and slips on a soiled floor. Schoberer et al. (2022) lists examples of PPE (e.g., gloves, masks, gowns) to protect healthcare workers from the spread of illness and transmission of bodily fluids. These forms of PPE are a vital resource when working with individuals diagnosed with ASD and intellectual developmental disabilities that may engage with their bodily fluids (e.g., emesis, enuresis, and encopresis). Examples of PPE that we recommend organizations have on site for staff conducting treatment of severe behavior include goggles, face masks, or face shields to protect the eyes and mouth from bodily fluids (e.g., spitting directed at a staff member). Additionally, disposable gowns, gloves, and shoe covers can protect staff clothing from being soiled by bodily fluids. Utilization of disposable bed pads, typically used as an incontinence product, to quickly soak up bodily fluids on the ground can prevent slipping hazards that may arise when bodily fluid elimination occurs in therapy spaces. When clients engage in severe behavior that is accompanied by bodily fluid elimination (e.g., spitting, fecal smearing), it is necessary for organizations to purchase and maintain supplies of all necessary types and sizes of PPE for the staff.

Two-Way Radio Communication

Two-way radio communication, with devices such as walkie-talkies, serves as a vital tool to minimize risk during severe behavior escalations (e.g., announcing transitions throughout the center to ensure a clear path). The use of walkie-talkies allows staff to provide immediate proactive and reactive support for one another and is an effective antecedent strategy to ensure streamlined communication to support safety. We recommend that each staff member have their own assigned walkie-talkie that they secure and test prior to each client shift. Using a hip clip for the walkie-talkie facilitates staff ability to keep it on their person and within reach. Clinicians should ensure that there is a procedure to confirm the walkie-talkies are charged each day and that all staff receive training in how to use the walkie-talkie (e.g., turning up/down volume, turning it on/off, setting the channel, what channel the center uses, and how to place in the dock for charging; Padmanabhan & Bakkialakshmi, 2023).

It is important to have two-way radio communication procedures established to protect privacy and increase efficiency (e.g., a coding system). Code systems can include a numerical or color system (e.g., Code 1, Code 2, Code 3; Code Green, Code Yellow, Code Red) and each code should correspond to the type of support that staff may need (e.g., check-in, supervisor support, crisis support).

Team Member Dress Code

The established and enforced dress code for staff also plays a large role in staff and client safety, beginning with clothing items. Well-fitted tops and bottoms versus loose clothing protect staff from clothing grabs, which can lead to other forms of aggression and injury. Sweatshirts with hoods may pose risk of a choking hazard if grabbed from behind, and jackets with zippers can pose risk of injury to clients' hands following clothing grabs. Hair should be tied up and securely fastened to avoid successful hair pulls, and staff should keep their fingernails short to protect clients from incidental scratches from staff when they may need to block aggressive or self-injurious behaviors. We recommend that loose or hanging jewelry, such as a necklace, earrings, and bracelets, is not worn when working with clients to avoid injury to both the client and staff members (e.g., scratches to clients from jewelry, injuries to staff ears if a client pulls an earring). Practitioners should consider various cultural or religious practices that may impact what PPP or clothing items an individual can wear and what modifications or additional PPP may be needed for individual staff. It is important to note that adherence to dress codes and guidelines regarding PPP and PPE is a proactive measure to prevent injury. We recommend that clinicians conduct and document regular integrity checks on staff adherence to dress code and PPP and PPE requirements. These proactive measures can significantly decrease the likelihood of injury to the staff and the client and decrease the need for more restrictive measures to maintain safety.

Responding Safely to Severe Behavior

To ensure staff and client safety, it is important to establish proactive plans to respond to episodes of severe behavior and ensure staff are trained on those plans (Winokur et al., 2018). Organizations should develop center protocols on how to respond to severe behavior that is individualized to the clinical population that the center serves. This section of the chapter will review recommended practices for establishing standard operating procedures surrounding communication systems, crisis management, and debriefing.

Communication Systems

An effective communication system includes the following components: (a) technology or environmental arrangements that allow for quick communication, (b) key phrases or code words to efficiently communicate support needs, (c) training on how to use the communication system, (d) resources to support the system, and (e) performance monitoring to ensure correct system use.

Clinicians (e.g., the client's board certified behavior analyst® [BCBA®]) should consider their environment and what tools could assist them with communicating in the event of a behavioral escalation. If the clinician is working in a small center with a few session rooms and an office that is within earshot, they may be able to arrange the environment to allow for verbal communication. For instance, they could remove doors from session rooms or use half doors to maintain open lines of communication. In larger centers, the clinician can enlist the use of technology to call for behavioral support (see Section on two-way radio communication for additional details). Additionally, team-messaging platforms allow for the creation of chat spaces for staff to request support on company devices (e.g., laptops, tablets) when a client demonstrates precursors to severe behavior (e.g., Padmanabhan & Bakkialakshmi, 2023).

Staff training on behavioral escalation procedures should include when and how to communicate during a behavioral escalation. The procedure should specify calling for support from a clinician at the first sign of a possible behavioral escalation. It can be helpful to identify common precursors in the client's BIP and directly state that the direct support staff will call for clinician support when they observe those behaviors. Clinicians should also train staff in the language the program uses when describing a behavioral escalation and when asking for assistance (e.g., a color or number code system). The specific code words that an organization chooses are less important than the all-staff training needed to implement this code system effectively. To minimize the need for training on code words, some organizations opt for plain language communication (Dauksewicz, 2019), that is, they clearly state what the need is using their communication system, for example, stating on the walkie-talkie, "behavior support in room 5." Whichever system the organization selects, it should ensure that all current staff and new hires are oriented to the system and that the system is used consistently. Clinicians should implement behavioral skills training (BST; Reid et al., 2021) to describe how to use the communication system, model correct use of the communication system, and provide feedback when staff use the system for nonrelated communication, fail to use the system for behavioral escalations, and correctly use the system to request support in the event of a behavioral escalation (Parsons et al., 2013).

Crisis Management

Supervision and Support

Centers should ensure that a trained clinician is available for behavior support and can arrive quickly whenever a staff member calls for support during a behavioral escalation (e.g., an increasing frequency and/or severity of severe behavior that increases imminent risk of harm to client or staff). One way that centers may do this is by assigning a specific clinician to be assigned to floor-support coverage. This clinician would ensure that they have access to the communication system and only schedule appointments that they can step away from in the event of a call for behavior support. Another consideration is to have a few direct support staff who are not directly assigned to a client and are available to assist in the event of a behavioral escalation or a team in need of additional PPP or PPE. Ensuring sufficient staff are present to support safety will help decrease client and staff injuries and increase staff satisfaction in their role (Ryan et al., 2019).

It is often helpful to have more than one clinician observe any behavioral escalations. Ideally, multiple additional clinicians would be available for in-person support; however, due to logistical barriers, it may not always be possible. Using telehealth to allow for remote observation can allow for other clinicians (e.g., leadership or clinicians at other sites) to support and provide recommendations to the on-site clinician to assist in de-escalating the client (O'Brien et al., 2021). It can be helpful to have direct-care staff trained in how to activate this level of support if the clinician is not able to step away from the behavioral escalation. For example, direct support staff might be added to behavioral escalation support chat spaces on group messaging platforms so that they can notify other clinicians of the need for remote support if the on-site clinician is directly supporting the client. We recommend that organizations develop a behavioral escalation support policy that outlines this increased supervision and support and how staff should notify leadership if they need additional support.

In the event of a more significant behavioral escalation, the behavioral escalation policy will outline possible differences in procedures for (a) minor staff and/or client injuries that can be addressed using basic first aid, (b) significant staff and/or client injuries that required medical attention, and (c) intervention from emergency services such as paramedics or police. A communication hierarchy can be helpful to ensure that teams have a resource to quickly escalate communication and how to decide when external support (e.g., emergency medical services) may be necessary.

If the clinical staff anticipate the possibility of a behavioral escalation with a new client or new protocol, they should review the BIP, protective equipment, and behavioral escalation plan with staff before the client arrives to ensure that all staff are prepared (Wright et al., 2024). If the staff are not available for a pre-session meeting, clinical staff should provide the direct support staff with a written BIP before the session and schedule overlap with the client at the start of the session to ensure the direct support staff is prepared to safely implement the session (Lin et al., 2024).

De-escalation

Clinicians should follow their agency-specific training and ethical obligation to use the least restrictive and most effective interventions to support de-escalation (Van Houten et al., 1988; Behavior Analyst Certification Board, 2020). The staff should remain calm and use a neutral tone of voice when communicating with the client. When managing escalated behavior, it is important to evade any aggressive behavior if staff can do so safely without concerns for other topographies of behavior (e.g., the need to be close to block dangerous SIB). While evading, the staff should continually move away from the client who is engaging in aggressive behavior while remaining mindful of any environmental dangers. The clinician should remove any items that could become a projectile if thrown, especially large or hard objects. Elopement is often a concern during an escalation, so the clinician should ensure they remain between the client and any unsafe locations (e.g., an exterior door that leads to a busy road, a hallway that other clients are walking through). If the client engages in SIB or destructive behavior, the clinician should block and redirect the behavior if necessary while wearing personal protective equipment or using blocking pads (Metoyer et al., 2020). It is the clinician's responsibility to ensure that they have taught or are teaching the client replacement skills such as functional communication, waiting, and tolerance skills. If the client's behavioral escalation indicates that the client has not mastered, maintained, or generalized those skills, the clinician should provide the functional reinforcer for the severe behavior (Wong et al., 2022) if necessary to maintain immediate safety prior to considering the use of a restrictive intervention (e.g., restraint). While reinforcing the target behavior may increase the probability of the behavior in the future, it allows the clinician to de-escalate the client in the moment using the least restrictive procedures, ensure staff and client safety, and take time to revisit their clinical programming to support the client to master the target skill. Clinicians should exhaust least restrictive interventions prior to using hands-on interventions. In the event of a more significant behavioral escalation, the behavioral escalation policy will outline procedures for (a) minor staff and/or client injuries that can be addressed using basic first aid, (b) significant staff and/or client injuries that required medical attention, and (c) intervention from emergency services such as paramedics or police.

Incident and Injury Reporting and Debriefing

Working with individuals with aggressive, self-injurious, and destructive behavior can result in physical injuries and induce stress on the client and the staff (Oster & Doyle, 2000). Following a bout of escalated behavior, we recommend a clinician conduct an in-the-moment debrief with the staff, a debrief with the client and/or their caregivers, documentation of the incident (e.g., incident report), and review of the incident report.

It is best practice to review the incident with the client in a way that aligns with their vocal-verbal capabilities. A clinician should lead the debrief alongside other staff who were part of the escalation. For example, the clinician may describe clearing the room of furniture and materials during an episode of property destruction by saying, "sometimes we have to move things out of our room, so everyone stays safe." It is also important that the clinician focuses on the safe and adaptive behavior going forward. For example, in a situation where severe behavior is maintained by escape from instructions, the clinician may say, "when you need a break, you can… (e.g., say 'I need a break')" and provide the client with the opportunity to practice the functional communication response. Clients with more robust expressive communication skills may be able to participate in a discussion of the antecedents, behaviors, and consequences and what everyone (i.e., client and staff) can do differently the next time to maintain safety and communicate needs.

Clinicians should notify caregivers as soon as possible after the escalation about what the behavior looked like, what led up to the behavior, and how the clinical team and client responded to the behavior and de-escalation strategies. If the client can participate in the debrief (described above), it can be helpful to first debrief with the caregiver and then have them observe or participate in the debrief with the client. If the escalation required the use of an approved emergency restrictive intervention (e.g., restraint), the clinician must inform the caregiver of the procedure(s) used, which staff were present, how long the procedure lasted, and if there were any adverse outcomes from the procedure. Specifically, staff should conduct a post-procedure assessment by looking at the visible skin to determine if the client sustained any markings or injuries following the procedure. With client and caregiver consent, it can be helpful to have two staff assess covered areas of skin (e.g., the client's biceps and thighs) that were held during restrictive intervention to determine if the client sustained any markings or injuries in those areas (Taha, 2013). The clinician should review the outcomes of the assessment and the use of physical intervention(s) with the caregivers the same day as the appointment and before the client goes home to ensure transparency with caregivers and provide timely communication (Taylor et al., 2018; Walton, 2011).

Following the debrief, the staff present for the behavioral escalation should document the event, any injuries that occurred, and if any emergency restrictive procedures were implemented. A documentation system allows for monitoring of staff and client injuries to assess for trends that could warrant BIP revisions or any necessary staff retraining. Staff should complete incident reports for any staff or client injury and should describe the injury, the events leading up to the incident, and the employee response to the incident, including the need for first aid, medical intervention, or emergency services. Staff should also complete incident reports for any emergency restrictive procedures (e.g., restraint). We recommend documenting several items when reporting the use of restraint, including (a) which procedure(s) were used, (b) the total duration of the procedure, (c) start time, and end time of the procedure(s), (d) which less restrictive procedures were implemented prior to using the restrictive procedure, (e) the duration of time spent attempting to de-escalate the client without the use of a restrictive procedure, (f) events or behaviors leading up to the event, (g) client response to the restrictive procedure, (h) criteria for ending the restrictive procedure (e.g., time based, calm criteria), and (i) results of the post-procedure assessment.

Organizations should develop an incident report policy that standardizes what events staff need to report, the timeline for submitting an incident report, the timeline for clinical leadership to review the incident report, and action items following incidents to decrease the probability that the incident will happen again. Clinicians should provide praise when staff submit incident reports and navigate any necessary feedback about the event or reporting delicately, as reprimands or performance coaching surrounding incidents could inadvertently punish reporting incidents and result in underreporting (Labrague, 2024).

We recommend using an electronic incident reporting system that is built in a way such that data on incidents are separated by type, person, and location are automatically graphed to allow clinicians to evaluate trends in the incident report data. Clinicians should regularly meet to review incident reports and discuss modifications that could prevent the incidents from occurring again. Some areas for consideration in the incident report review include (a) determining if a client has produced repeated injuries and what BIP changes are appropriate to best support improved safety, (b) determining if a staff has sustained repeated injuries and what additional training or PPP or PPE could support improved safety, and (c) what environmental changes the team could make to the treatment space, such as minimizing unsafe items or adding in large blocking pads to increase safety. We recommend that a clinical leader (e.g., clinical director) be assigned to review incident reports and summarize incidents to review with the organization's leadership team monthly. Some metrics that are helpful to take data on include the total number of incidents per category (e.g., client, staff), the number of days since the last injury, and the number of days since the last restrictive intervention (Arnetz et al., 2015). With these data, organizations can use objective data to define and measure progress toward goals in increasing client and staff safety. After the clinical leadership has reviewed the incident report data, it is important to ensure that they inform the direct support staff of the outcomes of the review and any actions they have added to ensure increased client and staff safety going forward.

Training Considerations for Delivering Severe Behavior Services

Organizations planning to deliver severe-behavior services should ensure that all staff receive training on relevant safety, assessment, and treatment procedures. This is essential for several reasons. First, BCBAs are ethically required to provide their supervisees with training and supervision relevant to procedures implemented while delivering behavior-analytic services (Behavior Analyst Certification Board, 2020). Additionally, Registered Behavior Technicians (RBTs) should only deliver behavior-analytic services after the supervisor confirms they have demonstrated competency of all procedures to be implemented (Behavior Analyst Certification Board, 2021). Second, this training, along with ongoing monitoring and performance feedback, supports the consistent high levels of procedural fidelity necessary to ensure sustainable, safe, and effective service delivery (Reid et al., 2021).

Organizations with an existing staff-training process can likely embed training content relevant to severe-behavior services during onboarding training for new staff members or ongoing staff development and supervisory activities for existing staff members. For example, existing training materials can be revised to include additional or more specific examples of how various interventions might be applied during severe-behavior services. However, other essential training components will require the development of additional or alternative materials, such as training on emergency or crisis response protocols that are not common or appropriate in other service settings. Training on these procedures as well as ongoing supervision should be conducted using evidence-based, competency-based strategies to ensure all staff can implement session protocols with a high level of fidelity throughout service delivery (i.e., BST; Reid et al., 2021). This section outlines specific recommendations for content that organizations should consider including in training for staff delivering severe-behavior services that will promote staff and client safety.

Training on Environmental Safety and the Use of PPP/PPE

Given that severe-behavior services inherently present a clinical environment where certain behavioral topographies (e.g., aggression) are more common and have an increased risk of causing injuries to both staff and clients or environmental damage, staff training should emphasize this characteristic of service delivery and describe strategies for minimizing the risk of injury or damage. Some general strategies for staff to decrease potential injuries from aggression include (a) remaining standing any time a client is standing, (b) remaining at or above the client's head level any time they are sitting, (c) remaining in a kneeling or lunging position that staff can easily return to a standing position from, rather than sitting fully on the floor, whenever the client is sitting on the floor, (d) requesting for another staff member to provide blocking support in the event a staff member needs to bend over in front of a client (e.g., when helping a client tie their shoes), (e) and always keeping the side of their body directed toward the client (i.e., never turning their back to the client).

Staff training should cover environmental safety strategies such as proactive safety sweeps that include removing any hazardous or broken materials (e.g., sharp, heavy, or blunt items and small items that may be easily ingested, or pose a choking hazard, for clients who engage in pica) from the therapeutic space prior to each session. Training should also cover how to use communication tools in the therapeutic space (e.g., walkie-talkies) and the protocol for requesting support when needed. For example, staff should receive instruction on ensuring they always carry their walkie-talkie with them to ensure they can quickly call for support either in the primary therapeutic space or during transitions around the building (e.g., arrival, departure, trips to the bathroom, leisure activities) as well as the code system for requesting support (e.g., "Code Green" for general questions, "Code Yellow" for behavioral support, and "Code Red" for medical emergencies). Appendix A provides an example of a two-way radio communication procedure visual that can support the training and consistent staff use of a code system (e.g., can be posted in therapeutic spaces for staff to reference).

As discussed above, there are many different pieces of PPP and PPE that staff can use to increase staff and client safety. All staff should experience training on how to properly hold or wear each piece of staff PPP and PPE and how to apply PPP and PPE intended to be worn by the client (e.g., padded helmet) as part of their individualized BIPs. We recommend including time for trainees to practice putting on each article of PPP and PPE on their body to ensure they demonstrate proper wearing and proper fit of all equipment.

In addition to general training on all articles of PPP and PPE used in the organization's severe-behavior services, all staff should receive training on the individualized PPP and PPE that they need to wear when working with each client served. For example, staff should be shown that the BIP for one client who engages in persistent upper-body and head-directed aggression toward others outlines that staff must wear PPP that covers their arms, chest, and head. For a client who engages in operant fluid elimination, the BIP should outline what PPE may be required, and staff should learn to apply fluid-resistant gowns, foot covers, and facial shields. Appendix B includes an example of a sign that can be placed in each client's therapy space to inform staff of what PPP and PPE are required to be worn prior to working with each client.

Additionally, staff should demonstrate competency of the criteria for the application and removal of a soft-shelled helmet to be worn by a client who engages in head-directed SIB (as prescribed and outlined in a BIP). If a client's BIP outlines the progressive application or removal of articles of staff-worn PPP and PPE, training should specifically incorporate this information. For example, staff should practice identifying the criterion for increasing the amount of PPP and PPE (e.g., putting a helmet on themselves) contingent upon a certain frequency, topography, or magnitude of a client's aggression (e.g., the client shifts topography of aggression from open-hand arm-directed to closed-fist head-directed hits).

Organizations should also include training on the use of PPP and PPE that is not directly worn on a staff member's or client's body, such as blocking pads. Staff should learn how to properly hold each size of blocking pad that could be used during appointments (i.e., how to hold both small, hand-sized pads as well as larger pads). The training on the use of these pads should focus on proper placement of the pad between (a) the staff member and the client if the pad is used to block instances of aggression or (b) the client's body and the surface toward which they are engaging in SIB. These pads provide protection to the staff member and client during episodes of severe behavior. Staff training should emphasize that these pads should *never* be used in a way that pushes or restricts the client's body. The improper use of a blocking pad to push or restrict a client's body could result in a variety of risks or negative outcomes, such as causing the client to fall backward and potentially injure themselves.

Healthy Session Contingencies

An important element of delivering severe-behavior services is the establishment and maintenance of a therapeutic environment for clients that is reinforcing, minimally restrictive, and unlikely to evoke the occurrence of severe behaviors outside of specific intervention activities (e.g., functional communication training; Carbone et al., 2007). Practitioners should direct staff on implementing healthy contingencies as an antecedent strategy for mitigating the risk of a behavioral escalation outside of specific intervention activities as well as de-escalation strategies following episodes of severe behavior. These healthy contingencies include the delivery of noncontingent reinforcement (NCR), frequent preference assessments to identify current motivations across appointments, differential reinforcement for all safe and adaptive responses whenever possible, the incorporation of teaching opportunities to teach and model adaptive replacement behaviors (e.g., practicing coping skills), as well as the frequent and ongoing opportunity to make choices throughout appointments. Each of these procedures is a common intervention component in behavior-analytic services and is included as competencies on task lists for RBTs and BCBAs (Behavior Analyst Certification Board, 2017, 2018). Thus, we recommend that the general training on these procedures in severe-behavior services be imbedded in the initial RBT training sequence. Practitioners can target specific refinements of these procedures for individual clients (e.g., identifying what types of NCR are relevant, forms of functional communication to prompt and deliver reinforcement following, etc.) in ongoing training and supervision activities.

Crisis De-escalation and Restrictive Interventions

The occurrence of severe behaviors that may increase the risk of injury to the client or those supporting them is inherent to the delivery of severe-behavior services. In certain situations, enhanced safety procedures that focus on the de-escalation of severe behavior and the application of emergency restrictive interventions (e.g., restraint) may be warranted or necessary to maintain the safety and well-being of both the client and their staff. Both the need and type of de-escalation or restrictive strategies are based on several variables, such as the topography of the severe behavior, the associated history or risk of injury caused by that behavior, and the age, size, and relative strength of the client.

In addition to training on antecedent strategies and interventions intended to decrease the likelihood or intensity of severe behaviors, all staff who provide severe-behavior services should receive comprehensive training on crisis de-escalation strategies as well as the implementation of emergency restrictive interventions. General examples of crisis de-escalation strategies are described below; however, organizations providing severe-behavior services should ensure that the crisis de-escalation and restrictive intervention protocols they choose follow all state and funder requirements. The legal use of some restrictive interventions, such as restraint and seclusion, varies state-to-state. That is, one state may legally permit both restraint and seclusion procedures, one may permit certain restraints but not seclusion, while another may not permit either type of procedure. For organizations providing severe-behavior services across multiple states, extra care should be taken in the development of service models to determine which procedures may be universally applied across all clinical locations and which need to be individualized for each state or location.

In addition to state legal requirements, organizations should also ensure compliance with specific funder requirements. That is, some funders may require specific packages of crisis de-escalation and emergency restrictive interventions to be implemented with any clients they fund. For example, a certain funder may require all staff working with their subscribers to be certified in a commercially available crisis management package like the Crisis Prevention Intervention (CPI) Training® or Safety-Care®, or emergency procedures such as CPR (Crisis Prevention Institute, 2024; Quality Behavior Solutions, 2024). Alternatively, funders may require specific learning modules to be completed prior to staff members delivering direct services, such as "positive behavior supports," commonly implemented in schools.

Supervision During Training and Ongoing Service Delivery

The supervision of initial training activities as well as ongoing service delivery is a critical, and required, component of behavior-analytic services (Behavior Analyst Certification Board, 2020, 2021). Supervision during initial training typically occurs during the completion of the RBT® Initial Competency Assessment and the concurrent or subsequent training for specific organization practices and client protocols (Behavior Analyst Certification Board, 2019). The duration of this initial training will likely vary between organizations but should continue until competency of all required skills is demonstrated (Reid et al., 2021).

The structure of ongoing supervision may be based on many factors. We recommend conducting an increased amount of supervision for severe-behavior services delivered relative to more standard behavior-analytic services. Depending on the funding source and authorized service code, constant supervision or the accessibility of a clinician to support session activities may even be required for the entire duration of the appointment. Regardless of the funder requirements for the purposes of billing for services, we recommend that at least one BCBA be present on site during all severe-behavior services to ensure ongoing supervision and quick accessibility to clinical support for frequent protocol modifications or crisis situations. Organizations should determine the number of required BCBAs on site by considering the number of clients served, the frequency and severity of the severe behaviors of those clients, and the number of clinical staff needed to safely and effectively manage escalated episodes of severe behavior. For example, the Council of Autism Service Providers (CASP) suggests in their *Applied Behavior Analysis Practice Guidelines for the Treatment of Autism Spectrum Disorder* that a full-time BCBA may be capable of providing 100–150 hours of case supervision per month to achieve a ratio of 10–20% of case supervision to direct therapy services (CASP, 2024). As an example, this case supervision ratio may be achieved in organizations providing early intensive behavioral interventions by assigning a caseload of 10 clients to each BCBA; however, BCBAs providing services for the assessment and treatment of severe behaviors will likely need to increase their case supervision ratios (e.g., double the amount of case supervision per client relative to an early-intervention client) in order to ensure proper oversight and support and meaningful treatment progress. Therefore, an example caseload for a full-time BCBA providing 100–150 hours of case supervision per month at a 20% case supervision to direct therapy services ratio might be five clients rather than ten. As the percentage of case supervision necessary to maintain safe and effective service delivery for a client or clients increases, caseloads should decrease.

Another factor that organizations should use to determine the appropriate and necessary amount of supervision is the complexity and severity of each client's topographies of severe behavior. That is, the necessary amount of supervision for an adult client that engages in high-frequency, high-intensity aggression with a necessary staffing ratio of 3:1 is likely higher than that required for a younger or smaller client who engages in relatively less frequent, less intense aggression with a necessary staffing ratio of 2:1. Similarly, a client with treatment goals targeting behavioral reductions and related skill acquisition targets across several behavioral topographies and functions may require a relatively higher amount of supervision and protocol modification relative to a client with relatively fewer or less complex treatment goals.

In addition to the supervision of staff implementation and client progress toward treatment goals, organizations should also plan to include fidelity checks for all crisis, de-escalation, and PPP and PPE procedures in place for each client. That is, supervisors should continuously monitor the accuracy of implementation of all safety procedures established for each client and should deliver ongoing feedback and necessary booster training for any procedures not implemented with high fidelity. The inclusion of these fidelity checks provides the opportunity for in-vivo feedback and for the clinical team to determine when more comprehensive retraining for one or more staff members may be necessary or when modifications may be needed to existing BIPs or session protocols to increase clarity of expectations.

In summary, service delivery surrounding the assessment and treatment of severe behavior can present unique complexities when it comes to maintaining staff and client safety. Organizations and practitioners in this service area should consider all safeguarding recommendations (e.g., antecedent strategies, staff training, crisis management and response, ongoing monitoring) to ensure that they are equipped to provide safe and effective care to the clients they serve, build a culture focused on the prevention of client and staff injuries, and establish policies, procedures, and resources to equip their providers to prioritize safety.

Appendix A

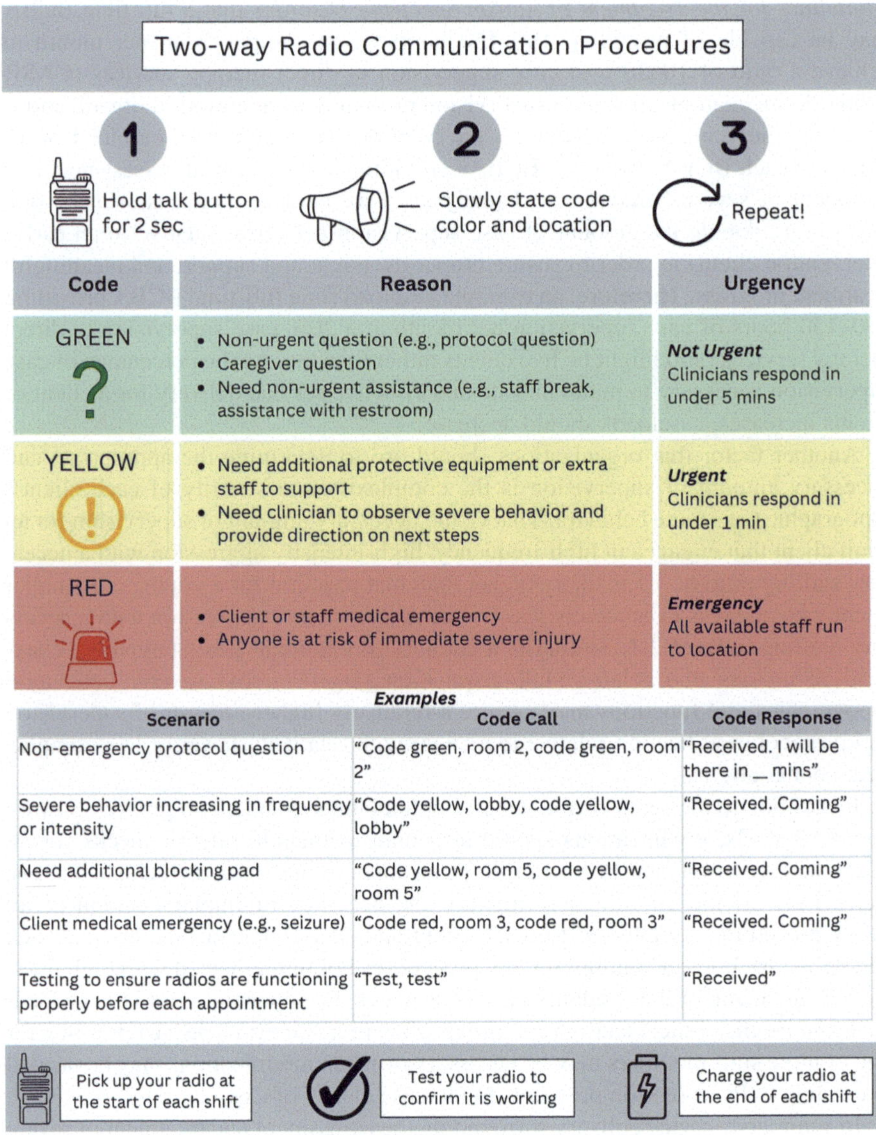

Two-way Radio Communication Procedures

1. Hold talk button for 2 sec
2. Slowly state code color and location
3. Repeat!

Code	Reason	Urgency
GREEN ?	• Non-urgent question (e.g., protocol question) • Caregiver question • Need non-urgent assistance (e.g., staff break, assistance with restroom)	***Not Urgent*** Clinicians respond in under 5 mins
YELLOW !	• Need additional protective equipment or extra staff to support • Need clinician to observe severe behavior and provide direction on next steps	***Urgent*** Clinicians respond in under 1 min
RED	• Client or staff medical emergency • Anyone is at risk of immediate severe injury	***Emergency*** All available staff run to location

Examples

Scenario	Code Call	Code Response
Non-emergency protocol question	"Code green, room 2, code green, room 2"	"Received. I will be there in __ mins"
Severe behavior increasing in frequency or intensity	"Code yellow, lobby, code yellow, lobby"	"Received. Coming"
Need additional blocking pad	"Code yellow, room 5, code yellow, room 5"	"Received. Coming"
Client medical emergency (e.g., seizure)	"Code red, room 3, code red, room 3"	"Received. Coming"
Testing to ensure radios are functioning properly before each appointment	"Test, test"	"Received"

Pick up your radio at the start of each shift

Test your radio to confirm it is working

Charge your radio at the end of each shift

Two-way radio communication procedures sign

Appendix B

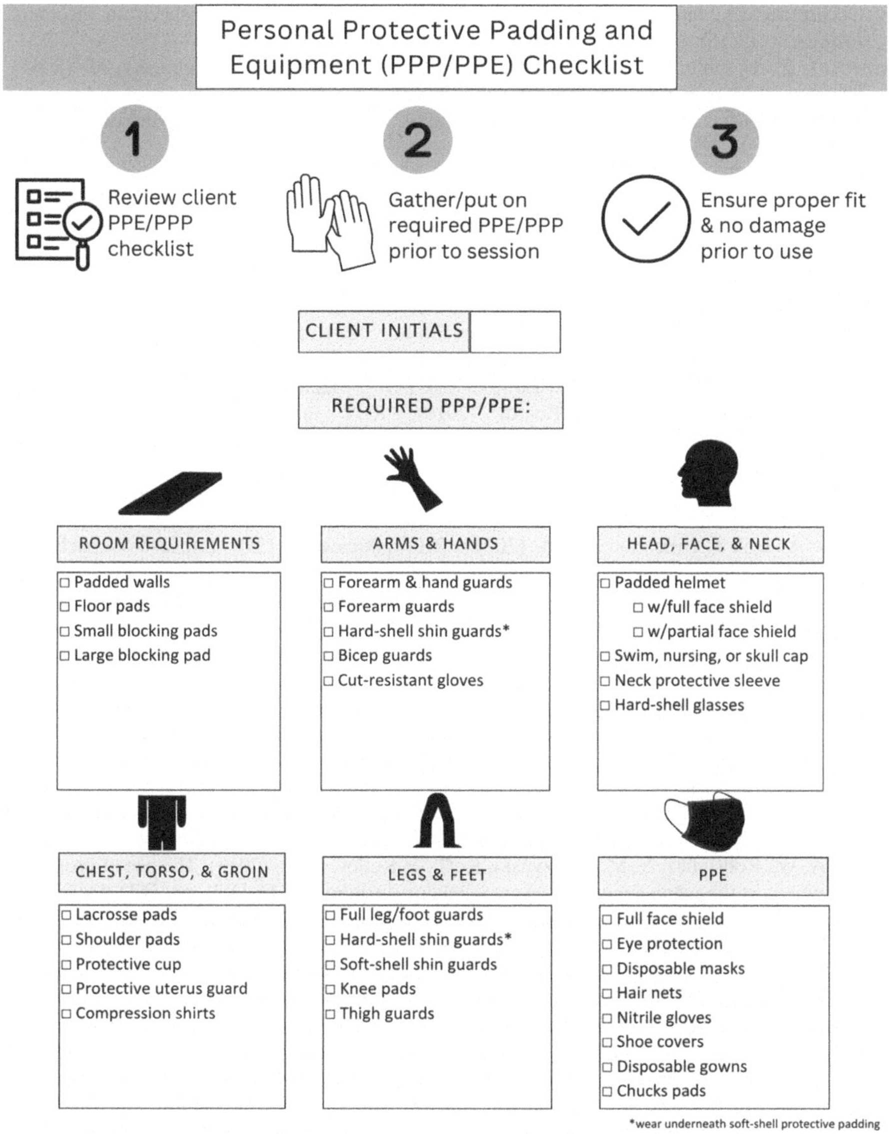

Personal protective padding and equipment sign

References

Anderson, C., Law, J. K., Daniels, A., Rice, C., Mandell, D. S., Hagopian, L., & Law, P. A. (2012). Occurrence and family impact of elopement in children with autism spectrum disorders. *Pediatrics, 130*(5), 870–877. https://doi.org/10.1542/peds.2012-0762

Arnetz, J. E., Hamblin, L., Essenmacher, L., Upfal, M. J., Ager, J., & Luborsky, M. (2015). Understanding patient-to-worker violence in hospitals: A qualitative analysis of documented incident reports. *Journal of Advanced Nursing, 71*(2), 338–348. https://doi.org/10.1111/jan.12494

Association of Professional Behavior Analysts. (2010). Position statement on the use of restraint and seclusion as interventions for dangerous and destructive behaviors: Supporting research and practice guidelines. https://cdn.ymaws.com/www.apbahome.net/resource/collection/1FDDBDD2-5CAF-4B2A-AB3F-DAE5E72111BF/Support_for_APBA_Pos_Stmt_-_Restraint_&_Seclusion.pdf.

Behavior Analyst Certification Board. (2017). *BCBA task list* (5th ed.). https://www.bacb.com/wp-content/uploads/2020/08/BCBA-task-list-5th-ed-240216-a.pdf

Behavior Analyst Certification Board. (2018). *RBT task list* (2nd ed.). https://www.bacb.com/wp-content/uploads/2020/05/RBT-2nd-Edition-Task-List_240220-a.pdf

Behavior Analyst Certification Board. (2019). RBT initial competency assessment. https://www.bacb.com/wp-content/uploads/2023/12/RBT_Competency_Assessment_Initial_2024-240612-a.pdf.

Behavior Analyst Certification Board. (2020). Ethics code for behavior analysts. https://bacb.com/wp-content/ethics-code-for-behavior-analysts/.

Behavior Analyst Certification Board. (2021). RBT ethics code (2.0). https://www.bacb.com/wp-content/rbt-ethics-code

Carbone, V. J., Morgenstern, B., Zecchin-Tirri, G., & Kolberg, L. (2007). The role of the reflexive conditioned motivating operation (CMO-R) during discrete trial instruction of children with autism. *Journal of Early Intensive Behavioral Intervention, 4*, 658–680. https://doi.org/10.1037/h0100399

Council of Autism Service Providers. (2024). *Applied behavior analysis practice guidelines for the treatment of autism spectrum disorder*. https://www.casproviders.org/asd-guidelines

Crisis Prevention Institute. (2024). Nonviolent crisis intervention® training program. https://www.crisisprevention.com/our-programs/nonviolent-crisis-intervention/

Dauksewicz, B. W. (2019). Hospitals should replace emergency codes with plain language. *Journal of Healthcare Risk Management, 38*, 32–41. https://doi.org/10.1002/jhrm.21346

Fisher, W. W., Rodriguez, N. M., Luczynski, K. C., & Kelley, M. E. (2013). The use of protective equipment in the management of severe behavior disorders. In D. D. Reed, F. D. DiGennaro Reed, & J. K. Luiselli (Eds.), *Handbook of crisis intervention for individuals with developmental disabilities* (pp. 87–105). Springer. https://doi.org/10.1007/978-1-4614-6531-7_6

Fisher, W. W., Piazza, C. C., & Fuhrman, A. M. (2022). Developing a severe behavior program: A tool kit. Retrieved from https://docs.autismspeaks.org/behavior-program/.

Haddock, J. N., & Hagopian, L. P. (2020). Self-injurious behavior in individuals with autism spectrum disorder. In S. W. White, B. B. Maddox, & C. A. Mazefsky (Eds.), *The Oxford handbook of autism and co-occurring psychiatric conditions* (pp. 327–348). Oxford University Press.

Hess, J., Matson, J., Neal, D., Mahan, S., Fodstad, J., Bamburg, J., & Holloway, J. (2010). A comparison of psychotropic drug side effect profiles in adults diagnosed with intellectual disabilities and autism spectrum disorders. *Journal of Mental Health Research in Intellectual Disabilities, 3*(2), 85–96. https://doi.org/10.1080/19315861003690588

Kalb, L. G., Stuart, E. A., Freedman, B., & Zablotsky, B. (2012). Emergency department visits among children with autism spectrum disorder. *Pediatrics, 130*(6), 1200–1208. https://doi.org/10.1097/PEC.0b013e3182767d96

Kanne, S. M., & Mazurek, M. O. (2011). Aggression in children and adolescents with ASD: Prevalence and risk factors. *Journal of Autism and Developmental Disorders, 41*(7), 926–937. https://doi.org/10.1007/s10803-010-1118-4

Labrague, L. J. (2024). Nurses' adherence to patient safety protocols and its relationship with adverse patient events. *Journal of Nursing Scholarship, 56*(2), 282–290. https://doi.org/10.1111/jnu.12942

Lin, E., Malhas, M., Bratsalis, E., Thomson, K., Hargreaves, F., Donner, K., Baig, H., Boateng, R., Swain, R., Benadict, M. B., & Busch, L. (2024). Behavioral skills training for teaching safety skills to mental health service providers compared to training-as-usual: A pragmatic randomized control trial. *BMC Health Services Research, 24*(1), 639. https://doi.org/10.1186/s12913-024-10994-1

Metoyer, C. N., Fritz, J. N., Hunt, J. C., & Fletcher, V. L. (2020). Teaching caregivers to respond safely during agitated states before aggression using simulation training. *Journal of Applied Behavior Analysis, 53*(4), 2250–2259. https://doi.org/10.1002/jaba.751

Mouridsen, S. E., Brønnum-Hansen, H., Rich, B., & Isager, T. (2008). Mortality and causes of death in autism spectrum disorders: An update. *Autism: The International Journal of Research and Practice, 12*(4), 403–414. https://doi.org/10.1177/1362361308091653

O'Brien, M. J., Schieltz, K. M., Berg, W. K., McComas, J. J., & Wacker, D. P. (2021). Delivering interventions via telehealth: Functional communication training with a child with autism as a case example. *Research and Practice for Persons with Severe Disabilities, 46*(1), 53–60. https://doi.org/10.1177/1540796920980452

Oster, N. S., & Doyle, C. J. (2000). Critical incident stress and challenges for the emergency workplace. *Emergency Medicine Clinics of North America, 18*(2), 339–3xi. https://doi.org/10.1016/s0733-8627(05)70129-2

Padmanabhan, L., & Bakkialakshmi, C. (2023). Augmented wireless technologies too employees ease access. *Humanities and Social Science Studies, 12*(2), 145–150.

Parsons, M. B., Rollyson, J. H., & Reid, D. H. (2013). Teaching practitioners to conduct behavioral skills training: A pyramidal approach for training multiple human service staff. *Behavior Analysis in Practice, 6*(2), 4–16. https://doi.org/10.1007/BF03391798

Plantiveau, C., Dounavi, K., & Virués-Ortega, J. (2018). High levels of burnout among early-career board-certified behavior analysts with low collegial support in the work environment. *European Journal of Behavior Analysis, 19*(2), 195–207. https://doi.org/10.1080/15021149.2018.1438339

Quality Behavior Solutions. (2024). Safety-care® crisis prevention training. https://qbs.com/safety-care-crisis-prevention-training/

Reid, D. H., Parsons, M. B., & Green, C. W. (2021). *The supervisor's guidebook: Evidence-based strategies for promoting work quality and enjoyment among human service staff.* Charles C Thomas Publisher.

Ryan, C., Bergin, M., & Wells, J. S. G. (2019). Work-related stress and well-being of direct care workers in intellectual disability services: A scoping review of the literature. *International Journal of Developmental Disabilities, 67*(1), 1–22. https://doi.org/10.1080/20473869.2019.1582907

Schoberer, D., Osmancevic, S., Reiter, L., Thonhofer, N., & Manuela, H. (2022). Rapid review and meta-analysis of the effectiveness of personal protective equipment for healthcare workers during the COVID-19 pandemic. *Public Health in Practice, 4*, 100280. https://doi.org/10.1016/j.puhip.2022.100280

Taha, N. (2013). Physical restraints in critical care units: Impact of a training program on nurses' knowledge and practice and on patients' outcomes. *Journal of Nursing & Care, 02*(02). https://doi.org/10.4172/2167-1168.1000135

Taylor, B. A., LeBlanc, L. A., & Nosik, M. R. (2018). Compassionate care in behavior analytic treatment: Can outcomes be enhanced by attending to relationships with caregivers? *Behavior Analysis in Practice, 12*(3), 654–666. https://doi.org/10.1007/s40617-018-00289-3

Van Houten, R., Axelrod, S., Bailey, J. S., Favell, J. E., Foxx, R. M., Iwata, B. A., & Lovaas, O. I. (1988). The right to effective behavioral treatment. *Journal of Applied Behavior Analysis, 21*(4), 381–384. https://doi.org/10.1901/jaba.1988.21-381

Walton, M. K. (2011). Supporting family caregivers: Communicating with family caregivers. *The American Journal of Nursing, 111*(12), 47–53. https://doi.org/10.1097/01.NAJ.0000408186.67511.b9

Winokur, E. J., Loucks, J., & Raup, G. H. (2018). Use of a standardized procedure to improve behavioral health patients' care: A quality improvement initiative. *Journal of Emergency Nursing, 44*(1), 26–32. https://doi.org/10.1016/j.jen.2017.07.008

Wong, K. K., Fienup, D. M., Richling, S. M., Keen, A., & Mackay, K. (2022). Systematic review of acquisition mastery criteria and statistical analysis of associations with response maintenance and generalization. *Behavioral Interventions, 37*(4), 993–1012. https://doi.org/10.1002/bin.1885

Wright, A. M., Snowdon, A., Saunders, M., & Trampas, D. (2024). The necessity of healthcare supply chain resilience for crisis preparedness. *Healthcare Management Forum, 37*(2), 95–100. https://doi.org/10.1177/08404704231207386

Chapter 10
Ensuring Successful Transfer of Treatment to Community Settings: Comprehensive Discharge Planning

Sophia Sodano, Adam M. Briggs, Brittany H. Loder-Lafferty, Samantha J. Zohr, Skylar DeWitt, and Omar M. Elwasli

Relief, excitement, and hope are just some of the feelings a caregiver might feel after they have successfully secured behavioral services for their autistic child. These feelings come after likely months of uncertainty, despair, and dread as they pursued expert opinions and a clinical diagnosis. Undoubtedly, the strain of making urgent calls navigating appointment scheduling, and enduring long waits for answers has placed an immeasurable emotional and mental burden. After what was once suspected is finally confirmed, another time-consuming and stressful period begins, which includes locating an appropriate behavioral service provider with the shortest waitlist to ensure their child receives the critical "early" and "intensive" behavioral services they have been reading about as soon as possible. Thus, following this overwhelming whirlwind, it is no wonder that families feel a sense of relief and hope that their child will finally receive the services they need. Although enrolling one's child in behavioral services may have been the family's initial goal, it marks the beginning of their therapeutic journey.

As behavioral service providers, our goal is to work with these families to learn about the child's strengths, identify areas for growth, and determine a behavioral intervention plan that aligns with the child's needs while also honoring the values of the family. It is also our responsibility to make the family aware that this treatment placement represents just a step in this journey and that the goal will be to eventually transition them to a setting that is less intensive once they have gained the skills needed to be more independent and successful in another environment. Therefore,

S. Sodano · A. M. Briggs (✉) · S. J. Zohr · S. DeWitt · O. M. Elwasli
Department of Psychology, Eastern Michigan University, Ypsilanti, MI, USA
e-mail: abrigg11@emich.edu

B. H. Loder-Lafferty
Severe Behavior Department, University of Nebraska Medical Center's Munroe-Meyer Institute, Omaha, NE, USA

M. P. Kranak (ed.), *Behavioral Treatments for Individuals with Autism*, Autism and Child Psychopathology Series,
https://doi.org/10.1007/978-3-031-91965-7_10

as difficult as it may be to forecast what the future holds for this child and their family at this moment, it is our responsibility to have these discussions—what are the family's hopes and aspirations for their child? What will their subsequent placement look like? What skills will they be expected to have to be successful in this environment? These conversations will need to be had early and often, as the information gained from them is essential so that the treatment team can keep these short- and long-term goals in mind while building a comprehensive therapeutic plan with suitable programming to address them.

This ongoing transition planning process occurs across several unique but interrelated phases: initial intake, throughout admission, and discharge. We will discuss the critical behavioral strategies required for successfully transferring treatment effects and preparing the child and their family for their eventual transition out of one placement and into another. We will also review the barriers (environmental and systemic) that might interfere with this progress and how to plan for and mitigate their impact. Finally, we discuss additional resources that ought to be considered to support a successful treatment transfer during transition.

Transition Planning

This section discusses the importance of transition planning for effectively transferring challenging behavior interventions to the everyday environment, the optimal timing to initiate transition planning, and the key variables and steps involved. It is essential to consider various factors at different stages of the admission process, including (a) initial planning, (b) ongoing care during admission, and (c) discharge planning. This section is organized into these three components to offer general recommendations and considerations for how and when to implement specific procedures to increase the likelihood of a successful transition and reduce the risk of future readmissions to more intensive placements.

Initial Planning

Although it may seem unusual to discuss transition planning before beginning services, these conversations should occur early on to gain information about the likely placement following the current services such that the components of the intervention plan are designed in a way that aligns with the skills and behavior reduction goals necessary for the individual to be successful in this subsequent setting (Stokes & Osnes, 1989; Osnes & Lieblein, 2003). Understanding these short- and long-term goals for a particular case helps to determine the behavior-change priorities, program sequencing, anticipated timelines, and general expectations for each case. Of course, these goals can shift and be modified throughout the process; however, it is essential to know the destination before you set out on the journey. For instance, if a goal is to teach functional communication as a replacement for challenging behavior, it is vital to gather information about their everyday life, including the different contexts they may encounter and the likelihood of a particular response being honored within and across these settings, as this will inform the appropriateness of the communication response selected. Gathering these details during the initial intake meeting through interviews and observations will directly inform these goals and help you determine which assessments and interventions must be conducted.

The initial intake process should involve structured interviews and direct observation. During these interviews, the behavior analyst should ask a caregiver or other involved party (e.g., teacher, referring clinician) specific questions related to the occurrence of the individual's challenging behavior and the context under which it occurs (e.g., Functional Assessment Interview; O'Neill et al., 1997), obtain information about the client's preferred items (e.g., Reinforcer Assessment for Individuals with Severe Disability; Fisher et al., 1996), conduct various skill assessments (e.g., The Verbal Behavior Milestones Assessment and Placement Program; Sundberg, 2014), and determine relevant daily routines the individual is expected to engage in within their home and community settings. In addition to providing information on the behavior and environment, the caregiver, or guardian, can also serve as a valuable resource for providing information on cultural considerations and any idiosyncrasies of the client and family to be incorporated into treatment (Ennis-Cole et al., 2013).

If it is reported that challenging behavior occurs in multiple settings (e.g., school and home), it may be beneficial to conduct multiple structured interviews with each involved party (e.g., teacher and caregiver) to gather pertinent information and details related to each setting. Before recruiting information from other involved parties, behavior analysts should obtain proper consent to release information. Once permission is obtained, the interview questions can be slightly altered to be relevant for any setting (see Fig. 10.1 for sample intake questions for assessing and treating challenging behavior).

Direct observation should also be conducted during the intake process to gain information about the individual's current skills and facilitate generalization and transition planning. This should occur in the individual's everyday environment (e.g., at home or school). Conducting observations of the individual across various contexts allows the behavior analyst to directly observe the individual interact with their environment to corroborate the information gained from others in order to gain a complete picture of the individual in these settings and understand additional aspects of the environment (e.g., structure and routines within each setting, items and activities engaged with), the client's skill and communication level within these environments, and the variables that may be influencing the occurrence of challenging behavior in these settings (i.e., antecedents, consequences). Gathering this information during the intake process is vital for determining the treatment goals that must be achieved throughout admission to prepare the individual to navigate these environments successfully following transition and discharge.

Sample Intake Questions

Target behavior

1. What are the topographies (i.e., forms) of challenging behavior that occur?
   a. How often does this behavior occur?
   b. Where does this behavior occur?
   c. With whom does this behavior occur?
2. What are the common triggers that occur prior to the behavior (i.e., what occurs before)?
   a. Can you provide a recent example?
3. How do you respond to the behavior when it occurs (i.e., what do you do right after)?
   a. Can you provide an example?

Individual's natural environment

4. Who lives in the setting with the individual?
5. Can you list some expectations throughout the day that might be placed on the client, including weekdays and weekends?
6. Does the individual attend school?
   a. What school do they attend?
   b. What grade are they in?
   c. What expectations are placed throughout the day?
   d. What is their skill level?

General

7. How does the client communicate?
8. What are some of the client's strengths?
9. What items (e.g., toys) or activities (e.g., basketball, board games) does the client like most?
10. What are some lower preferred items or activities that the client likes?
11. What type of attention does the client like most (e.g., tickles, hugs)?
12. What work tasks does the client dislike doing most (e.g., reading, math, brushing teeth)?
13. Does the engagement in challenging behavior prevent you from doing community outings?
    a. If so, what type of community outings do you wish to do?

Goals

14. List three goals related to the above-mentioned target behavior:
    a. Goal 1:
    b. Goal 2:
    c. Goal 3:
15. What are the plans following discharge (i.e., where is the client transitioning to)?

Fig. 10.1 Sample intake questions

Throughout Admission

Although individual treatment plans will vary as a function of client needs, there are necessary aspects that will be incorporated within and across programming throughout admission to increase the likelihood of a successful transition. In particular, it will be vital to establish stimulus control within programming and plan to generalize the newly acquired skills throughout admission. Establishing stimulus control is essential for teaching, managing, and generalizing behavior across contexts and behavior change agents. As such, it will enable the subsequent transfer of treatment effects when preparing for discharge. This section will discuss common approaches to establishing stimulus control and programming for generalization throughout admission.

Establishing Stimulus Control and Using Conditional Discriminations to Promote Sustained Behavior Change

When a behavior occurs more frequently in the presence of a discriminative stimulus (S^D) than in its absence (stimulus delta [S^Δ]), it is said to be under stimulus control (Cooper et al., 2020). Establishing stimulus control over behavior by teaching the learner the conditions under which specific behavior will be reinforced and when its occurrence will not be reinforced (i.e., conditional discrimination training) is necessary to promote sustained behavior change and ultimately serves as a critical tool for transitioning treatment effects.

For instance, Betz et al. (2013) established discriminative control over functional communication and challenging behavior by arranging contingencies for each that were associated with unique visual stimuli (i.e., using a multiple or chained schedule of reinforcement). That is, functional communication was reinforced under certain conditions (i.e., when a green-colored card was present, the S^D) and was not reinforced when another stimulus was present (i.e., a red-colored card was present, the S^Δ), and challenging behavior was never reinforced under these conditions. Once the individuals consistently engaged in communication under the S^D and not the S^Δ and challenging behavior remained at near-zero levels, discriminative control was established. A benefit of establishing stimulus control in this manner (i.e., using the green and red cards as condition-signaling stimuli) was that these stimuli could be used to promote schedule thinning as they prepared the individuals to transition from relatively dense schedules of reinforcement (e.g., 30 s of waiting without reinforcement before their communication would be reinforced for 30 s) to leaner schedules of reinforcement (e.g., 4 min of waiting without reinforcement before their communication would be reinforced for 1 min) in a relatively rapid manner. Thus, establishing stimulus control allowed for the transfer of treatment effects from dense-to-lean schedules relatively efficiently, allowing the individual to successfully tolerate reinforcement schedules that they were more likely to experience in their everyday environment. While these procedures (i.e., establishing stimulus control and using conditional discriminations) have been demonstrated to be effective in the above context, they also possess advantages when transferring treatment effects across settings and behavior change agents.

Transferring Stimulus Control to Promote the Spread of Treatment Effects

Once treatment effects are achieved in a controlled setting, programming for the transfer of stimulus control is critical as it promotes the spread of treatment effects (i.e., generalization), which aids in sustaining behavior change and mitigating treatment relapse. In particular, it is critical to transfer treatment effects to other behavior-change agents and across settings. This has been demonstrated in the literature by either (a) using schedule-correlated stimuli to transfer effects across people and settings or (b) bringing aspects of the everyday environment (e.g., caregivers, stimuli in the home) into the training setting to promote the transfer of treatment effects.

Using Schedule-Correlated Stimuli to Transfer Effects Across Contexts

Extending treatment effects to caregivers is crucial, as they often are or become the primary behavior-change agents (Hembree-Kigin & McNeil, 2013). This process can prove difficult, as initially, the presence of caregivers may serve as a discriminative stimulus (i.e., S^D) for social reinforcement for challenging or inappropriate behavior. This can result from lengthy histories of caregiver-delivered reinforcement following challenging behavior (Thompson & Iwata, 2001) who may do so to avoid or escape its aversive properties (e.g., Miller et al., 2010). As such, caregiver-led interventions may initially be challenging due to this history of reinforcement and the lack of association between the caregiver and the newly taught communication response (Greer et al., 2019). Further, the environmental conditions that can lead to treatment relapse may be of particular concern for caregivers outside of the clinic setting, where treatment adherence is often challenged (Mitteer et al., 2018). Therefore, the transfer of stimulus control is a delicate process that warrants special consideration.

Fisher et al. (2015) demonstrated that functional communication training (FCT) reduced challenging behavior and facilitated the transfer of stimulus control across settings using schedule-correlated stimuli. They found that multiple schedules of reinforcement when signaled (e.g., with a yellow wristband) led to differentiated rates of functional communication responses (FCRs) and low challenging behavior across contexts. Greer et al. (2019) expanded on this by showing the rapid transfer of FCT effects to caregivers using schedule-correlated stimuli, attributing the effectiveness to discriminative control and continued extinction of challenging behaviors. These studies highlight the importance of using schedule-correlated stimuli when transferring treatment effects across environments and individuals.

Fading Everyday Environment Stimuli into the Training Setting to Promote Treatment Transfer

Kelley et al. (2018) explored renewal effects in children with autism, demonstrating that pairing caregivers with trained therapists during escape extinction mitigated renewal and facilitated generalization across contexts. Another evidence-based method involves gradually fading contextual stimuli to increase the similarity between treatment and home contexts. For instance, Haney et al. (2021) extended Kelley et al. (2018) by using therapist-caregiver pairing and systematic fading for transferring stimulus control in seven participants with avoidant/restrictive food intake disorder. Therapists implemented function-based extinction, while caregivers received behavioral skills training. Therapist proximity and context similarity were faded, and participants returned to the original context where caregivers alone implemented extinction. Results suggest that systematic fading helps caregivers associate with extinction contingencies and reduces generalization failures, while programming common stimuli may enhance generalization. These studies highlight the importance of context pairing and fading in other relevant environmental stimuli when transferring treatment effects across contexts. Although this section covered different evidence-based approaches for transferring stimulus control across contexts (e.g., behavior-change agents and settings), the discriminative stimuli used to promote treatment transfer may still need to be faded out to some extent to promote long-term maintenance and generalization of the treatment effects.

Understanding Stimulus Fading to Promote Independent Performance

While the approaches described above promote behavior change and transfer of treatment effects, some are often impractical to implement in the natural environment over time. Thus, stimulus fading is vital in achieving more practical interventions and bringing the target response under the control of naturally occurring stimuli.

Stimulus fading involves modifying the physical properties of a stimulus while maintaining the stimulus control properties over the behavior (Martin & Pear, 1996). This approach is useful when fading out non-natural discriminative stimuli (e.g., activity schedules) such that the learner's performance is sustainable in the natural environment (e.g., in the absence of activity schedules). Brown et al. (2008) used script fading to promote verbal interactions in three children with ASD without relying on non-natural discriminative stimuli. After pre-teaching sessions to ensure participants learned the reinforcement system and associated stimuli, they were tested in a community setting where the target behavior (i.e., appropriate conversation) was measured. During the intervention, scripts were gradually faded, and participants progressed based on their independent engagement in appropriate conversation. When designing a stimulus fading protocol, behavior analysts must consider whether to manipulate the S^{Δ} or S^{D} (Markham et al., 2023). Schreibman and Charlop (1981) found that fading the S^{D} first led to more efficient learning with fewer errors. Behavior analysts must also ensure that each step in the fading sequence differs slightly from the previous one to ensure success and prevent relapse (Bishop et al., 2013). Ultimately, the sequence pacing should balance efficiency with avoiding unnecessary steps. Conducting probe sessions of the terminal step can help identify essential steps and ensure the effective acquisition and maintenance of treatment effects in an efficient manner (Kranak & Falligant, 2022; Schiff et al., 2011).

Programming and Assessing for Generalization and Maintenance

Generalization is one of the core concerns of developing treatment, as it ensures that the learned behavior is effective across settings, people, and time (Stokes & Baer, 1977). Learning to generalize skills is essential because, without it, individuals would be required to relearn skills for each new context, which would be inefficient and impractical. For an intervention to be effective, it must generalize to the individual's natural environment, maximizing the desired outcomes and ensuring the effective treatment transfer (Bahry et al., 2022; Codes 2.01 and 2.14; Behavior Analyst Certification Board, 2020). If behavior analysts neglect to effectively incorporate these strategies, they risk limiting the transfer of treatment effects and creating conditions where challenging behavior may reemerge (i.e., relapse). Given the critical role of generalization and maintenance in transition planning, an important question arises: "When should programming for generalization and maintenance begin?" Although it may seem logical to consider thinking about whether treatment effects will generalize and maintain as you approach discharge and transition planning, it is crucial that planning for both generalization and maintenance begins before admission and continues throughout admission to ensure the successful transfer of treatment effects. Thus, it is imperative that behavior analysts thoughtfully program and regularly assess for generalization and maintenance throughout the admission process.

Programming for Generalization

Treatment effects established during initial treatment often do not transfer to other contexts or therapists without direct programming (Stokes & Baer, 1977), so it is important to consider developing treatments with specific mechanisms to program for generalization and maintenance in mind (Baer et al., 1968). To effectively program for generalization, a behavior analyst must (1) select behaviors that are appropriate for the patient's environment (i.e., will meet natural contingencies of the natural environment) and (2) specify all desired variations of the target behavior and the contexts in which the behaviors should and should not occur (Cooper et al., 2020). This can be accomplished by strategies known as incorporating common stimuli and programming for generalization across contexts. Further, it will also be imperative to evaluate the effects of generalization programming throughout admission by assessing for the emergence of generalized and maintained responding. Below, we will review strategies for accomplishing this approach (see also Chap. 4, Grunewald et al., 2025 and Chap. 2, Norris et al., 2025).

Incorporating Common Stimuli

Programming for generalization by incorporating common stimuli is a strategy that involves making the learning environment similar to the everyday environment where the skill(s) will eventually be used. The mechanism that promotes generalization across contexts has been described to occur due to stimulus similarity, suggesting that generalization is more likely to occur when stimuli are present across both the learning environment and the new context (Carruthers et al., 2020). Stimuli, such as common instructional materials, vocal rules, specific individuals, programmed discriminative stimuli, and so on, can be thoughtfully incorporated into the training environment to establish stimulus control and promote the transfer of treatment effects (i.e., generalization) across other contexts (Stokes & Osnes, 1989).

Generalization Across Contexts

Neglecting to program for generalization across contexts (e.g., environments, people) can limit the transfer of appropriate skills following discharge from services and potentially result in the relapse of challenging behavior (i.e., resurgence, renewal; Kimball et al., 2023). Training diversely (Stokes & Baer, 1977; Stokes & Osnes, 1989) is a generalization and maintenance strategy that involves providing training across various contexts, thereby increasing the flexibility of the skill under different settings and circumstances (Brown & Odom, 1994).

Introduction to Natural Maintaining Contingencies

Behavior analysts ensure that behavior generalizes over time (i.e., maintenance) by preparing the behavior to be maintained under natural reinforcement contingencies through reinforcement schedule thinning (Briggs et al., 2023). Schedule thinning involves transitioning to reinforcement schedules similar to those in everyday environments (i.e., transitioning from continuous to intermittent schedules). In addition to promoting sustainable behavior change, transitioning to these schedules reduces caregiver burden and increases the likelihood of treatment adherence, which is an important consideration for behavior analysts seeking to discharge clients (Allen & Warzak, 2000). Understanding the contingencies available in one's environment is crucial in designing the schedule thinning progression and terminal goal, which must balance caregivers' input with specific learner characteristics (see Briggs et al., 2023).

Assessing for Generalization

Without a plan for regularly assessing generalization and maintenance, it will be unclear whether attempts to program for generalization and maintenance have been effective. Moreover, continuous assessment of generalization and maintenance can reduce the need for unnecessary intervention if desired effects are demonstrated early. Conversely, additional intervention may be necessary if generalization is assumed but has not actually occurred. This can be accomplished by conducting probe sessions across (a) novel behavior-change agents and settings, (b) unique contexts, and (c) terminal reinforcement schedules.

Summary

The critical importance of generalization and maintenance in behavioral interventions cannot be overstated. As Baer et al. (1968) highlighted, behavior change must appear across various individuals and environments and be durable over time to be considered effective. Ensuring that learned behaviors generalize and maintain over time reduces the likelihood of treatment relapse and the need for readmission, enhancing functional independence. Programming for generalization and assessing its occurrence throughout treatment ensures that clients can apply learned skills across various settings and conditions, ultimately promoting long-term success and reducing the need for continuous intervention. Effective treatment plans must include strategies for establishing stimulus control and programming for generalization and maintenance to ensure that clients can utilize their new skills in settings outside of the treatment setting.

Discharge Planning

This is the final phase in transitioning treatment effects from a more intensive setting to a less restrictive one. This section reviews the considerations related to discharge criteria, timing, and scheduling follow-up appointments.

Discharge Criteria and Timing

Discharge should typically occur once the treatment plan goals and objectives have been met and a safe and appropriate continuing care program is arranged and deployed (Fisher et al., 2022). Although not the focus of this chapter, there are instances in which an *unplanned* discharge may occur, such as the child no longer meeting intake criteria, the client not making progress toward goals, caregivers not participating in treatment or following program rules, or unplanned events (e.g., relocating, illness). In these instances, it is best to provide training and ensure that the family has a crisis plan if needed.

During planned discharge, once discharge criteria have been met and all involved parties are trained, the behavior analyst should communicate with the placement setting (e.g., school, residential setting, early intervention) to ensure a smooth, timely transition. Despite how much training we provide, there are bound to be questions and situations that arise following discharge regarding challenging behavior and treatment procedures. Therefore, clinicians should plan follow-ups to provide support and feedback and answer questions on treatment-related situations.

Follow-Up Check-Ins

These consist of an email or phone call simply inquiring about progress and any related questions the involved parties may have. Behavior analysts may also have involved parties collect data and report on the occurrence of challenging behavior during this time. It is suggested that these check-ins occur more frequently immediately following discharge and fade over time so long as treatment effects are maintained. For instance, check-ins may occur once a week for the month following discharge, followed by biweekly and eventually once a month before discontinuing on an "as needed" basis.

Transition planning is necessary to ensure clients' successful treatment transfer following challenging behavior services. Failure to adequately plan for transitioning can result in ineffective treatment, increase the risk of relapse, and lead to readmittance into more intensive or restrictive services. As behavior analysts, we must specifically program for transition, beginning early in the admission process and continuing until after discharge. Although we have briefly outlined this general process above, we recognize it is not without its challenges. Therefore, we review the barriers one may encounter and suggest strategies and considerations for overcoming them below.

Common Challenges and Barriers to Proper Treatment Transfer Planning

Proper treatment transfer planning often involves the initiation of continued care with another clinic, community agency, and/or within the home setting. Where and when treatment effects will be transferred should be considered early in the treatment process. Despite this advanced planning, many barriers exist to securing behavioral services and maintaining caregiver treatment implementation in the home setting. This section discusses common environmental and systemic barriers to treatment transfer planning. Each barrier will be defined, examples will be provided, and potential solutions will be explored. Finally, the section concludes by discussing what constitutes a successful treatment transfer.

Environmental Barriers to Treatment Transfer Planning

Environmental barriers to treatment transfer planning include factors the behavioral service provider can plan for and directly address. These include programming relapse mitigation strategies, preparing caregivers to adhere to treatment recommendations, and communicating with future placements.

Relapse (Resurgence, Renewal, and Reinstatement)

Treatment relapse refers to any instance in which treatment gains are lost when reinforcement conditions are worsened, which, as noted above, is an especially relevant consideration when a client transitions to a post-treatment environment following discharge. This is because behavioral interventions often cannot be implemented with the same degree of efficacy as they are in the treatment environment (e.g., a caregiver fails to reinforce an appropriate alternative response due to competing demands in the environment). As such, treatment relapse is a prevalent phenomenon studied extensively in the behavioral literature (Briggs et al., 2018; Falligant et al., 2021; Kranak & Falligant, 2021; Mitteer et al., 2022; Muething et al., 2021). Treatment relapse is generally understood to be transient in nature, so long as the environment does not reinforce the recurrence and adheres to treatment recommendations (Mitteer et al., 2018); however, although this may be manageable in a clinical setting with well-trained staff and a dense staff-to-client ratio, managing these phenomena is likely more difficult in less controlled everyday settings.

When planning for client discharge, it is important to understand that the typical treatment setting is unlike the post-treatment environments (e.g., homes, schools) in that they are dynamic, ever-changing, and less predictable. As a result, treatment gains will need to be durable, and the intervention will need to be designed in a manner that is adaptable and easily supported by the environment such that it can persist when it is inevitably challenged in the post-treatment environment. Otherwise, the risk of treatment relapse will be exceptionally high. For example, there will be instances where a trained response goes unreinforced (which may lead to resurgence), there will be context changes (which may lead to renewal), and challenging behavior will be inadvertently reinforced (which may lead to reinstatement). For a more thorough review of resurgence, renewal, and reinstatement, please refer to Chaps. 2, Norris et al. (2025), Chap. 4, Grunewald et al. (2025), and Chap. 6, Stephens et al. (2025), this volume.

Given that treatment relapse can be expected to occur in some form upon entering the post-treatment environment, it is critical to be prepared to address instances of relapse promptly. Implementing procedures with high procedural fidelity will decrease the magnitude and persistence of challenging behavior and reduce the risk of prolonged relapse. Additionally, recent research has outlined strategies for purposefully arranging treatment for challenging behavior such that it is more resistant to relapse later on (i.e., utilizing mitigation techniques throughout the treatment process), also known as *behavioral inoculation* (Kimball et al., 2023; Weinsztok & DeLeon, 2022). Relevant examples for various types of treatment relapse have been documented, such as generalization training to mitigate renewal (e.g., Podlesnik et al., 2017), discrimination training (Betz et al., 2013; Fisher et al., 2020a; Fuhrman et al., 2016), lag schedules (Falcomata et al., 2018), or serial DRA training to mitigate resurgence (e.g., Lambert et al., 2015, 2017), and use of DRA without extinction to mitigate reinstatement (Briggs et al., 2019). There is also evidence suggesting that some mitigation strategies are effective at reducing all three of these forms of treatment relapse, such as programming lean schedules of reinforcement for alternative response (see Kimball et al., 2023). Practitioners should consider informing caregivers of treatment relapse (i.e., what it is and that it can be expected to occur), the practices implemented to mitigate it throughout the treatment process, and how to carry on these practices in the post-treatment environment to the best of their ability.

Treatment Adherence

To maintain treatment outcomes, aftercare is transferred, the treatment must be implemented accurately and consistently within the home environment. Allen and Warzak (2000) describe many potential barriers to caregiver treatment adherence that may influence implementation. These barriers are primarily due to inefficiencies in caregiver training by the treatment team, which can be remedied by improving caregiver training procedures (please refer to Fig. 10.2 for a guide on training caregivers). In particular, specific areas related to establishing operations, stimulus generalization, response acquisition, and consequent events should be considered

Training Outline for Involved Parties
Safety and behavior management
1. General preventative strategies (antecedent and consequence strategies) 2. Environmental manipulations 3. Behavior management techniques a. blocking procedures b. hair and bite release procedures c. restraint and seclusion procedures 4. Crisis response plan 5. Helpful resources (e.g. safety equipment)
Introduction to behavior
6. What is behavior and how to describe it 7. Three-term contingency 8. Functions of behavior 9. Data collection
Reinforcement and punishment
10. Reinforcement 11. Punishment
Proactive strategies
12. Catching your child being good 13. Child led play 14. Setting the environment up for success
Reactive strategies
15. Differential reinforcement 16. Functional communication training 17. Three step prompting 18. Shaping 19. Attending and planned ignoring 20. Time out
Individualized treatment procedures
21. Treatment procedures

Fig. 10.2 Training outline for involved parties

and addressed (see Table 10.1 for a description of barriers to caregiver adherence). For example, a parent may be able to effectively implement an extinction intervention for tantrums (attention-seeking behavior) in the home environment yet be unsure of how to address inappropriate vocalizations (attention-seeking behavior) in similar contexts. This barrier to the caregiver's adherence to intervene with challenging behaviors in the home environment is due to insufficient training across multiple exemplars (*stimulus generalization*). In such a case, appropriate caregiver training might include exposure to multiple topographies of behaviors within the

Table 10.1 Common barriers to caregiver adherence

Establishing operations	*Failure to establish immediate outcomes as reinforcers*: Results from behavioral interventions take time, unlike medications which have more immediate effects. This delay in outcomes might deter caregivers from consistently implementing strategies in the home
	Failure to disestablish competing social approval as reinforcers: Some interventions, like ignoring tantrums in public, might not be approved by the caregivers' social communities. Disapproval from their social communities might lead to caregivers inconsistently implementing interventions
Stimulus generalization	*Trained insufficient exemplars:* If the range of behaviors caregivers are trained to intervene upon is too narrow, they will not generalize to the behaviors they need to address in the home and community environments
	Trained narrow range of stimuli: Similarly, a caregiver might be trained to implement interventions in the clinic or home environment, but this training might not generalize to other environments (e.g., school, public) in which challenging behaviors occur
	Weak rule following: Adherence might be lower among caregivers with histories of little reinforcement for rule following and/or when the rule following prescribed by BCBAs is highly technical and does not correspond with the caregivers' verbal behavior
Response acquisition	*Excessive skill complexity:* If a targeted intervention is too complex, caregiver adherence will be low
	Weak instructional technology: Caregiver training based solely on verbal or written instructions will lead to poor adherence. Training should include instructions, modeling, rehearsal, and feedback components
	Weak instructional environment: Distracting learning environments might limit caregivers' attention to training materials and may result in poor adherence to treatment implementation at home
Consequent events	*Competing punitive contingencies:* Caregivers providing reinforcement (e.g., attention) to desirable behaviors might see an increase in challenging behaviors that have also been reinforced by attention in the past. This increase in challenging behaviors might punish the caregivers' implementation of reinforcement in the future
	Competing reinforcing contingencies: Caregivers have multiple concurrent schedules of reinforcement that compete with the consistent implementation of interventions. Because of this, caregivers are more likely to engage in behaviors with a high rate of reinforcement provided immediately and behaviors with a lower response effort

Note. The information summarized in this table is adapted from Allen and Warzak (2000)

same functional class so that caregivers are more prepared to respond effectively to various behaviors in the home environment.

Moreover, a parent might not be able to implement a treatment at home because the procedures were very complex, and the clinic was noisy the day they learned the intervention (*response acquisition*). As a result, the intervention did not work as intended because they did not accurately recall and implement the necessary steps. In this case, appropriate caregiver training might entail repeated instruction for the caregiver, alongside opportunities for modeling, rehearsal, and feedback, so that after the training, the caregiver feels confident in implementing the intervention at home.

As caregivers often receive insufficient training to effectively implement behavioral interventions independently in the home setting, behavioral service providers should revise their approaches to caregiver training to address each of the barriers described by Allen and Warzak (2000). For example, to address barriers related to *stimulus generalization,* behavioral service providers could train caregivers how to implement specific interventions and teach them foundational information about behavior analytic principles and behavioral functions. This approach to caregiver training that provides instructions specific to their situation, as well as broader knowledge about behavior analytic principles (e.g., how to identify behaviors from a similar functional class that has differing topographies), might improve caregivers' abilities to apply interventions to varying challenging behaviors in the home and community environments.

Cooperation of Future Placements

Successful treatment transfer typically involves the continuity of care across novel settings (e.g., the community, other clinical placements, schools, and home environments). Before transferring care, the client-specific goals and expectations for implementing behavioral interventions in the novel environment should be discussed and agreed upon between the current providers and the person to whom care is being transferred. These goals should adhere to the criteria set forth by Kazdin (2011) for defining target behaviors (i.e., objectivity, clarity, and completeness) to ensure that the person to whom care is being transferred has a solid understanding of the types of behavior to be intervened upon and how to implement the desired intervention effectively.

Once the goals and expectations for the transfer of care have been established, sufficient training should be provided to the person to whom care is being transferred. Sufficient training includes behavioral skills training (BST), where the following steps are utilized: instructions, modeling, rehearsal, and feedback. Given that the use of BST is time and resource-intensive (Briggs et al., 2024), behavior analysts should consider using technology-based approaches that maintain the fidelity of the training but require less time with an actual trainer (e.g., self-instruction manuals, computer-based modules, and video modeling). Moreover, as described in Table 10.1, to enhance adherence to consistent implementation of the targeted interventions, such training should include sufficient target behaviors, stimuli, and environments (the community, other clinical placements, schools, and home environments) to ensure that generalization of the person's ability to effectively administer the behavioral interventions across behaviors, stimuli, and environments occurs (Allen & Warzak, 2000).

As described above, many barriers to consistent adherence to implementing behavioral interventions occur when transitioning care to a novel treatment team and environment. These barriers should be thoroughly assessed and addressed before initiating the transfer of care. This is especially important, as there is no way to monitor the effectiveness and durability of the treatment by the original provider once the transfer is completed. Thus, when assessing and addressing potential barriers to the future implementation of care, providers should consider how caregivers and future providers can monitor the efficacy of treatments being implemented so that they can best identify when changes to the treatment plan might be necessary.

Systemic Barriers to Treatment Transfer Planning

Systemic barriers to successful treatment transfer planning include factors that cannot be directly intervened upon by the behavioral service provider in charge of the transfer and are, therefore, more difficult for individual providers to address. These systemic barriers include (a) fees for services, (b) waitlists for services, and (c) multicultural factors.

Fees for Services

Currently, there are disparities in both the cost and quality of services depending on the type of insurance (i.e., private or public) a family has. Nationwide, families with private insurance are far more likely to incur out-of-pocket costs for behavioral services and are significantly less likely to obtain relevant services (e.g., speech, occupational, and behavioral therapies) than those with public insurance (Zhang & Baranek, 2016). However, while public insurance generally provides lower-cost access to a broader range of services, public services are reportedly perceived as lower quality by service recipients, with recipients citing delays to diagnosis and lack of family-centered care as reasons for dissatisfaction with services (Burkett et al., 2015; Čolić et al., 2022).

Offering scholarships from national or state-level funding sources to clients needing services might limit financial barriers to obtaining necessary services due to a lack of insurance coverage or financial constraints. If these scholarships were set in place, behavioral service providers could support the efforts by providing resources and instructions to families in their community aimed at helping families apply for funding to gain access to needed services. Moreover, national and state-level grant funding to develop and promote free or low-cost behavioral therapy services could also mitigate barriers to services based on cost alone. In addition to client-specific incentives, policy changes such as loan forgiveness programs and service scholarships can be offered to practicing behavioral service providers and those in training to incentivize service delivery in more remote areas (Scarpa et al., 2020).

Finally, some state-funded services exist, such as the Autism Program of Illinois, which provides access to a variety of services such as screening and diagnostics, various forms of education and training, intervention, and support groups; however, families living in rural areas might have more difficulty accessing providers from these entities (Stahmer et al., 2019). Some states have started to remedy this issue by developing mobile autism clinics, which serve families and schools located in remote areas with limited access to behavioral health providers (e.g., Hamrick & Lock, 2020). Similarly, since the onset of the COVID-19 pandemic, there has been an increase in the availability of telehealth services. Continuing to utilize telehealth services, even post-pandemic, may help reach traditionally underserved populations across the United States (Iacono et al., 2016).

Waitlists for Services

While the number of BCBAs in the United States increases annually, many counties nationwide still do not have access to a BCBA in their immediate or neighboring areas (Yingling et al., 2022). Such disparity tends to result in long waitlists for needed services, which, in some cases, is associated with worsening behavior problems or lapses in previously made treatment gains (Stephens et al., 2023). Thus, if clients are planning to transfer care to a new clinic, behavior analysts should support them in initiating services in these settings as soon as possible (e.g., as soon as they become aware of a planned discharge date) to decrease delays in the continuity of care during the treatment transfer process.

Systems-level solutions should be explored to increase caregivers' access to needed information while waiting for services. First, clinics should consider providing educational materials to families waiting for services. These materials may include descriptions and contact information for other services that may be beneficial during the waiting period for treatment (e.g., respite care), information on how to obtain in-school services (e.g., individualized education plans), and simple behavioral management strategies that caregivers can implement with little to no training (e.g., environmental adaptations, communication strategies, caregiver emotional coping strategies). Second, providing national and state-level grant funding opportunities for establishing more training programs and clinics—particularly in areas with limited access to behavior analysts—would significantly increase the population of trained service providers, thereby reducing waitlist times for nearby families. Third, policymakers should support adding insurance codes to provide coverage for caregiver training in behavioral management (Stephens et al., 2023). Relatedly, clinics/providers should seek to become credentialed with various insurance providers in addition to supporting private pay.

Multicultural Factors

Access to services is even lower among socially, geographically, and economically marginalized populations (Čolić et al., 2022; Dennison et al., 2019; Pickard & Ingersoll, 2016; Stahmer et al., 2019). These populations often experience a lack of access to information about autism and behavioral services, delayed or inaccurate diagnoses, higher rates of service rejections, limited access to providers in their community, and limited access to providers with similar racial, cultural, or lingual backgrounds (Čolić et al., 2022; Stahmer et al., 2019). Families of lower socioeconomic status are more likely to endorse needing access to services such as respite care, in-home services, and parent training and are less likely to report feeling satisfied with the services they are receiving compared to higher SES families (Pickard & Ingersoll, 2016). Linguistically diverse families may face added barriers in obtaining information and educational resources about behavioral services and its benefits, as much information from the field of behavior analysis is only available in English and usually contains highly technical jargon that might be difficult to translate (Dennison et al., 2019; Stahmer et al., 2019). Immigrant families may face additional, unique barriers to accessing services (e.g., need for translation services, fear of deportation if citizenship or residency status has not yet been achieved; Dennison et al., 2019; Wallace-Watkin et al., 2023) and may be unable to obtain the necessary insurance coverage to support services.

Many of the barriers to accessing services faced by traditionally underserved and marginalized populations are systems-level concerns. Some potential solutions include creating bilingual training programs, the inclusion of multiculturalism and cultural humility competencies in existing training programs, providing contingencies for current providers to pursue continued education and professional development opportunities focused on issues of diversity and implicit biases, utilizing interpreters to enhance communication between clients and providers when language barriers are present, making information about behavioral services and developmental disorders more readily available, and providing incentives for current practitioners to offer telehealth or in-person services in rural or underserved areas (Čolić et al., 2022; Dennison et al., 2019). For a more detailed discussion of the individual-level and systems-level barriers to services faced by marginalized populations, please see Čolić et al. (2022) and Dennison et al. (2019).

The Successful Transfer

There is no current consensus on what a "successful" treatment transfer looks like. Thus, we propose that a successful transfer must be socially valid across the three levels proposed by Wolf (1978): the treatment transfer must have socially significant goals, socially appropriate procedures, and socially important effects. First, to be "successful," treatment transfers must be socially meaningful to the client and the broader social community. For a treatment transfer to be successful, the transfer has to be the initial goal of the behavioral treatment. For example, if a treatment transfer were not a goal of the behavioral intervention, then the behavior analyst would not need to program a transfer into the treatment plan. However, in most instances, the ultimate goal of initiating high-cost behavioral health services is to see desired behavior change and to identify effective skills and interventions that caregivers or teachers can administer in the home and school environments to maintain that behavior change. Thus, these situations value the treatment transfer as an important treatment plan goal.

Second, the procedures for transferring treatment must be appropriate and acceptable to all individuals involved (e.g., current providers, clients, caregivers, broader social communities, novel providers; Wolf, 1978). The procedures must be feasible, meaning the effort involved must match the perceived benefits of the outcomes of the treatment transfer. Moreover, the transfer must be doable. If care is being transferred to the caregivers within the home environment, they need clear definitions and descriptions of what and how to implement all necessary interventions. If the caregiver finds the procedures of the treatment transfer to be too convoluted or complex, then their consistent implementation of the treatment within the home environment is unlikely.

Lastly, for a treatment transfer to be deemed "successful," the effects must be important to the individual and their community (Wolf, 1978). As mentioned earlier, desired behavior changes are typically the most obvious goal of an intervention. Additionally, individuals want to see the maintenance of behavioral changes resulting from an intervention over time and across contexts. Thus, a "successful" treatment transfer would be one in which the treatment was effectively re-initiated in the novel setting (e.g., in the home environment, administered by caregivers) and the behavior change is maintained over time.

Access to Resources

As described in this section, it has been demonstrated that many barriers exist to consistently implementing prescribed behavior change procedures. For a "successful" treatment transfer to occur, we must ensure that the caregiver and other providers have access to the tools and resources needed to adhere to the treatment plan.

Respite Care

Due to the competing demands of caregivers, respite care is often needed to reduce stress and help cope with their child's challenging behavior (Cooke et al., 2020). Respite care involves short-term relief or support provided by others (e.g., agency staff) so that caregivers can step away from providing direct support to their child and instead attend to other needs. Respite care is associated with other positive outcomes, such as decreased acute hospitalizations (Mandell, 2012). However, many families are unable to access respite care. Barriers to accessing respite care include limited access to information about available respite care services, limited respite care services available (mainly in rural areas), high costs for services, need for transportation to and from the respite care facility, waitlists, and long wait times (Cooke et al., 2020). Programs such as Michigan's Family Support Subsidy Program, which provides families of children with developmental disabilities with financial assistance that may be used for relevant services (e.g., respite care, therapy, special equipment), may help to increase access to needed services for low-income families.

Funds for Protective Equipment

For children with severe challenging behavior (e.g., self-injurious behavior, aggression, property destruction), protective equipment might need to be obtained before the transfer of care (Irwin Helvey et al., 2024). Many barriers to accessing protective equipment exist, such as knowledge about what type of equipment to obtain and how to use it, as well as the initial cost of protective equipment. Before initiating the transfer, clinicians should inform caregivers, staff, or teachers of the specific equipment needed and potential funding sources available (e.g., insurance, care management organizations, and community funding agencies) to help offset the cost of purchasing protective equipment.

Concluding Remarks

Our goal for this chapter was to provide a general overview of the transition planning process, which begins during the initial intake, proceeds throughout admission, and concludes during discharge. We covered some critical behavioral strategies required for successfully transferring treatment effects (i.e., establishing stimulus control, programming and assessing for generalization and maintenance) and preparing the child and their family to transition from one placement to another. We identified potential barriers behavior analysts and caregivers likely encounter, including environmental and systemic, and provided some strategies for mitigating or circumventing them throughout the transition planning process. Finally, we discussed some additional resources that should be considered to support a successful treatment transfer during discharge and transition. We hope this overview serves as a helpful resource to behavior analysts and caregivers as they navigate the transition planning process so that it supports the successful transfer of treatment effects across contexts.

References

Allen, K. D., & Warzak, W. J. (2000). The problem of parental nonadherence in clinical behavior analysis: Effective treatment is not enough. *Journal of Applied Behavior Analysis, 33*(3), 373–391. https://doi.org/10.1901/jaba.2000.33-373

Baer, D. M., Wolf, M. M., & Risley, T. R. (1968). Some current dimensions of applied behavior analysis. *Journal of Applied Behavior Analysis, 1*(1), 91–97. https://doi.org/10.1901/jaba.1968.1-91

Bahry, S., Gerhardt, P. F., Weiss, M. J., Leaf, J. B., Putnam, R. F., & Bondy, A. (2022). The ethics of actually helping people: Targeting skill acquisition goals that promote meaningful outcomes for individuals with autism spectrum disorder. *Behavior Analysis in Practice, 16*(3), 672–695. https://doi.org/10.1007/s40617-022-00757-x

Behavior Analyst Certification Board. (2020). Ethics code for behavior analysts. https://bacb.com/wp-content/ethics-code-for-behavior-analysts/

Betz, A. M., Fisher, W. W., Roane, H. S., Mintz, J. C., & Owen, T. M. (2013). A component analysis of schedule thinning during functional communication training. *Journal of Applied Behavior Analysis, 46*(1), 219–241.

Bishop, M. R., Kenzer, A. L., Coffman, C. M., Tarbox, C. M., Tarbox, J., & Lanagan, T. M. (2013). Using stimulus fading without escape extinction to increase compliance with toothbrushing in children with autism. *Research in Autism Spectrum Disorders, 7*(6), 680–686.

Briggs, A. M., Fisher, W. W., Greer, B. D., & Kimball, R. T. (2018). Prevalence of resurgence of destructive behavior when thinning reinforcement schedules during functional communication training. *Journal of Applied Behavior Analysis, 51*(3), 620–633. https://doi.org/10.1002/jaba.472

Briggs, A. M., Dozier, C. L., Lessor, A. N., Kamana, B. U., & Jess, R. L. (2019). Further investigation of differential reinforcement of alternative behavior without extinction for escape-maintained destructive behavior. *Journal of Applied Behavior Analysis, 52*(4), 956–973. https://doi.org/10.1002/jaba.648

Briggs, A. M., Mitteer, D. R., Bergmann, S., & Greer, B. D. (2023). Reinforcer thinning: General approaches and considerations for maintaining skills and mitigating relapse. In J. L. Matson (Ed.), *Handbook of applied behavior analysis* (pp. 105–122). Springer International Publishing. https://doi.org/10.1007/978-3-031-19964-6_6

Briggs, A. M., Zohr, S. J., & Harvey, O. B. (2024). Training individuals to implement discrete-trial teaching procedures using behavioral skills training: A scoping review with implications for practice and research. *Journal of Applied Behavior Analysis, 57*(1), 86–103. https://doi.org/10.1002/jaba.1024

Brown, W. H., & Odom, S. L. (1994). Strategies and tactics for promoting generalization and maintenance of young children's social behavior. *Research in Developmental Disabilities, 15*(2), 99–118. https://doi.org/10.1016/0891-4222(94)90016-7

Brown, J. L., Krantz, P. J., McClannahan, L. E., & Poulson, C. L. (2008). Using script fading to promote natural environment stimulus control of verbal interactions among youths with autism. *Research in Autism Spectrum Disorders, 2*(3), 480–497.

Burkett, K., Morris, E., Manning-Courtney, P., Anthony, J., & Shambley-Ebron, D. (2015). African American families on autism diagnosis and treatment: The influence of culture. *Journal of Autism and Developmental Disorders, 45*(10), 3244–3254. https://doi.org/10.1007/s10803-015-2482-x

Carruthers, S., Pickles, A., Slonims, V., Howlin, P., & Charman, T. (2020). Beyond intervention into daily life: A systematic review of generalisation following social communication interventions for young children with autism. *Autism Research, 13*(4), 506–522. https://doi.org/10.1002/aur.2264

Čolić, M., Araiba, S., Lovelace, T. S., & Dababnah, S. (2022). Black caregivers' perspectives on racism in ASD services: Toward culturally responsive ABA practice. *Behavior Analysis in Practice, 15*(4), 1032–1041. https://doi.org/10.1007/s40617-021-00577-5

Cooke, E., Smith, V., & Brenner, M. (2020). Parents' experiences of accessing respite care for children with autism spectrum disorder (ASD) at the acute and primary care interface: A systematic review. *BMC Pediatrics, 20*(1), 244. https://doi.org/10.1186/s12887-020-02045-5

Cooper, J. O., Heron, T. E., & Heward, W. L. (2020). *Applied behavior analysis* (3rd ed.). Pearson.

Dennison, A., Lund, E. M., Brodhead, M. T., Mejia, L., Armenta, A., & Leal, J. (2019). Delivering home-supported applied behavior analysis therapies to culturally and linguistically diverse families. *Behavior Analysis in Practice, 12*(4), 887–898. https://doi.org/10.1007/s40617-019-00374-1

Ennis-Cole, D., Durodoye, B. A., & Harris, H. L. (2013). The impact of culture on autism diagnosis and treatment: Considerations for counselors and other professionals. *The Family Journal, 21*(3), 279–287. https://doi-org.ezproxy.emich.edu/10.1177/1066480713476834

Falcomata, T. S., Muething, C. S., Silbaugh, B. C., Adami, S., Hoffman, K., Shpall, C., & Ringdahl, J. E. (2018). Lag schedules and functional communication training: Persistence of mands and relapse of problem behavior. *Behavior Modification, 42*(3), 314–334. https://doi.org/10.1177/0145445517741475

Falligant, J. M., Kranak, M. P., McNulty, M. K., Schmidt, J. D., Hausman, N. L., & Rooker, G. W. (2021). Prevalence of renewal of problem behavior: Replication and extension to an inpatient setting. *Journal of Applied Behavior Analysis, 54*(1), 367–373. https://doi.org/10.1002/jaba.740

Fisher, W. W., Piazza, C. C., Bowman, L. G., & Amari, A. (1996). Integrating caregiver report with systematic choice assessment to enhance reinforcer identification. *American Journal of Mental Retardation: AJMR, 101*(1), 15–25.

Fisher, W. W., Greer, B. D., Fuhrman, A. M., & Querim, A. C. (2015). Using multiple schedules during functional communication training to promote rapid transfer of treatment effects. *Journal of Applied Behavior Analysis, 48*(4), 713–733. https://doi.org/10.1002/jaba.254

Fisher, W. W., Fuhrman, A. M., Greer, B. D., Mitteer, D. R., & Piazza, C. C. (2020a). Mitigating resurgence of destructive behavior using the discriminative stimuli of a multiple schedule. *Journal of the Experimental Analysis of Behavior, 113*(1), 263–277. https://doi.org/10.1002/jeab.552

Fisher, W. W., Luczynski, K. C., Blowers, A. P., Vosters, M. E., Pisman, M. D., Craig, A. R., … & Piazza, C. C. (2020b). A randomized clinical trial of a virtual-training program for teaching applied-behavior-analysis skills to parents of children with autism spectrum disorder. *Journal of Applied Behavior Analysis, 53*(4), 1856–1875. https://doi.org/10.1002/jaba.778

Fisher, W. W., Piazza, C. C., & Fuhrman, A. M. (2022). *Developing a severe behavior program: A tool kit.* Autism Speaks. https://docs.autismspeaks.org/behavior-program/

Fuhrman, A. M., Fisher, W. W., & Greer, B. D. (2016). A preliminary investigation on improving functional communication training by mitigating resurgence of destructive behavior. *Journal of Applied Behavior Analysis, 49*(4), 884–899. https://doi.org/10.1002/jaba.338

Greer, B. D., Fisher, W. W., Briggs, A. M., Lichtblau, K. R., Phillips, L. A., & Mitteer, D. R. (2019). Using schedule-correlated stimuli during functional communication training to promote the rapid transfer of treatment effects. *Behavioral Development, 24*(2), 100.

Grunewald, K., King, H. C., Phillips, S., H., Spink, C., Falligant, J. M., & Kranak, M. P. (2025). Renewal in clinical practice: Implications and mitigation strategies. In M. P. Kranak (Ed.), *Behavioral treatments for individuals with autism: Promoting longevity and durability.* Springer.

Hamrick, J., & Lock, R. H. (2020). Providing behavior analytic supports and services: A unique approach to rural service delivery. *Delta Kappa Gamma Bulletin, 87*(1), 63–68. http://ezproxy.emich.edu/login?url=https://www.proquest.com/scholarly-journals/providing-behavior-analytic-supports-services/docview/2457214703/se-2

Haney, S. D., Piazza, C. C., Peterson, K. M., & Greer, B. D. (2021). An evaluation of a renewal-mitigation procedure for inappropriate mealtime behavior. *Journal of Applied Behavior Analysis, 54*(3), 903–927.

Hembree-Kigin, T. L., & McNeil, C. B. (2013). *Parent – Child interaction therapy.* Springer Science & Business Media.

Iacono, T., Dissanayake, C., Trembath, D., Hudry, K., Erickson, S., & Spong, J. (2016). Family and practitioner perspectives on telehealth for services to young children with autism. *Studies in Health Technology and Informatics, 231*, 63–73.

Irwin Helvey, C., Fisher, W. W., Mitteer, D. R., Fuhrman, A. M., & Greer, B. D. (2024). Protective equipment in clinical intervention. In J. K. Luiselli, F. L. Bird, H. Maguire, & R. M. Gardner (Eds.), *Behavior safety and clinical practice in intellectual and developmental disabilities* (pp. 139–168). Springer Nature Switzerland. https://doi.org/10.1007/978-3-031-54923-6_7

Kazdin, A. E. (2011). *Single-case research designs: Methods for clinical and applied settings* (2nd ed.). Oxford University Press.

Kelley, M. E., Jimenez-Gomez, C., Podlesnik, C. A., & Morgan, A. (2018). Evaluation of renewal mitigation of negatively reinforced socially significant operant behavior. *Learning and Motivation, 63*, 133–141.

Kimball, R. T., Greer, B. D., Fuhrman, A. M., & Lambert, J. M. (2023). Relapse and its mitigation: Toward behavioral inoculation. *Journal of Applied Behavior Analysis, 56*(2), 282–301. https://doi.org/10.1002/jaba.971

Kranak, M. P., & Falligant, J. M. (2021). Further investigation of resurgence following schedule thinning: Extension to an inpatient setting. *Behavioral Interventions, 36*(4), 1003–1012. https://doi.org/10.1002/bin.1831

Kranak, M. P., & Falligant, J. M. (2022). Analysis of terminal schedule probes and schedule thinning effects following functional communication training. *Behavioral Interventions, 37*(2), 323–333. https://doi.org/10.1002/bin.1842

Lambert, J. M., Bloom, S. E., Samaha, A. L., Dayton, E., & Rodewald, A. M. (2015). Serial alternative response training as intervention for target response resurgence. *Journal of Applied Behavior Analysis, 48*(4), 765–780. https://doi.org/10.1002/jaba.253

Lambert, J. M., Bloom, S. E., Samaha, A. L., & Dayton, E. (2017). Serial functional communication training: Extending serial DRA to mands and problem behavior. *Behavioral Interventions, 32*(4), 311–325. https://doi.org/10.1002/bin.1493

Mandell, D. S. (2012). The interplay of outpatient services and psychiatric hospitalization among medicaid-enrolled children with autism spectrum disorders. *Archives of Pediatrics & Adolescent Medicine, 166*(1), 68. https://doi.org/10.1001/archpediatrics.2011.714

Markham, V., Austin, J., Roderique-Davies, G., & May, R. (2023). A comparison of stimulus fading and stimulus shaping on perceptual category learning. *Quarterly Journal of Experimental Psychology, 77*(8), 1662–1677. https://doi.org/10.1177/17470218231210446

Martin, G., & Pear, J. (1996). *Behavior modification: What it is and how to do it* (5th ed.). Prentice-Hall, Inc.

Miller, J. R., Lerman, D. C., & Fritz, J. N. (2010). An experimental analysis of negative reinforcement contingencies for adult-delivered reprimands. *Journal of Applied Behavior Analysis, 43*, 769–773. https://doi.org/10.1901/jaba.2010.43-769

Mitteer, D. R., Greer, B. D., Fisher, W. W., Briggs, A. M., & Wacker, D. P. (2018). A laboratory model for evaluating relapse of undesirable caregiver behavior. *Journal of the Experimental Analysis of Behavior, 110*(2), 252–266. https://doi.org/10.1002/jeab.462

Mitteer, D. R., Greer, B. D., Randall, K. R., & Haney, S. D. (2022). On the scope and characteristics of relapse when treating severe destructive behavior. *Journal of Applied Behavior Analysis, 55*(3), 688–703. https://doi.org/10.1002/jaba.912

Muething, C., Pavlov, A., Call, N., Ringdahl, J., & Gillespie, S. (2021). Prevalence of resurgence during thinning of multiple schedules of reinforcement following functional communication training. *Journal of Applied Behavior Analysis, 54*(2), 813–823. https://doi.org/10.1002/jaba.791

Norris, H. M., Mitteer, D. R., Irwin Helvey, C., & Greer, B. D. (2025). Applied research on mitigating resurgence. In M. P. Kranak (Ed.), *Behavioral treatments for individuals with autism: Promoting longevity and durability*. Springer.

O'Neill, R. E., Horner, R. H., Albin, R. W., Sprague, J. R., Storey, K., & Newton, J. S. (1997). *Functional assessment and program development for problem behavior: A practical handbook*. Brooks/Cole Publishing.

Osnes, P. G., & Lieblein, T. (2003). An explicit technology of generalization. *The Behavior Analyst Today, 3*(4), 364–374. https://doi.org/10.1037/h0099994

Pickard, K. E., & Ingersoll, B. R. (2016). Quality versus quantity: The role of socioeconomic status on parent-reported service knowledge, service use, unmet service needs, and barriers to service use. *Autism, 20*(1), 106–115. https://doi.org/10.1177/1362361315569745

Podlesnik, C. A., Kelley, M. E., Jimenez-Gomez, C., & Bouton, M. E. (2017). Renewed behavior produced by context change and its implications for treatment maintenance: A review. *Journal of Applied Behavior Analysis, 50*(3), 675–697. https://doi.org/10.1002/jaba.400

Scarpa, A., Jensen, L. S., Gracanin, D., Ramey, S. L., Dahiya, A. V., Ingram, L. M., Albright, J., Gatto, A. J., Scott, J. P., & Ruble, L. (2020). Access to autism spectrum disorder services for rural appalachian citizens. *Journal of Appalachian Health, 2*(1), 25–40. https://doi.org/10.13023/JAH.0201.04

Schiff, A., Tarbox, J., Lanagan, T., & Farag, P. (2011). Establishing compliance with liquid medication administration in a child with autism. *Journal of Applied Behavior Analysis, 44*(2), 381–385.

Schreibman, L., & Charlop, M. H. (1981). S+ versus S− fading in prompting procedures with autistic children. *Journal of Experimental Child Psychology, 31*(3), 508–520.

Stahmer, A. C., Vejnoska, S., Iadarola, S., Straiton, D., Segovia, F. R., Luelmo, P., Morgan, E. H., Lee, H. S., Javed, A., Bronstein, B., Hochheimer, S., Cho, E., Aranbarri, A., Mandell, D., Hassrick, E. M., Smith, T., & Kasari, C. (2019). Caregiver voices: Cross-cultural input on improving access to autism services. *Journal of Racial and Ethnic Health Disparities, 6*(4), 752–773. https://doi.org/10.1007/s40615-019-00575-y

Stephens, A. M., Briggs, A. M., Loder, B. H., Barr, J., & Miller, A. (2023). Delays to behavioral therapy in Michigan for children diagnosed with autism: A summary of needs assessment outcomes to inform public policy advocacy initiatives. *Behavior Analysis in Practice*. https://doi.org/10.1007/s40617-023-00896-9

Stephens, M., Wessel, M., Falligant, J. M., & Kranak, M. P. (2025). Reacquisition and reinstatement of problem behavior: Knowns and unknowns. In M. P. Kranak (Ed.), *Behavioral treatments for individuals with autism: Promoting longevity and durability*. Springer.

Stokes, T. F., & Baer, D. M. (1977). An implicit technology of generalization. *Journal of Applied Behavior Analysis, 10*(2), 349–367. https://doi.org/10.1901/jaba.1977.10-349

Stokes, T. F., & Osnes, P. G. (1989). An operant pursuit of generalization. *Behavior Therapy, 20*(3), 337–355. https://doi.org/10.1016/S0005-7894(89)80054-1

Sundberg, M. L. (2014). *The verbal behavior milestones assessment and placement program: The VB-MAPP* (2nd ed.). Concord, CA: AVB Press.

Thompson, R. H., & Iwata, B. A. (2001). A descriptive analysis of social consequences following problem behavior. *Journal of Applied Behavior Analysis, 34*(2), 169–178.

Wallace-Watkin, C., Sigafoos, J., & Waddington, H. (2023). Barriers and facilitators for obtaining support services among underserved families with an autistic child: A systematic qualitative review. *Autism, 27*(3), 588–601. https://doi.org/10.1177/13623613221123712

Weinsztok, S. C., & DeLeon, I. G. (2022). The mitigating effects of enhanced reinforcer magnitude and quality on treatment degradation. *Journal of Applied Behavior Analysis, 55*(2), 547–571. https://doi.org/10.1002/jaba.910

Wolf, M. M. (1978). Social validity: The case for subjective measurement or how applied behavior analysis is finding its heart. *Journal of Applied Behavior Analysis, 11*(2), 203–214. https://doi.org/10.1901/jaba.1978.11-203

Yingling, M. E., Ruther, M. H., & Dubuque, E. M. (2022). Trends in geographic access to Board Certified Behavior Analysts among children with autism spectrum disorder, 2018–2021. *Journal of Autism and Developmental Disorders, 52*(12), 5483–5490. https://doi.org/10.1007/s10803-021-05402-0

Zhang, W., & Baranek, G. (2016). The impact of insurance coverage types on access to and utilization of health services for U.S. Children with autism. *Psychiatric Services, 67*(8), 908–911. https://doi.org/10.1176/appi.ps.201500206

Index

M. P. Kranak (ed.), *Behavioral Treatments for Individuals with Autism*, Autism and Child Psychopathology Series, https://doi.org/10.1007/978-3-031-91965-7

The manufacturer's authorised representative in the EU is Springer
Nature Customer Service Centre GmbH, Europaplatz 3, 69115 Heidelberg,
Germany. If you have any concerns regarding our products, please
contact ProductSafety@springernature.com

Printed and bound by CPI Group (UK) Ltd, Croydon, CR0 4YY
30/09/2026
02225564-0003